Biomechanics-Based Motion Analysis, Volume II

Biomechanics-Based Motion Analysis, Volume II

Guest Editors

Christina Zong-Hao Ma
Hong Fu

MDPI

Basel • Beijing • Wuhan • Barcelona • Belgrade • Novi Sad • Cluj • Manchester

Guest Editors

Christina Zong-Hao Ma
Department of Biomedical Engineering
The Hong Kong Polytechnic University
Hong Kong
China

Hong Fu
Department of Mathematics and Information Technology
The Education University of Hong Kong
Hong Kong
China

Editorial Office

MDPI AG
Grosspeteranlage 5
4052 Basel, Switzerland

This is a reprint of the Special Issue, published open access by the journal *Bioengineering* (ISSN 2306-5354), freely accessible at: https://www.mdpi.com/journal/bioengineering/special_issues/5198F4Y195.

For citation purposes, cite each article independently as indicated on the article page online and as indicated below:

Lastname, A.A.; Lastname, B.B. Article Title. *Journal Name* **Year**, *Volume Number*, Page Range.

ISBN 978-3-7258-6434-8 (Hbk)
ISBN 978-3-7258-6435-5 (PDF)
https://doi.org/10.3390/books978-3-7258-6435-5

Contents

About the Editors

Christina Zong-Hao Ma

Christina Zong-Hao Ma is an Assistant Professor, a Certified Prosthetist and Orthotist (CPO, ISPO Category I), and a Certified Rehabilitation Therapist (CRT) at the Department of Biomedical Engineering, The Hong Kong Polytechnic University (PolyU). Before her appointment at PolyU, she served as a Lecturer, later promoted to Assistant Professor (permanent position), in Prosthetics and Orthotics at the Department of Rehabilitation, Jönköping University, Sweden, from 2018 to 2020. She received her PhD from the Faculty of Engineering, the Hong Kong Polytechnic University (2018), and her BSc from the West China School of Medicine, Sichuan University (2012). She also used to work as a Certified Prosthetist and Orthotist and a Clinical Instructor at the China Rehabilitation Research Center (permanent employment, 2012–2013) and as a Visiting Research Scholar in Mechanical Engineering at the University of Michigan, Ann Arbor (2017). Dr. Ma's research focuses on (1) investigating the mechanisms of human posture and motion control; (2) promoting physical activity and active health; and (3) developing solutions for improving balance and preventing falls in older/disabled people. Her research has been supported by the Health and Medical Research Fund (HMRF) Research Fellowship Scheme, the Chinese Association of Rehabilitation Medicine, and the Hong Kong Research Grants Council (RGC) Early Career Scheme (ECS).

Hong Fu

Hong Fu is an Associate Professor at the Department of Mathematics and Information Technology, the Education University of Hong Kong. She received her PhD from the Hong Kong Polytechnic University (2007) and her M.Eng (2003) and B.Eng and B.Mgt (2000) from Xi'an Jiaotong University. Dr. Fu's research focuses on computer vision algorithms, artificial intelligence in healthcare and education, eye tracking, and motion detection. Her research has been recognized by a number of awards, including a Gold Medal from the International Exhibition of Inventions of Geneva 2023, a Gold Medal and Jury's Choice Award from the International Invention Innovation Competition in Canada (iCAN) 2023, a Silver Medal from the 3rd Asia Exhibition of Innovations and Inventions (2023), and a Bronze Medal from the International Exhibitions of Inventions Geneva 2025.

bioengineering MDPI

Editorial

Advancing Biomechanics-Based Motion Analysis from Methodology to Application

Chen He [1], Hong Fu [2] and Christina Zong-Hao Ma [3,4,*]

1 School of Health Science and Engineering, University of Shanghai for Science and Technology, Shanghai 200093, China; hechen@usst.edu.cn
2 Department of Mathematics and Information Technology, The Education University of Hong Kong, Hong Kong SAR 999077, China; hfu@eduhk.hk
3 Department of Biomedical Engineering, The Hong Kong Polytechnic University, Hong Kong SAR 999077, China
4 Research Institute for Smart Ageing, The Hong Kong Polytechnic University, Hong Kong SAR 999077, China
* Correspondence: czh.ma@polyu.edu.hk; Tel.: +852-2766-7671; Fax: +852-2334-2429

1. Introduction

Biomechanics-based motion analysis provides the foundation for understanding human movement, from diagnosing pathological gait to optimizing athletic performance. The field is now evolving from traditional subjective observation to objective data-driven analysis, through advanced technologies in real-world environments. This special issue compiles ten original research articles that not only refine measurement methodologies but also demonstrate their significant impact on addressing clinical and sports-related challenges. The contributions examine two complementary areas: advanced methodology development and their practical implementation. Through technologies such as deep learning, wearable sensors, and computational modeling, these studies collectively enhance the precision, accessibility, and ecological validity of motion analysis across diverse movement contexts.

2. Contributions to This Special Issue

2.1. Methodological Innovations in Motion Analysis

A prominent focus in motion analysis is the continuous improvement of the tools and techniques for data acquisition and analysis, which prioritizes accuracy, accessibility, and applicability. Several studies in this Special Issue showcase significant progress in measurement technologies and computational modeling. Torvinen et al. [1] validated a deep learning-based 3D markerless motion capture system for skate skiing, demonstrating high agreement with marker-based systems. This system provides a promising tool for performance analysis and technique monitoring in sports. Similarly, Buckley et al. [2] validated the wearable Inertial Measurement Units (IMUs) against the clinical standard of overnight videography for assessing sleep biomechanics, confirming their reliability for efficient, home-based sleep monitoring.

Furthermore, Del Vecchio et al. [3] identified and mitigated movement artifacts in chronic pallidal local field potential recordings using IMU regression, which is a critical step to ensure the fidelity of neural biomarkers in adaptive deep brain stimulation. In parallel, Liang et al. [4] utilized a finite element model incorporating Hill-type muscle dynamics to simulate forearm flexion. Their simulations identified reduced fast-twitch fiber percentage, muscle strength, and neural excitation as key factors to diminished forearm mobility in the aging population, providing a computational framework to diagnose movement disorders.

2.2. Applications in Clinical and Sports Science

The ultimate value of biomechanical analysis lies in its application to address clinical and performance challenges. Some studies provide critical insights into pathophysiology, rehabilitation, and injury prevention through motion analysis. Ablove et al. [5] demonstrated that standing position produces the lowest pelvic floor pressures, with peak pressure localized at the symphysis. These biomechanical patterns explain both the protective nature of upright posture and the predisposition for anterior compartment prolapse. Meanwhile, Triantafyllou et al. [6] reported that IMU-based kinematic analysis during lumbar bridge tests were different in patients with chronic low back pain and healthy controls, which provides quantifiable diagnostics for evaluating rehabilitation efficacy. Further advancing neurorehabilitation, Joshi et al. [7] illustrated the potential of targeted neuromodulation, showing that trunk-specific spinal cord epidural stimulation can restore upright postural control in individuals with spinal cord injury.

In sports science, Zhang et al. [8] identified lower leg and knee stiffness in female athletes during a badminton landing task. The reduced dynamic stiffness indicated diminished joint stability and presented a biomechanical mechanism for the possible gender-related differences in non-contact anterior cruciate ligament injuries. Complementing this, Tong et al. [9] investigated the neuromuscular responses during standing balance challenges, and found that agonist muscles, particularly ankle muscles, activated fastest to counter perturbations, with muscle reaction speeds scaling with perturbation intensity. This hierarchy of control provides valuable insights for developing evidence-based fall-prevention protocols. Shim et al. [10] examined motor control in the absence of visual feedback, and demonstrated the remarkable capacity of the proprioceptive system to maintain bilateral symmetry and execute precise reaching movements under elastic loads, providing important implications for visual-deprived rehabilitation protocols.

3. Conclusions

This Special Issue presents a collection of studies that bridge advanced measurement technologies with critical applications in rehabilitation and sports science. These developments point toward increasingly personalized, data-driven approaches that translate biomechanical insights into optimized rehabilitation protocols and enhanced performance outcomes, thereby advancing both human health and athletic achievement.

Author Contributions: Conceptualization, C.H., H.F. and C.Z.-H.M.; writing—original draft preparation, C.H.; writing—review and editing, H.F. and C.Z.-H.M. All authors have read and agreed to the published version of the manuscript.

Funding: This research received no external funding.

Conflicts of Interest: The authors declare no conflicts of interest.

References

1. Torvinen, P.; Ruotsalainen, K.S.; Zhao, S.; Cronin, N.; Ohtonen, O.; Linnamo, V. Evaluation of 3D Markerless Motion Capture System Accuracy during Skate Skiing on a Treadmill. *Bioengineering* **2024**, *11*, 136. [CrossRef]
2. Buckley, N.; Davey, P.; Jensen, L.; Baptist, K.; Jacques, A.; Jansen, B.; Campbell, A.; Downs, J. A Comparison of Inertial Measurement Units and Overnight Videography to Assess Sleep Biomechanics. *Bioengineering* **2023**, *10*, 408. [CrossRef]
3. Vecchio, J.D.V.D.; Hanafi, I.; Pozzi, N.G.; Capetian, P.; Isaias, I.U.; Haufe, S.; Palmisano, C. Pallidal Recordings in Chronically Implanted Dystonic Patients: Mitigation of Tremor-Related Artifacts. *Bioengineering* **2023**, *10*, 476. [CrossRef] [PubMed]
4. Liang, C.; Jiang, F.; Kawaguchi, D.; Chen, X. A Biomechanical Simulation of Forearm Flexion Using the Finite Element Approach. *Bioengineering* **2024**, *11*, 23. [CrossRef] [PubMed]
5. Ablove, T.; DeRosa, A.; Lewis, S.; Benson, K.; Mendel, F.; Doyle, S. Pelvic Floor Pressures Differ Based on Location in the Pelvis and Body Position: A Cadaver Mode. *Bioengineering* **2023**, *10*, 329. [CrossRef] [PubMed]

6. Triantafyllou, A.; Papagiannis, G.; Stasi, S.; Gkrilias, P.; Kyriakidou, M.; Kampouroglou, E.; Skouras, A.-Z.; Tsolakis, C.; Georgoudis, G.; Savvidou, O.; et al. Lumbar Kinematics Assessment of Patients with Chronic Low Back Pain in Three Bridge Tests Using Miniaturized Sensors. *Bioengineering* **2023**, *10*, 339. [CrossRef] [PubMed]
7. Joshi, K.; Rejc, E.; Ugiliweneza, B.; Harkema, S.J.; Angeli, C.A. Spinal Cord Epidural Stimulation Improves Lower Spine Sitting Posture Following Severe Cervical Spinal Cord Injury. *Bioengineering* **2023**, *10*, 1065. [CrossRef] [PubMed]
8. Zhang, Y.; Hu, Z.; Li, B.; Qiu, X.; Li, M.; Meng, X.; Kim, S.; Kim, Y. Gender Differences in Lower Extremity Stiffness during a Single-Leg Landing Motion in Badminton. *Bioengineering* **2023**, *10*, 631. [CrossRef] [PubMed]
9. Tong, C.Y.; Zhu, R.T.-L.; Ling, Y.T.; Scheeren, E.M.; Lam, F.M.H.; Fu, H.; Ma, C.Z.-H. Muscular and Kinematic Responses to Unexpected Translational Balance Perturbation: A Pilot Study in Healthy Young Adults. *Bioengineering* **2023**, *10*, 831. [CrossRef] [PubMed]
10. Shim, G.; Yang, D.; Cho, W.; Kim, J.; Ryu, H.; Choi, W.; Kim, J. Elastic Resistance and Shoulder Movement Patterns: An Analysis of Reaching Tasks Based on Proprioception. *Bioengineering* **2024**, *11*, 1. [CrossRef] [PubMed]

bioengineering

MDPI

Article

Evaluation of 3D Markerless Motion Capture System Accuracy during Skate Skiing on a Treadmill

Petra Torvinen *, Keijo S. Ruotsalainen, Shuang Zhao, Neil Cronin, Olli Ohtonen and Vesa Linnamo

Faculty of Sport and Health Sciences, University of Jyväskylä, 88610 Jyväskylä, Finland;
keijo.s.ruotsalainen@jyu.fi (K.S.R.); zhaoshuangzs@hotmail.com (S.Z.); neil.j.cronin@jyu.fi (N.C.);
olli.ohtonen@jyu.fi (O.O.); vesa.linnamo@jyu.fi (V.L.)
* Correspondence: petra.l.m.torvinen@jyu.fi

Abstract: In this study, we developed a deep learning-based 3D markerless motion capture system for skate skiing on a treadmill and evaluated its accuracy against marker-based motion capture during G1 and G3 skating techniques. Participants performed roller skiing trials on a skiing treadmill. Trials were recorded with two synchronized video cameras (100 Hz). We then trained a custom model using DeepLabCut, and the skiing movements were analyzed using both DeepLabCut-based markerless motion capture and marker-based motion capture systems. We statistically compared joint centers and joint vector angles between the methods. The results demonstrated a high level of agreement for joint vector angles, with mean differences ranging from −2.47° to 3.69°. For joint center positions and toe placements, mean differences ranged from 24.0 to 40.8 mm. This level of accuracy suggests that our markerless approach could be useful as a skiing coaching tool. The method presents interesting opportunities for capturing and extracting value from large amounts of data without the need for markers attached to the skier and expensive cameras.

Keywords: kinematics; motion analysis; artificial intelligence; treadmill skiing; markerless motion capture

1. Introduction

Marker-based motion capture systems have been used extensively in biomechanics research. Infrared marker-based systems are considered an accurate method, but with some challenges and disadvantages. Traditionally, marker-based systems are time-consuming, often limited to laboratory environments, and require expensive equipment and high-level expertise. It is challenging or impossible to use marker-based motion capture systems in several cases, for example, in sports competitions or games. There are also challenges related to the use of markers, such as soft tissue artifact and marker placement errors [1–3]. Moreover, marker-based systems show errors when compared with biplanar videoradiography [1,2]. For example, root mean squared error (RMSE) angular differences ranging between 1.06° and 8.31° have been observed during walking and running [2].

Deep learning-based human pose estimation methods have been extensively studied in the computer vision literature, especially during the past 10 years [4], and this provides opportunities for applying these methods to multiple use cases like markerless motion capture. Nowadays, several deep learning-based markerless methods provide opportunities for detecting human movements with moderate accuracy [5,6]. Markerless methods can facilitate the understanding of human movement in different contexts, for example, in sports biomechanics, sports medicine, injury risk assessment, and rehabilitation [7,8]. There are several open-source pose estimation algorithms available such as OpenPose [9] and DeepLabCut [10], and also some commercial products such as Theia3D (Theia Markerless Inc., Kingston, ON, Canada) and Microsoft Kinect V2. Naturally, there are some challenges with markerless methods, such as mistakes in manual labelling during model training and issues related to the training data quantity and quality [11].

Several studies have used markerless open-source deep learning-based methods to perform 2D kinematic analyses using a single-camera view [12–15]. For example, high Pearson correlations (>0.97) were found for shoulder and knee angles during static hold arm-raises and squats when evaluated against marker-based motion capture [14]. With multiple calibrated cameras, 2D open-source pose estimation methods can be used to successfully detect the 3D position of human joint centers, joint angles, and segment angles [16–20]. When compared with marker-based motion capture data, differences in joint center locations were approximately 15–50 mm for activities such as throwing, walking, running, and jumping [16–18]. Some differences were also found between different pose estimation algorithms such as OpenPose, AlphaPose, and DeepLabCut during walking, running, and jumping [17]. The characteristics of markerless video cameras were also found to have small effects on the results [16]. In some studies, lower limb joint angles and segment angles were primarily calculated when evaluating markerless motion analyses against marker-based systems [18,19]. In a fully automated 3D markerless motion capture workflow with OpenPose, lower limb joint angles were detected with mean differences ranging between −3.9° and 10.5°, and RMSEs ranging between 1.2° and 7.4° for hip, knee, and ankle joint rotations during jumping, walking, and running [19]. In a clinical approach, lower limb joint angles were detected with an RMSE ranging between 3.16° and 11.90° [18]. In addition, studies using the commercial markerless product Theia3D obtained quite similar results than with open-source methods [21–23]. For example, RMSDs were less than 2.5 cm for joint centers except the hip, and less than 5.5° for segment angles when comparing Theia3D markerless to marker-based motion capture during treadmill walking [22].

Cross-country skiing and especially skate skiing is a complex movement involving both lower and upper body muscles and skiing equipment. To date, studies have focused on the biomechanics of skiing when skiers need to quickly modify skiing techniques at different speeds and on different terrains [24]. It would be of interest to study whether a markerless system would be accurate enough to analyze and provide feedback on a skier's skiing technique.

This study presents a DeepLabCut-based method that can be used for the 3D kinematic analysis of skate skiing on a treadmill. The method was used to determine joint centers and joint angles. The aim of this study was to compare our markerless motion capture system with a marker-based system in terms of skate skiing on a treadmill. It was hypothesized that our markerless motion capture system would be able to detect the joint centers and joint angles with about the same level of accuracy as previous similar studies, i.e., mean differences less than 50 mm for joint centers and mean differences between −5° and 5° for joint angles.

2. Materials and Methods

2.1. Participants and Experimental Protocol

Data from 13 female [Age: 21.7 ± 4.6 years] and 19 male [Age: 20.6 ± 7.5 years] athletes roller skiing with the G3 skating technique on a skiing treadmill were used to train the markerless model. The athletes were part of the Finnish junior national teams in cross-country skiing, biathlon and Nordic combined, and some were part of Vuokatti-Ruka sport academy. The athletes provided their consent to use their skiing videos in the development of the markerless models. Training data were collected during the athletes' normal training sessions. The angle of the skiing treadmill ranged between two and three degrees, and the speed ranged between 12 and 30 km per hour in the training sessions. Two 20 s videos were recorded with two cameras from each athlete.

A total of 10 experienced skiers who were familiar with roller skiing on a skiing treadmill (5 females [Age: 21.0 ± 3.1 years; height: 1.73 ± 0.49 m; weight: 63.9 ± 7.3 kg] and 5 males [Age: 24.4 ± 10.7 years; height: 1.85 ± 0.69 m; weight: 81.0 ± 4.1 kg]) volunteered in the evaluation study and provided written informed consent. The participants used the same pair of roller skis (Marwe, Skating 620 XC, wheel No. 0) and poles of suitable length (Swix, Triac 3.0). Each participant had a single testing session, which included a static calibration where the participant stood still on the skiing treadmill to make sure that all markers were visible, and that the systems were working correctly. Then, the participant performed four roller skiing trials with the G1 skating technique (two for both sides), and three roller skiing trials with the G3 skating technique. The G1 skating technique is "a skating form of the diagonal stride technique of classic skiing, in which the leg and arm are employed diagonally, with a single pole-push with each contra-lateral leg-push in a skating-like fashion" [25]. With the G3 skating technique, the skier performs "one double-pole together with every leg push" [25]. Each roller skiing trial started when the skier struck the treadmill with the ski pole to enable the systems to be synchronized, and then included at least thirty seconds of skiing. G1 trials included about 20 skiing cycles, and G3 trials included at least 15 skiing cycles. A skate skiing cycle includes each leg pushing once. A G1 cycle includes one impact of the poles, and G3 cycle includes two impacts of the poles. The roller skiing trial protocol is shown in Table 1.

Table 1. Protocol of roller skiing trials, including the skiing technique, speed of treadmill, and angle of treadmill for each trial. Note that for G3, treadmill speeds differed for males (m) and females (f).

Trial	Skiing Technique	Speed of Treadmill (km/h)	Angle of Treadmill (deg)
1	G1	8	5
2	G1	6	8
3	G1	8	5
4	G1	6	8
5	G3	12 f/14 m	2
6	G3	18 f/20 m	2
7	G3	24 f/26 m	2

2.2. Motion Capture Systems and Laboratory Configuration

This study was conducted at the Skiing Laboratory of the University of Jyväskylä in Vuokatti, which is equipped with a 2.7 m × 3.5 m skiing treadmill (RL3500E, Rodby Innovation AB, Vänge, Sweden). In this study, we used two motion capture systems concurrently. Marker-based data were captured using an infrared 8-camera marker-based motion capture system (100 Hz, Vicon, Oxford, UK) and NEXUS 2.8.1 software (Vicon, Oxford, UK). The cameras were positioned around the skiing treadmill on the ceiling at a height of about 2.5 m. In addition, the Skiing Laboratory was equipped with video cameras (LILIN, Taiwei, New Taipei City, Taiwan) and a Coachtech online measurement and feedback system [26]. In this study, two video cameras capable of capturing 1280 × 720 resolution videos at 100 Hz were used for markerless motion capture. Videos were recorded using the Coachtech system. A sampling frequency of 100 Hz was used in both motion capture systems, as this was the maximum rate possible for the video cameras. The video cameras were positioned to the right side (Cam0, perpendicular to skiing direction) and right obliquely (Cam1, 45 degrees to skiing direction) from the skiing treadmill. Cam0 was at a height of 1.05 m and a distance of 2.00 m from the skiing treadmill. Cam1 was at a height of 2.5 m and a distance of 1.90 m from the skiing treadmill. The Skiing Laboratory configuration and both system's camera placements are shown in Figure 1.

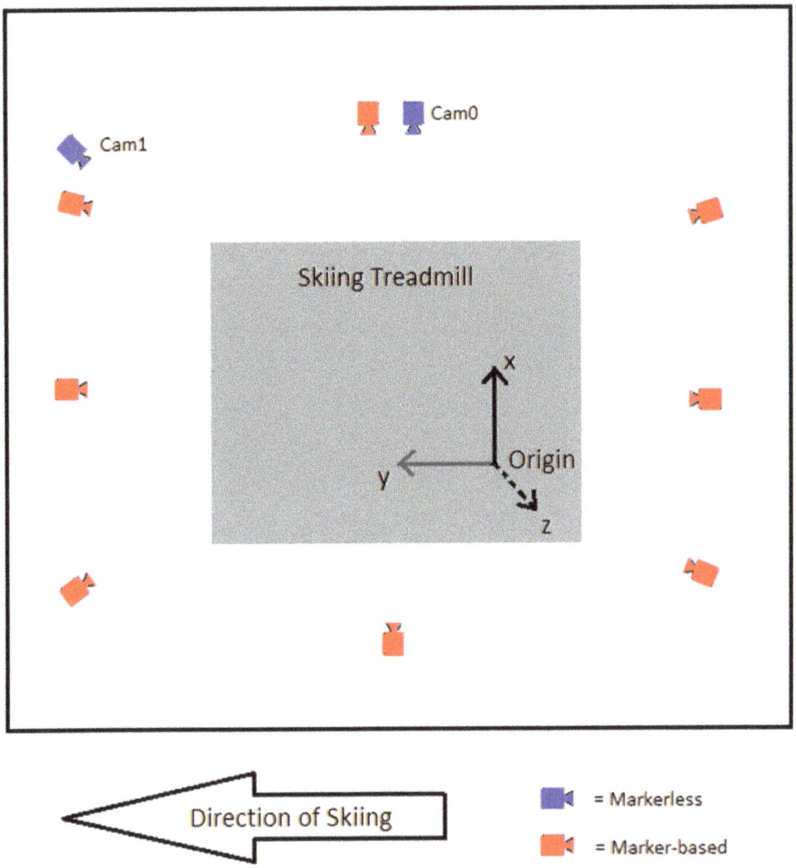

Figure 1. Skiing Laboratory configuration, camera placements, and coordinate system configuration.

2.3. Markerless Model Development

A total of 64 videos from both markerless video cameras were used in the development of the markerless model. Markerless 3D models were developed using DeepLabCut, which is an open-source pose estimation method based on transfer learning with deep neural networks [10]. Two-dimensional models were trained for both video cameras separately using DeepLabCut, and pixel coordinates were later transformed to global 3D coordinates using the Direct Linear Transformation (DLT) algorithm [27]. Training images were selected randomly from the videos using DeepLabCut's frame extraction method and imgaug algorithm. From each video, 15–20 images were selected, and about 1000 images per camera were used to train each 2D model. The images were manually labeled using DeepLabCut's graphical user interface. Manually labeled markers were placed on the joint centers of the wrist, elbow, shoulder, hip, knee, and ankle. In addition, the tip of the skiing boot was labeled to reflect toe position. In the 2D models, only the right side of the skier was detected, as well as the right pole and right roller ski. Examples of the output of both 2D models are shown in Figure 2.

The labeled images were then used to train deep neural networks. Labeled images were collected and divided randomly into a 95% training and 5% test split using DeepLabCut's training set creation method and imgaug algorithm. DeepLabCut's default network configuration parameters were used. ResNet50 models for both video cameras were initialized with weights trained on ImageNet, and the cross-entropy loss between the predicted score map and the ground truth score map was minimized using stochastic gradient descent. The deep neural networks were trained with 700,000 iterations, and after training, the 2D models were evaluated using the 5% test split. The mean training error was 1.80 pixels (approximately 0.61 cm), and the mean test error was 2.27 pixels (approximately 0.77 cm) for the model of Cam0. The mean training error was 2.10 pixels (approximately 0.72 cm), and the mean test error was 2.63 pixels (approximately 0.89 cm) for the model of Cam1.

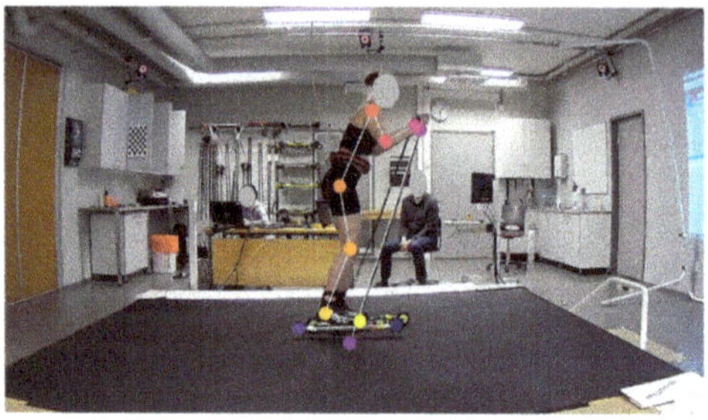

(a)

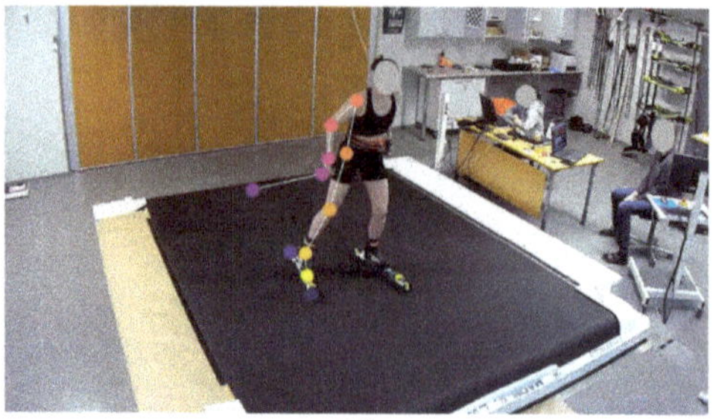

(b)

Figure 2. Examples of images labeled by our 2D models: (**a**) from Cam0 and (**b**) from Cam1.

2.4. System Calibration Procedure

Both motion capture systems were calibrated before the measurements. The same origin and axis directions were used for both systems. The configuration of the coordinate system is shown in Figure 1. The origin was defined at the left side of the skiing treadmill. The x-axis (black in Figure 1) was defined as the latitudinal axis of the treadmill, the y-axis (gray in Figure 1) as the longitudinal axis of the treadmill, and the z-axis (black dashed line in Figure 1) as perpendicular to the treadmill, pointing upward.

With the markerless system, a calibration procedure was performed using an aluminum calibration cube that was 2 m long in each dimension. The calibration cube was placed on the skiing treadmill with one corner placed at the origin. The placements of the calibration cube and origin are shown in Figure 3. Eight points were selected, marked, and measured from the calibration cube. The selected points were used as calibration points resulting in eight known 3D coordinates. These calibration points were manually digitized from both markerless video cameras. Using these calibration coordinates, both video camera's x- and y-coordinates were transformed to global 3D coordinates using the DLT algorithm [27].

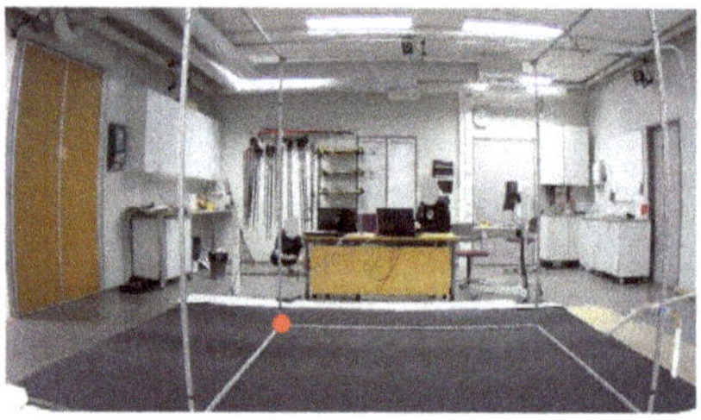

(a)

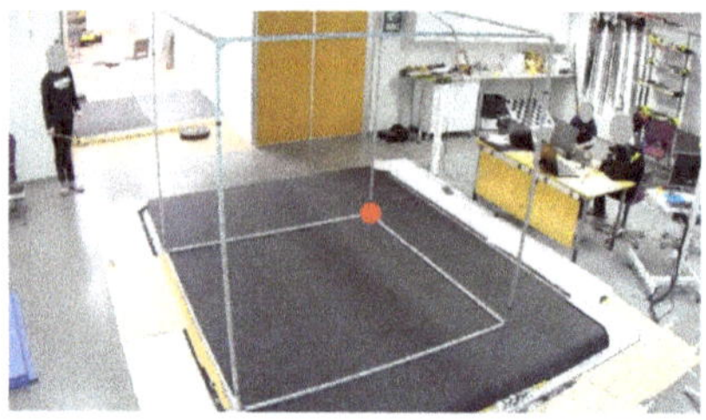

(b)

Figure 3. Placements of the calibration cube and origin (red circle) in the Skiing Laboratory: (**a**) from Cam0 and (**b**) from Cam1.

For the marker-based system, the coordinate system was defined by placing a Vicon L-Frame on the treadmill, allowing the coordinate system origin and axis directions to be defined. The marker-based system calibration was performed using Vicon NEXUS 2.8.1 software.

2.5. Data Collecting and Processing

In the evaluation study, markerless data were captured using the Coachtech system with two video cameras. Videos were analyzed using the developed 2D models, and markerless data were filtered using a 4th order low-pass Butterworth filter (cut-off frequency, 12 Hz). The synchronization of the videos was ensured using the strokes of the pole on the treadmill from the beginning of each trial. The pixel coordinates were transformed to global 3D coordinates with the DLT algorithm. These 3D coordinates were further filtered with a 4th order low-pass Butterworth filter (cut-off frequency, 6 Hz). The filtering and coordinate transformation were performed using Matlab (v2021b, MathWorks, Inc., Natick, MA, USA).

Marker-based data were captured using a modified marker set comprising 39 individual passive reflective markers on the participant and 12 markers on the skiing equipment: three markers on both roller skis and three markers on both poles. The marker set is shown in Appendix A. The recorded data were labeled and visually verified using Vicon NEXUS 2.8.1 software. Marker trajectory data gap filling and marker-based data filtering with a 4th order low-pass Butterworth filter (cut-off frequency, 6 Hz) were performed using Vicon NEXUS 2.8.1 software. The joint centers of the wrist, elbow, knee, and ankle were computed from the mid-points of the lateral and medial markers. The shoulder joint center was computed from the mid-points of the anterior and posterior shoulder markers. The hip joint center was calculated using the method described by Bell et al. (1989) [28]. Toe markers were placed on top of the skiing boots due to the movement of the skiing boots and roller skis during skiing, so the toe marker positions slightly differed from the points detected by the markerless system. The toe marker placements for both systems are shown Figure 4. Static calibrations were used to determine the difference in each participant's right toe placement between systems, and this was considered before statistical analysis. The joint center calculation and defining displacements of the right toe placement between systems were performed using Matlab.

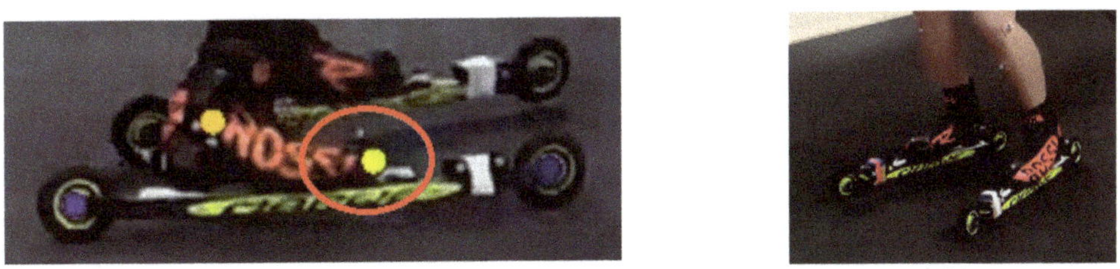

(**a**) (**b**)

Figure 4. (**a**) Toe marker placements for both the markerless and marker-based systems are shown in the red circle. The markerless toe marker is indicated by the yellow circle, and the marker-based marker appears as a gray circle. (**b**) Marker-based toe marker placement viewed from a different direction.

From each skiing trial, 10 skiing cycles were selected and time normalized. The skiing cycles were defined using the right pole markers. The start of each skiing cycle was defined as the point at which the right pole touched the treadmill. To compare the performance of the markerless and marker-based systems, the 3D Euclidean distances of each right-side joint center and toe placement at each time point were calculated. In addition, the vector angles at the elbow, shoulder, hip, knee, and ankle were calculated from both systems to describe the movements of skiing. The elbow angle was defined as the supplement of the angle between the two 3D vectors connecting the elbow position to the wrist and shoulder positions. The hip angle was defined as the supplement of the angle between the two 3D vectors connecting the hip position to the shoulder and knee positions. The knee angle was defined as the supplement of the angle between the two 3D vectors connecting the knee position to the hip and ankle positions. These are thus a simplified proxy for the elbow, hip, and knee flexion angles. The shoulder angle was defined as the angle between the two vectors connecting the shoulder position to the elbow and hip positions. The shoulder angle thus reflects the angle between the upper arm and the upper body. The ankle angle was defined as the complement of the angle between the two vectors connecting the ankle position to the knee and toe positions. The ankle angle is thus a simplified proxy for the ankle plantar/dorsiflexion angle. All angles were calculated using Matlab.

2.6. Statistical Analysis

The systems were compared using Bland–Altman analyses [29]. For the joint centers and toe placements, the mean difference (bias), standard deviation (SD) and 95% limits of agreement (LoA) were calculated with a one-sample *t*-test. For the vector angles, the bias, SD, and LoA were calculated with a paired-sample *t*-test. Additionally, for the vector angles, the root mean squared errors (RMSE), Pearson correlations (r), and intra-class correlation coefficient (ICC) were computed to indicate validity between systems. For the Pearson correlations, coefficients were interpreted with values of <0.30, 0.30–0.50, 0.50–0.70, 0.70–0.90, and >0.90 representing negligent, low, moderate, high, and very high correlations, respectively [30]. The ICCs for absolute agreement were estimated based on a single measurement and two-way mixed effects model. The ICCs were used to indicate the agreement, with values of <0.50, 0.50–0.75, 0.75–0.90, and >0.90 representing the quality thresholds for poor, moderate, good, and excellent validity, respectively [31]. The statistical analyses were performed using SPSS 28.0.1.1 (IBM Corporation, Armonk, NY, USA), and the significance level was set at $p \leq 0.05$.

3. Results

A total of 70 trials with 700 skiing cycles were compared between the markerless and marker-based systems: 40 trials with the G1 technique and 30 trials with the G3 technique. The results from the participants' right sides are reported below.

3.1. Joint Centers and Toe Placements

The results of the comparisons between the systems for joint centers and toe placements are shown in Table 2.

Table 2. Mean difference, standard deviation, and 95% limits of agreement for joint centers and toe placements.

Detected Point	Skiing Technique	Mean Difference (Bias) [mm]	±SD [mm]	95% LoA Lower/Upper
Wrist	G1	40.3	30.1	40.4/40.5
	G3	38.3	22.6	38.1/38.5
Elbow	G1	33.6	28.9	33.3/33.8
	G3	29.5	17.5	29.4/29.7
Shoulder	G1	26.6	19.7	26.4/26.8
	G3	24.0	14.1	23.9/24.1
Hip	G1	31.9	14.9	31.8/32.0
	G3	31.3	16.1	31.2/31.5
Knee	G1	30.5	16.6	30.4/30.7
	G3	30.2	20.2	30.0/30.4
Ankle	G1	31.5	17.0	31.4/31.6
	G3	32.4	22.9	32.2/32.6
Toe	G1	40.8	21.3	40.6/41.0
	G3	39.4	29.7	39.1/39.7

For all participants, the mean difference ranged from 24 to 41 mm at the wrist, elbow, shoulder, hip, knee, and ankle joint centers and toe positions. For both techniques, the smallest systematic differences and LoA were observed at the shoulder joint center (G1: 26.6 mm; G3: 24.0 mm) with standard deviations of 19.7 mm (G1) and 14.1 mm (G3). The wrist joint center and toe placement displayed the largest systematic differences with the highest standard deviation and LoA with both techniques. The elbow, hip, knee, and ankle joint center mean differences were typically larger than those at the shoulder but smaller than that at the wrist or toe with their standard deviation and LoA following the same trend.

For both techniques, the mean (black) ± SD (gray, shaded area) time-series differences in the joint centers and toe placements are shown for a single participant in Figure 5. Two trials were selected from both techniques, so 20 time-normalized skiing cycles are included for each.

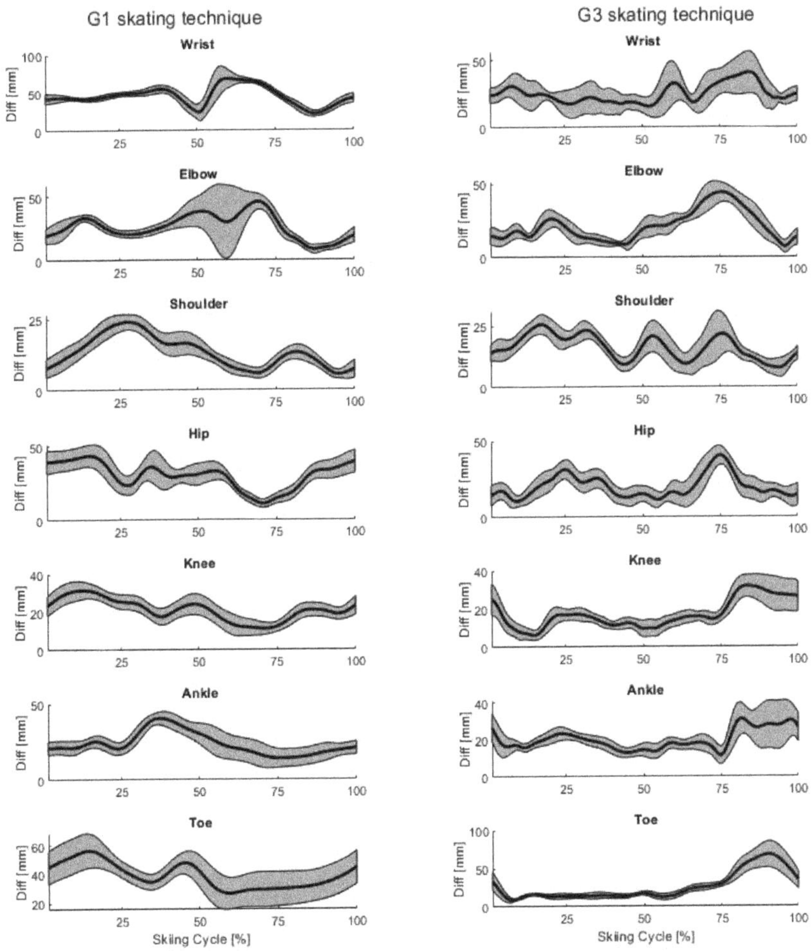

Figure 5. Example mean ± SD differences between markerless and marker-based joint centers and toe placements of a single participant (P03) during G1 and G3 skating technique cycles. The mean difference is shown as a black line, and the standard deviation as the shaded gray area.

3.2. Joint Vector Angles

The results of the comparisons between the systems for joint vector angles are shown in Table 3.

Table 3. Mean difference, standard deviation, 95% limits of agreement, RMSE, Pearson correlation, and intra-class correlation coefficient for joint vector angles.

Angle	Skiing Technique	Mean Difference (Bias) [deg]	±SD [deg]	95% LoA Lower/Upper	RMSE [deg]	r Pearson Correlation	p-Value	ICC [Mean (95% Confidence Interval)]
Elbow	G1	0.99	7.16	0.94/1.06	7.23	0.96	<0.001	0.96 (0.95/0.96)
	G3	0.60	5.69	0.55/0.66	5.72	0.97	<0.001	0.97 (0.96/0.97)
Shoulder	G1	3.69	3.84	3.66/3.72	5.33	0.94	<0.001	0.92 (0.87/0.97)
	G3	2.71	3.76	2.68/2.74	4.64	0.96	<0.001	0.97 (0.95/0.98)
Hip	G1	1.08	4.06	1.05/1.12	4.21	0.94	<0.001	0.94 (0.92/0.95)
	G3	0.74	3.48	0.72/0.78	3.56	0.97	<0.001	0.97 (0.96/0.97)
Knee	G1	1.15	3.06	1.13/1.18	3.27	0.96	<0.001	0.95 (0.93/0.97)
	G3	0.82	2.89	0.80/0.85	3.01	0.96	<0.001	0.96 (0.95/0.97)
Ankle	G1	−2.47	4.31	−2.51/−2.44	4.96	0.82	<0.001	0.77 (0.59/0.86)
	G3	−2.03	4.23	−2.07/−1.99	4.69	0.84	<0.001	0.80 (0.68/0.86)

Good levels of agreement were observed between the markerless and marker-based results. The Pearson correlations showed high to very high agreement between systems with the highest agreement in the elbow (0.97) and hip (0.97) angles for the G3 technique. The lowest Pearson correlations were observed for ankle angles with r-values of 0.82 and 0.84. The Pearson correlations were statistically significant ($p < 0.001$) for all joint vector angles and for both techniques. The ICC values also showed good to excellent validity between systems with the highest agreements in the elbow (0.97), shoulder (0.97), and hip (0.97) angles for the G3 technique. The lowest ICCs were observed for ankle angles with values of 0.80 and 0.77.

The mean differences in joint vector angles ranged between −2.47 and 3.69 degrees. The lowest systematic differences were observed at the elbow (<1°), but the standard deviation was the largest (>5°). For hip and knee angles, good agreement was observed with low mean differences (<1.1°) and a low standard deviation (<4°). The largest mean differences were observed for shoulder angles, most notably with the G1 technique with a mean difference and standard deviation of 3.69° ± 3.84°.

RMSE values ranged between 3.01 and 7.23 degrees for the joint vector angles. The lowest RMSE values were observed at the knee (<3.5°). For hip and knee angles, quite good agreement was observed with RMSE values < 5°. The largest RMSE values were observed for elbow angles (>5°).

For both skating techniques, time-normalized markerless (blue) and marker-based (red) joint vector angles and mean (black) ± SD (gray, shaded area) time-series differences for a single participant (P03) from a single skiing trial are shown in Figure 6. For both techniques, two trials and 20 skiing cycles are included.

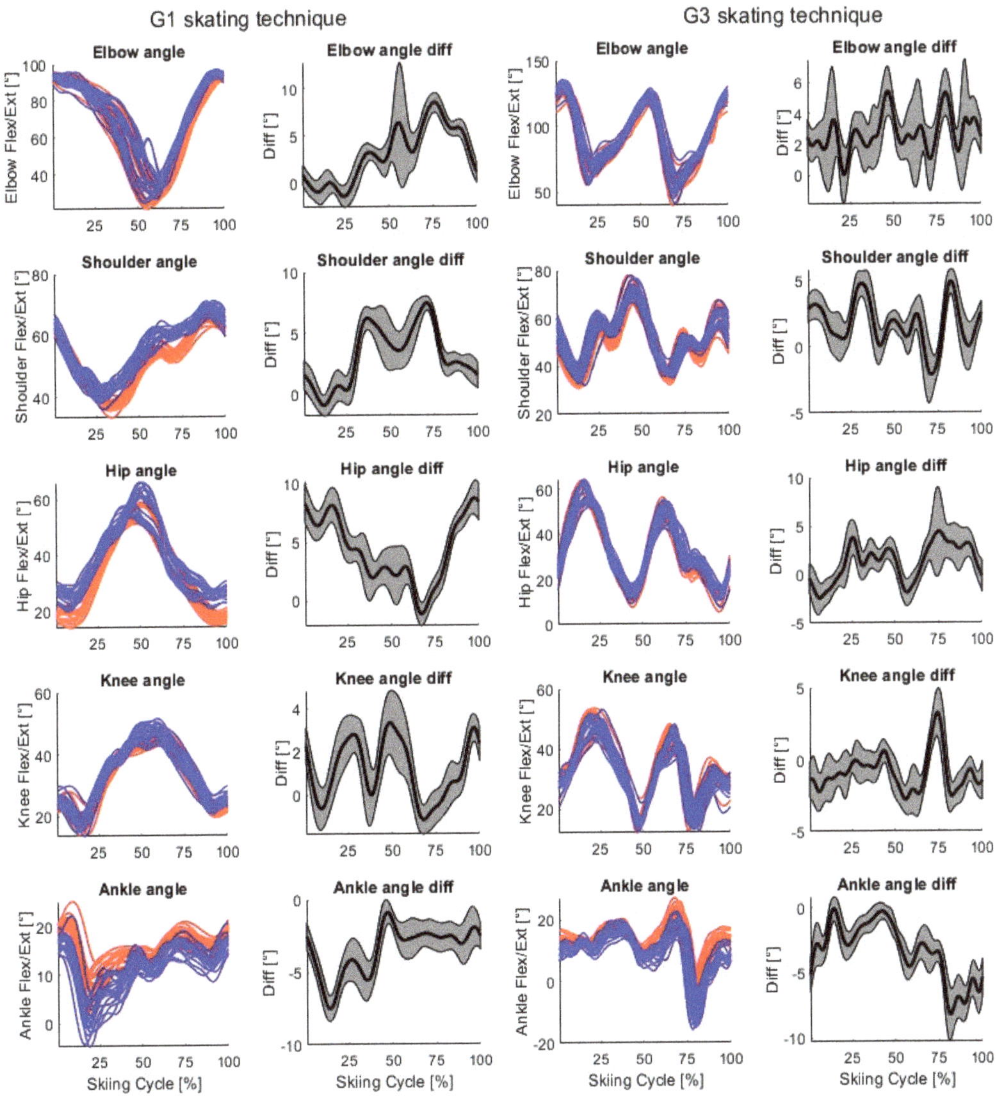

Figure 6. Columns 1 and 3—Example time-normalized markerless (blue) and marker-based (red) joint vector angles for a single participant (P03) during G1 and G3 skating technique cycles. Columns 2 and 4—Mean (black) and ± SD (gray, shaded area) differences for each calculated joint vector angle during G1 and G3 skating technique cycles. For both skating techniques, two skiing trials are included, so 20 skiing cycles are visualized.

4. Discussion

This study presents an evaluation of a 3D markerless motion capture system for skate skiing on a treadmill, focusing on the skier's right-side joint centers and joint vector angles. Our markerless motion capture system was able to detect 3D kinematics with a good level of agreement relative to the marker-based motion analysis, most notably for the joint vector angles (Table 3).

Our markerless motion capture system can correctly detect joint centers during skate skiing (Table 2). The mean differences and standard deviations were generally lower with the G3 skating technique compared to with the G1 technique, which is probably because the markerless model was developed using videos from the G3 skating technique. It is noteworthy that during the skiing cycle, the accuracy of the markerless method varied slightly, even for the same participant (Figure 5). These results are in line with earlier studies, where the joint centers were detected using open-source markerless methods and marker-based systems during throwing, jumping, walking, and running [16–18]. Quite similar results were observed in an earlier study in detecting joint centers using OpenPose, AlphaPose, and DeepLabCut during walking, running, and jumping, with mean differences between 14 and 58 mm [17]. Similar results were also obtained in another previous study, where joint centers were detected using OpenPose with multiple synchronized video cameras during walking, countermovement jumping, and ball throwing, with mean absolute errors (MAE) of less than 30 mm in 80% of the trials [16]. Compared to a commercial markerless product, Theia3D, the results of joint center detection are also quite similar to those obtained with open-source markerless methods. For example, Theia3D detected lower limb joint centers with a root mean square of the 3D distances (RMSD) between 20 and 30 mm during countermovement jumping [21]. In another study, Theia3D detected lower and upper limb joint centers with average 3D Euclidean distances between 11 and 36 mm [22].

In the present study, the elbow, shoulder, hip, and knee joint vector angles consistently demonstrated very high levels of agreement between the markerless and marker-based systems, while the ankle joint vector angles demonstrated high levels of agreement (Table 3). These findings demonstrate that our 3D markerless motion capture system can correctly reproduce the movements of skate skiing. Additionally, the calculated joint vector angles differ slightly between systems during the skiing cycle (Figure 6), because joint center detection varies between systems (Figure 5). Our joint angle results are quite similar to those of previous studies using open-source markerless methods and commercial markerless products [19,23,32]. For example, joint angles have been detected using OpenPose during jumping, walking, and running with higher mean differences (between −3.9° and 10.5°) but lower standard deviations (between 1.8° and 4.4°) than in this study [19]. In another study, lower limb joint angles during gait in clinical patients were detected using Theia3D with RMSDs generally less than 6° [23]. Upper limb joint angles have been detected during static postures and basic movements (holding boxes) using Microsoft Kinect V2 with MAEs from 2.5° to 12.9° and using the Captiv system (L7000) with MAEs from 1.9° to 14.9° when compared to a goniometer [32]. The results of our study are therefore in line with those of previous studies related to open-source markerless methods and commercial markerless products.

The results of this evaluation study are highly promising, and the differences between systems typically fell within the known uncertainties of marker-based motion capture. The development process of the markerless model influences the system's accuracy because the training images were labeled by a human and may thus include errors of judgement. In addition, the number, placements, and characteristics of the video cameras can affect the accuracy of a markerless motion capture system. However, marker-based systems also have inherent errors, which are mainly due to skin artifact. In previous studies, errors of up to ~8° have been reported when comparing marker-based motion capture to biplanar videoradiography for ankle joint rotations during walking and running [2], and knee flexion/extension angles during jumping [1]. Additionally, one previous study reported marker displacements of up to ~20 mm due to the effects of soft tissue artefacts at the knee during stair ascent using 3D fluoroscopy and a marker-based system [3]. It is noteworthy that the accuracies of marker-based systems also vary during the detected cycles (walking, running, jumping, and throwing) [1–3].

The differences observed in this study generally fall within the known challenges of marker-based motion capture, and it seems that our markerless motion capture system could be used especially as a skiing coaching tool. Cross-country skiing is developing all the time, with new modifications of subtechniques such as the "double-push" skating technique [33]. Race speeds have also increased, and this increases the importance of both skiing technique and skiing equipment [24]. Our markerless motion capture system presents interesting opportunities for cross-country skiing technique research and coaching. The markerless system combined with Coachtech system provides the results automatically [26], so changes in skiing technique could be viewed during training. There are several possibilities for using the markerless system from the coaching perspective. For example, the system provides possibilities for analyzing several parameters connected to technique in addition to joint angles, like body position and forward lean. Typically, the coach provides some instructions to the skier to change the skiing technique during training. With this markerless system, it can be determined whether the athlete has modified their skiing technique accordingly. In addition, it can be monitored how these technique changes influence, for example, the skiing economy and/or maximal skiing performance. In addition, this approach provides opportunities for capturing large amounts of skiing technique data. In the future, we could develop markerless models for other skating techniques (G4 and G5) and classic skiing.

Previous studies have provided information about propulsive forces during skiing [34,35]. In addition, the analysis of propulsive forces is important in the biomechanics of cross-country skiing, because it significantly affects the skiing speed. In the future, our markerless motion capture system could be used simultaneously with force sensors, for example, with the recently developed force measurement roller skis [36]. Thus, a more comprehensive analysis of the biomechanics of cross-country skiing could be obtained without additional equipment or markers.

In conclusion, we present and validate a markerless motion capture system that is low cost and easy to use for researchers and coaches. This markerless motion capture system could be used as a real-time coaching tool to monitor and improve skiing techniques.

Author Contributions: Conceptualization, P.T., S.Z., K.S.R., N.C., O.O. and V.L.; methodology, P.T., S.Z., K.S.R., N.C., O.O. and V.L.; software, P.T.; validation, P.T., K.S.R. and S.Z.; formal analysis, P.T.; investigation, P.T., K.S.R. and S.Z.; resources, P.T., K.S.R. and S.Z.; data curation, P.T.; writing—original draft preparation, P.T.; writing—review and editing, P.T., K.S.R., S.Z., N.C., O.O. and V.L.; visualization, P.T.; supervision, V.L.; project administration, V.L.; funding acquisition, V.L. All authors have read and agreed to the published version of the manuscript.

Funding: Research was funded partly by the "Smart Track" project (ERDF, 11853/09 020101/2021 Kainuu).

Institutional Review Board Statement: Ethical review and approval were waived for this study because the Human Sciences Ethics Committee of the University of Jyväskylä concluded that an ethical review, in this case, was not required.

Informed Consent Statement: Informed consent was obtained from all subjects involved in the study.

Data Availability Statement: The data are not publicly available because ethical restrictions were placed upon this data. In the informed consent form that was approved by the Research Ethical Committee, we stated that all data are confidential and will not be provided to third parties. Since it may be possible to identify individuals even after the anonymization of these data, our data cannot be shared publicly. Possible requests for limited data should be sent either to petra.l.m.torvinen@jyu.fi, to vesa.linnamo@jyu.fi, or to the Secretary of the University of Jyvaskyla Ethical Committee at secretary-ethicomm@jyu.fi.

Acknowledgments: The authors would like to thank Timo Rantalainen for helping out in the coding process and all the athletes for participating.

Conflicts of Interest: The authors declare no conflicts of interest.

Appendix A

The marker set that was used in the evaluation study is shown in Table A1.

Table A1. Names, definitions, and positions for markers.

Marker Name	Definition	Position on Participant/Skiing Equipment
OFFSET	Right back	Anywhere over the right scapula
LSHO	Left shoulder	On the acromioclavicular joint
LSHF	Left shoulder front	Humerus lesser tubercle
LSHB	Left shoulder back	Same position as LSHF on the posterior side
LUPA	Left upper arm	On the upper lateral 1/3 surface of the left arm (placed asymmetrically with RUPA)
LELB	Left elbow	On the lateral epicondyle
LELBM	Left elbow medial	On the medial epicondyle
LFRM	Left forearm	On the lower lateral 1/3 surface of the left forearm (placed asymmetrically with RFRM)
LWRA	Left wrist marker A	At the thumb side of a bar attached to a wristband on the posterior of the left wrist, as close to the wrist joint center as possible. Loose markers can be used, but for better tracking of the axial rotations, a bar is recommended.
LWRB	Left wrist marker B	At the little finger side of a bar attached to a wristband on the posterior of the left wrist, as close to the wrist joint center as possible. Loose markers can be used, but for better tracking of the axial rotations, a bar is recommended.
RSHO	Right shoulder	On the acromioclavicular joint
RSHF	Right shoulder front	Humerus lesser tubercle
RSHB	Right shoulder back	Same position as RSHF on the posterior side
RUPA	Right upper arm	On the lower lateral 1/3 surface of the right arm (placed asymmetrically with LUPA)
RELB	Right elbow	On the lateral epicondyle approximating the elbow joint axis
RELB	Right elbow	On the lateral epicondyle
RFRM	Right forearm	On the lower lateral 1/3 surface of the right forearm (placed asymmetrically with LFRM)
RWRA	Right wrist marker A	At the thumb side of a bar attached symmetrically with a wristband on the posterior of the right wrist, as close to the wrist joint center as possible
RWRB	Right wrist marker B	At the little finger side of a bar attached symmetrically with a wristband on the posterior of the right wrist, as close to the wrist joint center as possible
RPSI	Right PSIS	Right posterior superior iliac spine (immediately below the sacroiliac joints, at the point where the spine joins the pelvis)
RASI	Right ASIS	Right anterior superior iliac spine
LPSI	Left PSIS	Left posterior superior iliac spine (immediately below the sacroiliac joints, at the point where the spine joins the pelvis)
LASI	Left ASIS	Left anterior superior iliac spine
LTHI	Left thigh	Over the lower lateral 1/3 surface of the left thigh
LKNE	Left knee	On the flexion–extension axis of the left knee
LTIB	Left tibia	Over the lower 1/3 surface of the left shank
LANK	Left ankle	On the lateral malleolus along an imaginary line that passes through the transmalleolar axis

Table A1. *Cont.*

Marker Name	Definition	Position on Participant/Skiing Equipment
LHEE	Left heel	On the calcaneus at the same height above the plantar surface of the foot as the toe marker
LTOE	Left toe	Over the second metatarsal head, on the mid-foot side of the equinus break between forefoot and mid-foot
RTHI	Right thigh	Over the upper lateral 1/3 surface of the right thigh
RKNE	Right knee	On the flexion–extension axis of the right knee.
RTIB	Right tibia	Over the upper 1/3 surface of the right shank
RANK	Right ankle	On the lateral malleolus along an imaginary line that passes through the transmalleolar axis
RHEE	Right heel	On the calcaneus at the same height above the plantar surface of the foot as the toe marker
RTOE	Right toe	Over the second metatarsal head, on the mid-foot side of the equinus break between forefoot and mid-foot
LKNEM	Left knee medial	Left medial femur condyles
RKNEM	Right knee medial	Right medial femur condyles
LANKM	Left ankle medial	Left medial malleolus
RANKM	Right ankle medial	Right medial malleolus
LSKI1	Left Ski 1	On the front side of the binding of the left roller ski, on the left edge, on the front side of LSKI2
LSKI2	Left Ski 2	On the front side of the binding of the left roller ski, on the left edge, on the back side of LSKI1
LSKI3	Left Ski 3	On the front side of the binding of the left roller ski, on the right edge, placed asymmetrically with LSKI1
RSKI1	Right Ski 1	On the front side of the binding of the right roller ski, on the right edge, on the front side of RSKI2
RSKI2	Right Ski 2	On the front side of the binding of the right roller ski, on the right edge, on the back side of RSKI1
RSKI3	Right Ski 3	On the front side of the binding of the right roller ski, on the left edge, placed asymmetrically with RSKI1
LPOLE1	Left Pole 1	At the top of the left pole, below the handle of the pole
LPOLE2	Left Pole 2	In the middle of the left pole, below LPOLE1
LPOLE3	Left Pole 3	At the bottom of the left pole, below LPOLE2
RPOLE1	Right Pole 1	At the top of the right pole, below the handle of the pole
RPOLE2	Right Pole 2	In the middle of the right pole, below RPOLE1
RPOLE3	Right Pole 3	At the bottom of the left pole, below RPOLE2

References

1. Miranda, D.L.; Rainbow, M.J.; Crisco, J.J.; Fleming, B.C. Kinematic Differences between Optical Motion Capture and Biplanar Videoradiography during a Jump–Cut Maneuver. *J. Biomech.* **2013**, *46*, 567–573. [CrossRef]
2. Kessler, S.E.; Rainbow, M.J.; Lichtwark, G.A.; Cresswell, A.G.; D'andrea, S.E.; Konow, N.; Kelly, L.A. A Direct Comparison of Biplanar Videoradiography and Optical Motion Capture for Foot and Ankle Kinematics. *Front. Bioeng. Biotechnol.* **2019**, *7*, 474006. [CrossRef]
3. Tsai, T.-Y.; Lu, T.-W.; Kuo, M.-Y.; Lin, C.-C. Effects of Soft Tissue Artifacts on the Calculated Kinematics and Kinetics of the Knee during Stair-Ascent. *J. Biomech.* **2011**, *44*, 1182–1188. [CrossRef]
4. Zheng, C.; Chen, C.; Yang, T.; Zhu, S.; Shah, M.; Wu, W.; Shen, J.; Kehtarnavaz, N.; Zheng, C.; Wu, W.; et al. Deep Learning-Based Human Pose Estimation: A Survey. *J. ACM* **2023**, *56*, 1–37. [CrossRef]

5. Wang, J.; Tan, S.; Zhen, X.; Xu, S.; Zheng, F.; He, Z.; Shao, L. Deep 3D Human Pose Estimation: A Review. *Comput. Vis. Image Underst.* **2021**, *210*, 103225. [CrossRef]
6. Desmarais, Y.; Mottet, D.; Slangen, P.; Montesinos, P. A Review of 3D Human Pose Estimation Algorithms for Markerless Motion Capture. *Comput. Vis. Image Underst.* **2021**, *212*, 103275. [CrossRef]
7. Mündermann, L.; Corazza, S.; Andriacchi, T.P. The Evolution of Methods for the Capture of Human Movement Leading to Markerless Motion Capture for Biomechanical Applications. *J. Neuroeng. Rehabil.* **2006**, *3*, 6. [CrossRef] [PubMed]
8. Colyer, S.L.; Evans, M.; Cosker, D.P.; Salo, A.I.T. A Review of the Evolution of Vision-Based Motion Analysis and the Integration of Advanced Computer Vision Methods Towards Developing a Markerless System. *Sport. Med. Open* **2018**, *4*, 24. [CrossRef] [PubMed]
9. Cao, Z.; Hidalgo, G.; Simon, T.; Wei, S.E.; Sheikh, Y. OpenPose: Realtime Multi-Person 2D Pose Estimation Using Part Affinity Fields. *IEEE Trans. Pattern. Anal. Mach. Intell.* **2021**, *43*, 172–186. [CrossRef] [PubMed]
10. Mathis, A.; Mamidanna, P.; Cury, K.M.; Abe, T.; Murthy, V.N.; Mathis, M.W.; Bethge, M. DeepLabCut: Markerless Pose Estimation of User-Defined Body Parts with Deep Learning. *Nat. Neurosci.* **2018**, *21*, 1281–1289. [CrossRef] [PubMed]
11. Cronin, N.J. Using Deep Neural Networks for Kinematic Analysis: Challenges and Opportunities. *J. Biomech.* **2021**, *123*, 110460. [CrossRef] [PubMed]
12. Cronin, N.J.; Rantalainen, T.; Ahtiainen, J.P.; Hynynen, E.; Waller, B. Markerless 2D Kinematic Analysis of Underwater Running: A Deep Learning Approach. *J. Biomech.* **2019**, *87*, 75–82. [CrossRef] [PubMed]
13. Vonstad, E.K.; Su, X.; Vereijken, B.; Bach, K.; Nilsen, J.H. Comparison of a Deep Learning-Based Pose Estimation System to Marker-Based and Kinect Systems in Exergaming for Balance Training. *Sensors* **2020**, *20*, 6940. [CrossRef] [PubMed]
14. Slowik, J.S.; McCutcheon, T.W.; Lerch, B.G.; Fleisig, G.S. Comparison of a Single-View Image-Based System to a Multi-Camera Marker-Based System for Human Static Pose Estimation. *J. Biomech.* **2023**, *159*, 111746. [CrossRef] [PubMed]
15. Kidziński, Ł.; Yang, B.; Hicks, J.L.; Rajagopal, A.; Delp, S.L.; Schwartz, M.H. Deep Neural Networks Enable Quantitative Movement Analysis Using Single-Camera Videos. *Nat. Commun.* **2020**, *11*, 4054. [CrossRef]
16. Nakano, N.; Sakura, T.; Ueda, K.; Omura, L.; Kimura, A.; Iino, Y.; Fukashiro, S.; Yoshioka, S. Evaluation of 3D Markerless Motion Capture Accuracy Using OpenPose With Multiple Video Cameras. *Front. Sport Act. Living* **2020**, *2*, 538330. [CrossRef] [PubMed]
17. Needham, L.; Evans, M.; Cosker, D.P.; Wade, L.; McGuigan, P.M.; Bilzon, J.L.; Colyer, S.L. The Accuracy of Several Pose Estimation Methods for 3D Joint Centre Localisation. *Sci. Rep.* **2021**, *11*, 20673. [CrossRef]
18. Ripic, Z.; Nienhuis, M.; Signorile, J.F.; Best, T.M.; Jacobs, K.A.; Eltoukhy, M. A Comparison of Three-Dimensional Kinematics between Markerless and Marker-Based Motion Capture in Overground Gait. *J. Biomech.* **2023**, *159*, 111793. [CrossRef]
19. Needham, L.; Evans, M.; Wade, L.; Cosker, D.P.; McGuigan, M.P.; Bilzon, J.L.; Colyer, S.L. The Development and Evaluation of a Fully Automated Markerless Motion Capture Workflow. *J. Biomech.* **2022**, *144*, 111338. [CrossRef]
20. Ripic, Z.; Theodorakos, I.; Andersen, M.S.; Signorile, J.F.; Best, T.M.; Jacobs, K.A.; Eltoukhy, M. Prediction of Gait Kinetics Using Markerless-Driven Musculoskeletal Modeling. *J. Biomech.* **2023**, *157*, 111712. [CrossRef]
21. Strutzenberger, G.; Kanko, R.; Selbie, S.; Schwameder, H.; Deluzio, K. Assessment of Kinematic CMJ Data using a Deep Learning Algorithm-Based Markerless Motion Capture System. *ISBS Proc. Arch.* **2021**, *39*, 61.
22. Kanko, R.M.; Laende, E.K.; Davis, E.M.; Selbie, W.S.; Deluzio, K.J. Concurrent Assessment of Gait Kinematics Using Marker-Based and Markerless Motion Capture. *J. Biomech.* **2021**, *127*, 110665. [CrossRef] [PubMed]
23. Wren, T.A.L.; Isakov, P.; Rethlefsen, S.A. Comparison of Kinematics between Theia Markerless and Conventional Marker-Based Gait Analysis in Clinical Patients. *Gait Posture* **2023**, *104*, 9–14. [CrossRef] [PubMed]
24. Sandbakk, Ø.; Holmberg, H.-C. A Reappraisal of Success Factors for Olympic Cross-Country Skiing. *Int. J. Sport Physiol. Perform.* **2014**, *9*, 117–121. [CrossRef] [PubMed]
25. Pellegrini, B.; Sandbakk, Ø.; Stöggl, T.; Supej, M.; Ørtenblad, N.; Schürer, A.; Steiner, T.; Lunina, A.; Manhard, C.; Liu, H.; et al. Methodological Guidelines Designed to Improve the Quality of Research on Cross-Country Skiing. *J. Sci. Sport Exerc.* **2021**, *3*, 207–223. [CrossRef]
26. Ohtonen, O.; Ruotsalainen, K.; Mikkonen, P.; Heikkinen, T.; Hakkarainen, A.; Leppävuori, A.; Linnamo, V. Online Feedback System for Athletes and Coaches. In Proceedings of the 3rd International Congress on Science and Nordic Skiing, Vuokatti, Finland, 5 June 2015; p. 35.
27. Abdel-aziz, Y.; Karara, H. Direct Linear Transformation from Comparator to Object Space Coordinates in Close-Range Pho-Togramme. *Photogramm. Eng. Remote Sens.* **2015**, *81*, 103–107. [CrossRef]
28. Bell, A.L.; Brand, R.A.; Pedersen, D.R. Prediction of Hip Joint Centre Location from External Landmarks. *Hum. Mov. Sci.* **1989**, *8*, 3–16. [CrossRef]
29. Bland, J.M.; Altman, D.G. Measuring Agreement in Method Comparison Studies. *Stat. Methods Med. Res.* **1999**, *8*, 135–160. [CrossRef]
30. Mukaka, M. Statistics Corner: A Guide to Appropriate Use of Correlation Coefficient in Medical Research. *Malawi Med. J.* **2012**, *24*, 69–71.
31. Koo, T.K.; Li, M.Y. A Guideline of Selecting and Reporting Intraclass Correlation Coefficients for Reliability Research. *J. Chiropr. Med.* **2016**, *15*, 155–163. [CrossRef]
32. Steinebach, T.; Grosse, E.; Glock, C.; Wakula, J.; Lunin, A. Accuracy Evaluation of Two Markerless Motion Capture Systems for Measurement of Upper Extremities: Kinect V2 and Captiv. *Hum. Factors Ergon. Manuf. Serv. Ind.* **2020**, *30*, 291–302. [CrossRef]

33. Stöggl, T.; Müller, E.; Lindinger, S. Biomechanical Comparison of the Double-Push Technique and the Conventional Skate Skiing Technique in Cross-Country Sprint Skiing. *J. Sport Sci.* **2008**, *26*, 1225–1233. [CrossRef] [PubMed]
34. Stöggl, T.; Holmberg, H.-C. Three-Dimensional Force and Kinematic Interactions in V1 Skating at High Speeds. *Med. Sci. Sport Exerc.* **2015**, *47*, 1232–1242. [CrossRef] [PubMed]
35. Göpfert, C.; Pohjola, M.V.; Linnamo, V.; Ohtonen, O.; Rapp, W.; Lindinger, S.J. Forward Acceleration of the Centre of Mass during Ski Skating Calculated from Force and Motion Capture Data. *Sport Eng.* **2017**, *20*, 141–153. [CrossRef]
36. Zhao, S.; Linnamo, V.; Ruotsalainen, K.; Lindinger, S.; Kananen, T.; Koponen, P.; Ohtonen, O. Validation of 2D Force Measurement Roller Ski and Practical Application. *Sensors* **2022**, *22*, 9856. [CrossRef]

bioengineering

MDPI

Article

A Biomechanical Simulation of Forearm Flexion Using the Finite Element Approach

Chenyang Liang, Fei Jiang *, Daisuke Kawaguchi and Xian Chen

Department of Mechanical Engineering, Graduate School of Sciences and Technology for Innovation, Yamaguchi University, Tokiwadai, Ube 7558611, Yamaguchi, Japan; c505wdw@yamaguchi-u.ac.jp (C.L.); b026vd@yamaguchi-u.ac.jp (D.K.); xchen@yamaguchi-u.ac.jp (X.C.)

* Correspondence: fjiang@yamaguchi-u.ac.jp

Abstract: Upper limb movement is vital in daily life. A biomechanical simulation of the forearm with consideration of the physiological characteristics of the muscles is instrumental in gaining deeper insights into the upper limb motion mechanisms. In this study, we established a finite element model of the forearm, including the radius, biceps brachii, and tendons. We simulated the motion of the forearm resulting from the contraction of the biceps brachii by using a Hill-type transversely isotropic hyperelastic muscle model. We adjusted the contraction velocity of the biceps brachii muscle in the simulation and found that a slower muscle contraction velocity facilitated forearm flexion. Then, we changed the percentage of fast-twitch fibers, the maximum muscle strength, and the neural excitation values of the biceps brachii muscle to investigate the forearm flexion of elderly individuals. Our results indicated that reduced fast-twitch fiber percentage, maximum muscle strength, and neural excitation contributed to the decline in forearm motion capability in elderly individuals. Additionally, there is a threshold for neural excitation, below which, motion capability sharply declines. Our model aids in understanding the role of the biceps brachii in forearm flexion and identifying the causes of upper limb movement disorders, which is able to provide guidance for enhancing upper limb performance.

Keywords: upper limb; forearm flexion; muscle contraction; Hill-type transversely isotropic hyperelastic material; finite element method

1. Introduction

Upper limb movement is an essential part of daily life. Biomechanical simulations of the forearm, incorporating the salient physiological attributes of the upper limb muscles, serve as a pivotal tool for acquiring profound insights into the mechanisms governing upper limb motion. Many researchers have employed various methods for biomechanical simulations related to the upper limb. Ambrosio et al. [1] developed a multibody biomechanical model of the upper limb and conducted simulations to predict the muscle forces during humeral elevation. Teran et al. [2] developed a comprehensive upper limb model using finite volume methods and the finite element method, and conducted an inverse dynamics analysis. However, they adopted a simple constitutive model for muscle without consideration of the force-velocity relationship. Dereshgi et al. (2022) [3] investigated the mechanical behaviors of muscle fibers during dumbbell curl exercises with varying dumbbell weights. Later, they investigated the rest-pause biceps curl exercise effect on the biceps brachii muscles of women [4]. However, they simplified the upper limb model into basic geometric shapes, failing to accurately depict the true structural characteristics of the upper limb. Chen et al. [5] constructed a realistic upper limb model from MRI images and simulated forearm movements using the finite element method. However, the accuracy of the results was low due to the small number of elements used in their simulation. Blemker et al. [6] utilized the finite element method to simulate the contraction of the biceps brachii muscle and investigated the nonuniform shortening behavior of the biceps brachii muscle.

The finite element method is a common approach for simulating upper limb movements. In finite element modeling, the paramount component governing the kinetics of forearm flexion resides in the biceps brachii muscles. In general, muscular contraction is initiated through the cerebral transmission of neural excitation to the muscle fibers. [7,8]. After muscle contraction, tendons transmit tension to the bones, enabling joint movement and the motion of flexion. Muscles exhibit complex mechanical behavior, and they are usually regarded as incompressible transversely isotropic hyperelastic materials [9]. Additionally, there is a strain rate effect on the mechanical response of the muscle tissue [10,11]. The modeling of the biomechanical behavior of muscles is the key point for the finite element simulation, which includes both passive and active behavior. Passive behavior pertains to the intrinsic elasticity and compliance of both muscle fibers and the isotropic matrix. These properties enable muscles to undergo elongation and subsequently revert to their initial length in response to externally applied forces. This passive behavior can be delineated by nonlinear hyperelasticity, which elucidates the connection between muscle forces and the degree of stretching. On the other hand, active behavior represents the contractile characteristics of muscle fibers driven by neural excitation. The muscle forces generated by active behavior are associated with muscle contraction velocity and neural excitation level. The biomechanical behavior of muscles encompasses dynamic interactions between passive and active components. Therefore, the muscle force is a function of contraction velocity, neural excitation from the active part and stretch ratio from the passive part. The mathematical modeling of muscles needs to carefully consider these factors [12].

The Hill-type muscle model integrates both active and passive behaviors of muscles, and it is widely applied in biomechanical research [12,13]. However, the original Hill-type model is one-dimensional. Its applicability to real muscles, characterized by intricate three-dimensional (3D) structures, is limited. Many researchers have extended the one-dimensional Hill-type model to three dimensions to simulate the mechanical properties of various muscle tissues with real geometries [13–18]. Kojic et al. [14] proposed a 3D Hill-type model in which passive elastic behavior was simplified to be 3D linear elastic and isotropic, without considering the hyperelastic behavior of muscles. Furthermore, they did not consider the incompressibility of muscle tissue. Tang et al. [15] used this model to simulate the mechanical behavior of skeletal muscles considering fatigue factors. In contrast, Johansson et al. [16] proposed a 3D Hill-type model that considered the incompressibility of muscles. However, the passive behaviors of muscle fibers and the matrix that embeds these fibers were conflated in this model. Martins et al. [17] introduced an incompressible, transversely isotropic hyperelastic 3D muscle model that included both active and passive muscle behavior. However, this model did not consider the strain rate effects of muscles. Subsequently, Martins et al. [18] improved this model by incorporating the effects of strain rate on muscles. This muscle model appeared to simulate muscle contraction under real conditions. However, muscle fiber types, in terms of fast-twitch and slow-twitch fibers, have not been considered yet in this model. Research about the effect of muscle fiber composition on motion ability remains limited. Additionally, sarcopenia, defined as the loss of muscle mass and strength with age, is recognized as a major cause of disability and morbidity in elderly individuals, such as IADL (instrumental activities of daily living) disability [19]. Sarcopenia results from a combination of changes in muscle fiber composition, reduced muscle strength associated with muscle atrophy, and neurological dysfunction [20,21]. These factors have not been quantitatively investigated. The objective of this study was to extend the improved Hill-type muscle model [18] and employ the finite element method to simulate the effect of sarcopenia on forearm flexion movements.

2. Materials and Methods

2.1. Forearm Finite Element Model

We utilized CT images and the image processing software ScanIP (simpleware ScanIP, version M-2019.06; Synopsys Inc., Mountain View, CA, USA) to construct a 3D model of the forearm, which included the biceps brachii, tendon, and radius bone. The radius bone was automatically segmented using a single threshold segmentation method, while the biceps brachii muscle and tendon were manually segmented. Subsequently, a smoothing procedure was applied to the entire forearm model. Finally, we used the meshing software HyperMesh (Altair HyperMesh, version 2019.1.2; Altair Engineering Inc., Troy, MI, USA) to create a mesh for the forearm model (Figure 1a). The forearm finite element model comprises 16,001 tetrahedral elements and 4580 nodes. In this study, we considered a simplified model only composed of the radius bone, the biceps brachii, and tendon, which is enough to reproduce the forearm flexion motion.

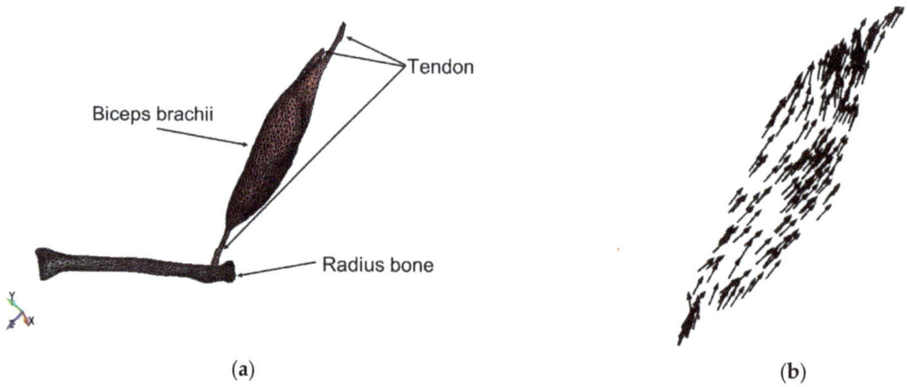

Figure 1. Finite element model of the forearm: (**a**) tetrahedral mesh elements of the model and (**b**) muscle fiber direction of the biceps brachii.

To reproduce the contraction motion of the biceps brachii muscle, the muscle fibers' direction information is necessary. As described later, the active contractile force will be generated along the fibers' direction. Therefore, we solved a Laplace's equation to determine the direction of the biceps brachii muscle fibers. The direction of the resulting gradient is assumed to be able to mimic the direction of the muscle fibers (Figure 1b). The obtained fiber directions (Figure 1b) exhibit a reasonable concordance with the anatomical literature [22].

2.2. Constitutive Models of the Muscle, Bone, and Tendon

The muscle was modeled as a fiber-reinforced composite in which the strain energy density function includes the contribution from the isotropic matrix embedding the muscle fiber and the contribution from the muscle fibers [23]. The strain energy density function of the muscle contains the following terms:

$$U = U_V + U_I + U_f \tag{1}$$

where U_I represents the strain energy in the isotropic matrix embedding the muscle fiber and U_f represents the strain energy of the muscle fiber. U_V means the strain energy related to the volume change, given as:

$$U_V = 2(J-1) \tag{2}$$

where J represents the determinant of the deformation gradient $\boldsymbol{F}$ ($J = det\boldsymbol{F}$).

As for U_I, we used the constitutive model proposed by Humphrey et al. [24]:

$$U_I = cexp^{b(\widetilde{I}_C - 3)} - 1 \quad (3)$$

where $\widetilde{I}_C$ is the first reducing invariant of the right Cauchy–Green deformation tensor C, defined as $\widetilde{I}_C = J^{-2/3} trC$. The right Cauchy–Green deformation tensor C is defined as $C = 2E + I$, where E and I are the Green–Lagrange deformation tensor and the identity tensor, respectively. c and b are the constants of this model. In this study, we used $c = 3.795 \times 10^{-4}$ Mpa and $b = 23.46$ [24].

As for U_f, we employed the skeletal muscle fiber strain energy function proposed by Martins et al. [18]. This function utilizes the Hill-type three-element model (Figure 2), incorporating a realistic representation of muscle mechanics. The Hill-type model comprises three core components: a Contractile Element (CE), a Series Element (SE), and a Parallel Element (PE). The CE is responsible for generating contractile force during muscle activation and does not contribute to passive forces when subjected to passive stretching. It is typically recognized as the sliding actin and myosin filaments. The SE, linked in series with the CE, behaves as a non-linear spring and is attributed to the inherent elasticity found within the myofilaments and cross-bridges. The PE, connected in parallel with the CE, functions as another non-linear spring. It is associated with the elasticity of connective tissues (epimysium, perimysium, and endomysium), as well as the sarcolemma.

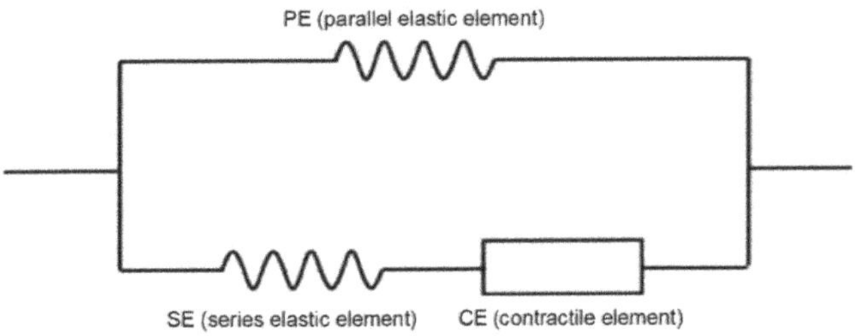

Figure 2. Hill-type three-element model of the muscle.

The total nominal stress T along the muscle fiber direction can be considered as the sum of the nominal stress produced by the PE and either the CE or SE elements.

$$T = T^{PE} + T^{SE} = T^{PE} + T^{CE} \quad (4)$$

The stress T^{PE} related to the PE elements is defined as follows:

$$T^{PE} = T_0^M f_{PE}\left(\widetilde{\lambda}_f\right) \quad (5)$$

$$f_{PE}\left(\widetilde{\lambda}_f\right) = \begin{cases} 2aA\exp\left[a\left(\widetilde{\lambda}_f - 1\right)^2\right]\left(\widetilde{\lambda}_f - 1\right) & \widetilde{\lambda}_f > 1.0 \\ 0 & \text{other} \end{cases} \quad (6)$$

where $\widetilde{\lambda}_f$ is the stretch ratio in the direction of the muscle fibers, which is calculated by $\widetilde{\lambda}_f = \left[J^{-2/3}\, \mathbf{C} : (\mathbf{N_m} \otimes \mathbf{N_m})\right]^{1/2}$. $\mathbf{N_m}$ is the initial direction of the muscle fibers. T_o^M is the maximum nominal stress of the muscle fibers, using the values $T_o^M = 0.535$ Mpa. A and a are material constants. In this study, we used the values $A = 8.568 \times 10^{-4}$ and $a = 12.43$ [18].

The stress T^{CE} of the CE element comprises three components: (1) the stretch-ratio-related part f_L^{CE}, which is a function of the stretch ratio of the muscle fibers $\widetilde{\lambda}_f$, (2) the contraction-velocity-related part f_V^{CE}, which is a function of the contraction velocity of the muscle fibers $\dot{\tilde{\lambda}}_f$, and (3) the activation level α, which is a function of the time t:

$$T^{CE}\left(\tilde{\lambda}_f, \dot{\tilde{\lambda}}_f, \alpha(t)\right) = T_o^M f_L^{CE}\left(\tilde{\lambda}_f\right) f_V^{CE}\left(\dot{\tilde{\lambda}}_f\right)\alpha(t) \tag{7}$$

The stretch-ratio-related function f_L^{CE} and the contraction-velocity-related function f_V^{CE} are defined as follows:

$$f_L^{CE}\left(\tilde{\lambda}_f\right) = \begin{cases} -4\left(\tilde{\lambda}_f - 1\right)^2 + 1 & 0.5 \le \tilde{\lambda}_f \le 1.5 \\ 0 & \text{other} \end{cases} \tag{8}$$

$$f_V^{CE}\left(\dot{\tilde{\lambda}}_f\right) = \begin{cases} 0 & \dot{\tilde{\lambda}}_f \le -10s^{-1} \\ -\frac{1}{\operatorname{atan}(5)}\operatorname{atan}\left(-0.5\dot{\tilde{\lambda}}_f\right) + 1 & -10s^{-1} \le \dot{\tilde{\lambda}}_f \le 2s^{-1} \\ \frac{\pi}{4\operatorname{atan}(5)} + 1 & \dot{\tilde{\lambda}}_f > 2s^{-1} \end{cases} \tag{9}$$

where $\dot{\tilde{\lambda}}_f > 0$ during muscle fiber lengthening and $\dot{\tilde{\lambda}}_f < 0$ during muscle fiber contraction. The absolute value of $\dot{\tilde{\lambda}}_f$ represents the rate of muscle fiber lengthening or contraction. The activation level α controls the muscle contraction intensity. Our study adopted the same activation formula as Pandy et al. [25], and its expression is as follows:

$$\alpha = \frac{\frac{u}{\tau_{\text{rise}}} + \frac{1}{\tau_{\text{fall}}}\alpha_{\min}(1-u)}{\frac{u}{\tau_{\text{rise}}} + \frac{1}{\tau_{\text{fall}}}(1-u)} \cdot \left(1 - e^{-t\left[\frac{u}{\tau_{\text{rise}}} + \frac{1}{\tau_{\text{fall}}}(1-u)\right]}\right) \tag{10}$$

where τ_{rise} and τ_{fall} represent the characteristic time constants governing the activation and deactivation processes of the muscle, respectively. They determine how quickly the muscle reaches its peak activation level and how rapidly it returns to its resting state after activation. The experimental values $\tau_{\text{rise}} = 0.02$ and $\tau_{\text{fall}} = 0.2$ were provided by Pandy et al. [25]. u represents the neural excitation, taking values from 0 to 0.5.

The strain energy produced by the muscle fibers can be written as follows:

$$U_f\left(\tilde{\lambda}_f, \dot{\tilde{\lambda}}_f, \alpha\right) = U_{PE}\left(\tilde{\lambda}_f\right) + U_{CE}\left(\tilde{\lambda}_f, \dot{\tilde{\lambda}}_f, \alpha\right) \tag{11}$$

where,

$$U_{PE}\left(\tilde{\lambda}_f\right) = T_o^M \int_1^{\tilde{\lambda}_f} f_{PE}\left(\tilde{\lambda}_f\right) d\tilde{\lambda}_f \tag{12}$$

$$U_{CE}\left(\tilde{\lambda}_f, \dot{\tilde{\lambda}}_f, \alpha\right) = \alpha \cdot T_o^M \int_1^{\tilde{\lambda}_f} f_L^{CE}\left(\tilde{\lambda}_f\right) f_V^{CE}\left(\dot{\tilde{\lambda}}_f\right) d\tilde{\lambda}_f \tag{13}$$

In summary, the biceps brachii muscle can be regarded as an incompressible, transversely isotropic, hyperelastic material which is assumed to be governed by a constitutive law linking the second Piola–Kirchhoff stress tensor $\boldsymbol{S}$ and the Green–Lagrange deformation tensor $\boldsymbol{E}$. The final second Piola–Kirchhoff stress tensor of the biceps brachii muscle is as follows:

$$\begin{aligned} S &= \frac{\partial U}{\partial E} = \frac{\partial U_J}{\partial E} + \frac{\partial U_I}{\partial E} + \frac{\partial U_f}{\partial E} = \frac{\partial U_J}{\partial J}\frac{\partial J}{\partial E} + \frac{\partial U_I}{\partial \widetilde{I}_C}\frac{\partial \widetilde{I}_C}{\partial E} + \frac{\partial U_f}{\partial \widetilde{\lambda}_f}\frac{\partial \widetilde{\lambda}_f}{\partial E} \\ &= 2JC^{-1} + \left\{bce^{b(\widetilde{I}_C-3)}\right\}\left(2J^{-3/2}I - \tfrac{2}{3}\widetilde{I}_C C^{-1}\right) + \frac{\partial U_f}{\partial \widetilde{\lambda}_f}\left(J^{-2/3}\widetilde{\lambda}_f^{-1}(N_m \otimes N_m) - \tfrac{1}{3}\widetilde{\lambda}_f C^{-1}\right) \end{aligned} \quad (14)$$

Furthermore, the radius bone and the tendon were treated as isotropic elastic materials, and the constitutive equation can be written as:

$$S = \lambda_m tr(E) + 2\mu E \quad (15)$$

where tr means the trace. The Lame parameters μ and λ_m were 6154 and 9231 MPa, respectively, for the radius bone, and 56 and 9296 MPa, respectively, for the tendon [26,27].

2.3. Finite Element Discretization

Skeletal muscles are typically regarded as incompressible materials [13]. We employed the Lagrange multiplier method to constrain the volumetric changes in the muscle. The incompressibility condition was treated by introducing a constraint function $W = J^2 - 1$. The total potential energy of the muscle can be expressed as a function concerning the displacement u and the Lagrange multiplier λ:

$$\Phi(u, \lambda) = \int_\Omega U\Omega + \int_\Omega \lambda W d\Omega - \int_\Gamma t \cdot u dS \quad (16)$$

where Ω and Γ indicate the volume and boundary surface, respectively. t represents the external conservative force on the boundary. The Lagrange multiplier λ is responsible for enforcing the incompressible constraint. According to the principle of minimum potential energy, the variation in the total potential energy Φ is equal to zero:

$$\delta\Phi = \int_\Omega \frac{\partial U}{\partial E}\delta E d\Omega + \int_\Omega \left(\lambda \frac{\partial W}{\partial E}\delta E + \delta\lambda W\right) d\Omega - \int_\Gamma t \cdot \delta u dS = 0 \quad (17)$$

The necessary condition for the satisfaction of Equation (17) with arbitrary δu and $\delta\lambda$ is:

$$\begin{cases} \int_\Omega \delta E : S_{inc}\Omega = \int_\Gamma t \cdot \delta u S \\ \int_\Omega \delta\lambda W d\Omega = 0 \end{cases} \quad (18)$$

where the second Piola–Kirchhoff stress tensor under incompressible conditions can be written as:

$$S_{inc} = \frac{\partial U}{\partial E} + \lambda \frac{\partial W}{\partial E} \quad (19)$$

The Galerkin procedure was adopted for spatial discretization. The shape function matrix for displacement u and virtual displacement δu is denoted as N. Similarly, the shape function matrix for Lagrange multiplier λ and virtual Lagrange multiplier $\delta\lambda$ is denoted as M. The discretization of u, δu, λ, and $\delta\lambda$ within each element is as follows:

$$u = Nu^{(n)} \qquad \delta u = N\delta u^{(n)} \quad (20)$$

$$\lambda = M\lambda^{(m)} \qquad \delta\lambda = M\delta\lambda^{(m)} \quad (21)$$

where n and m are the number of nodes and the number of the Lagrange multipliers within each element, respectively. The final discretized equation can be expressed as follows:

$$\begin{cases} \{\delta u\}^T \int_\Omega [B]^T \{S_{inc}\} d\Omega = \{\delta u\}^T \int_\Gamma [N]^T \{t\} dS \\ \{\delta\lambda\}^T \int_\Omega [M]^T W d\Omega = 0 \end{cases} \quad (22)$$

where $[B]$ is the strain–displacement matrix for a large deformation problem [28].

Our finite element model was validated by performing uniaxial passive stretching and active contraction simulations. More details can be referred to in Appendix A.

3. Results and Discussion

3.1. The Effect of Biceps Brachii Contraction Velocity on Forearm Flexion

Analyzing the elbow joint flexion angle under certain load condition offers valuable insights into the forearm's mobility and muscle performance [29,30]. Our developed finite element model can reproduce the forearm flexion motion (Video S1). The elbow joint flexion angle is defined as the difference between the final joint angle (right side of Figure 3) and the initial joint angle (left side of Figure 3).

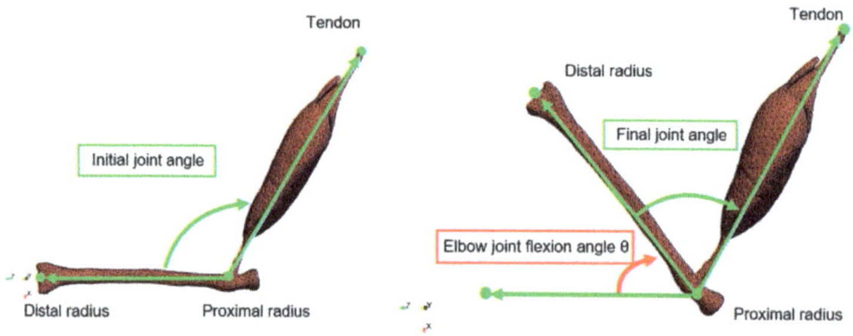

Figure 3. The definition of elbow joint flexion angle.

The maximum contraction velocity of muscles is related to their activation level [31]. A more rapid increase in muscle activation level results in a quicker muscle contraction velocity. Therefore, we controlled the muscle's contraction velocity by changing the activation level increase rates (Figure 4). We simulated the impacts of the contraction velocities (fast, medium, and slow) on the forearm flexion by using the linearly increasing activation level with different rates, as shown in Figure 4. The temporal duration for attaining the pinnacle of activation, denoted as α_{max}, within the fast, medium, and slow cases, amounted to 0.05 s, 0.20 s, and 1.00 s, correspondingly. For the boundary conditions, we imposed full constraints on the long head of the biceps brachii tendon and the proximal end of the radius. To restrict the supination of the forearm, we also constrained the Y-axis displacement of the nodes near both ends of the radius. Additionally, a vertically downward load was applied at the anterior end of the radius (Figure 5). This load was gradually applied from zero to the maximum value (100 N) along with the increase in the activation level.

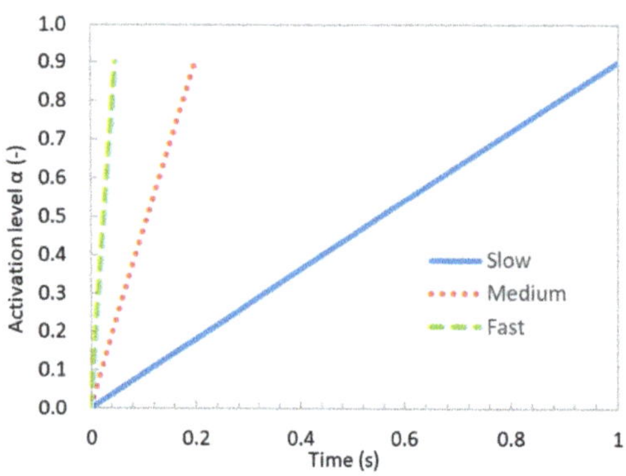

Figure 4. Temporal variations in muscle activation level with different increasing rates (fast, medium, and slow). The uniformity of the maximum activation level was maintained for each case ($\alpha_{max} = 0.91$).

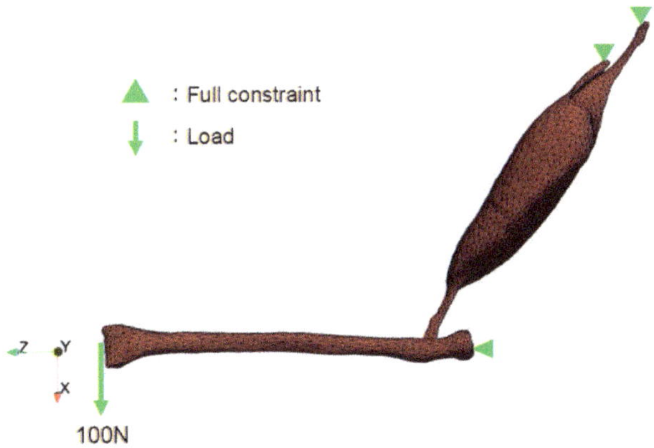

Figure 5. Forearm simulation boundary conditions: complete constraints were imposed on the nodes located at the distal extremities of the biceps brachii tendon heads, as well as the single node at the proximal end of the radius; displacement along the Y-axis was restricted at both ends of the radius; a vertical downward force, with a maximum magnitude of 100 N, was applied at the anterior end of the radius.

The results showed that the elbow joint flexion angle increased over time until the activation level reached its maximum value in all cases (Figures 6 and 7). In the medium and slow cases, the rate of increase in the elbow joint flexion angle gradually decreased over time. The highest degrees of elbow joint flexion achieved in the fast, medium, and slow cases were recorded as 28.47, 62.10, and 65.35 degrees, respectively. The force–velocity (F-V) curve of the skeletal muscles during concentric contraction demonstrates that muscle force decreases with an increasing contraction velocity [32]. This decrease in muscle force leads to a reduction in the elbow joint flexion angle. In other words, an increase in the contraction velocity leads to a diminishing maximum elbow joint flexion angle. Our results agreed with the F-V curve.

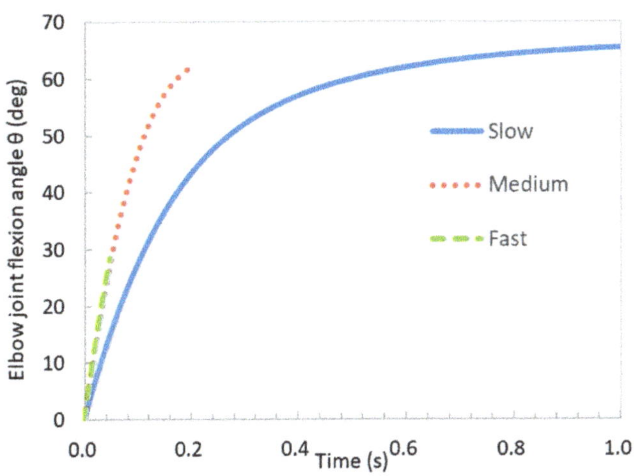

Figure 6. Temporal variations in elbow joint flexion angle for different muscle contraction velocities.

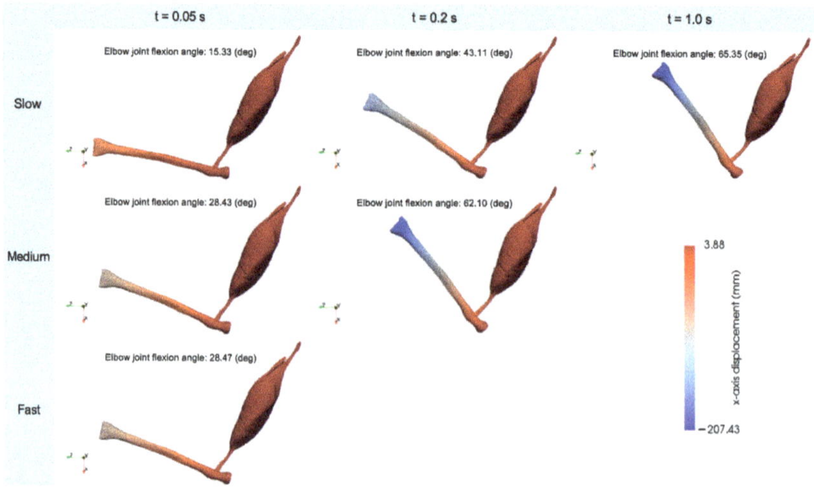

Figure 7. The displacements of the forearm along the *x*-axis and the elbow joint flexion angles at various times (fast: t = 0.05 s, medium: t = 0.05 s and t = 0.2 s, and slow: t = 0.05 s, t = 0.2 s, and t = 1.0 s).

From these results, we observed that larger contraction velocities of the biceps brachii muscle are less advantageous for promoting forearm flexion. When $\dot{\tilde{\lambda}}_f < -10$, the strain energy produced by the CE element remains constant at zero (Equations (9) and (13)), leading to diminished contraction stress (Equation (14)) of the muscle fibers, ultimately resulting in a reduction in the elbow joint flexion angle. According to Alcazar et al. [33], standard subjects exhibit a negative relationship between muscle force and contraction velocity during forearm flexion. When the velocity of muscle contraction surpasses a critical threshold, the muscle becomes incapable of exerting substantial force under a particular load [33]. Our simulation results matched with this previous finding. Therefore, we confirmed that our forearm model can reasonably reproduce the forearm's flexion movement.

3.2. *Simulation of Forearm Flexion Movement in Elderly Individuals*

Sarcopenia (muscle loss with aging) is a common disease in elderly individuals, leading to functional decline, disability, frailty, and falls. Changes in muscle fiber composition, muscle strength decline, and neurological dysfunction are the characteristics of sarcopenia [21,34,35]. By adjusting the relevant parameters of the biceps brachii model, we quantitatively investigated the influences of sarcopenia on functional decline by simulating the forearm's flexion movement: (1) changing the composition of the muscle fibers, i.e., the percentage of fast-twitch muscle fibers (refer to Section 3.2.1); (2) adjusting the maximum nominal stress T_0^M to reproduce muscle strength decline; and (3) modifying the neural excitation u to mimic neurological dysfunction. We further conducted a comparative analysis of the influence of these parameters on the forearm flexion motion. All simulation boundary conditions remained consistent with those detailed in the preceding section, except that the load (100 N) was constantly applied throughout the simulation period, mimicking the condition of the dumbbell curl exercise.

3.2.1. Changes in Muscle Fiber Composition

Muscles consist of two primary types of fibers: fast-twitch (Type II) and slow-twitch (Type I) fibers. Slow-twitch fibers contract slowly and are fatigue-resistant, making them well-suited for endurance activities such as long-distance running or maintaining posture.

Conversely, fast-twitch fibers contract rapidly but fatigue more quickly. The number of fast-twitch motor units have been found to decrease with human aging [36]. The proportion of slow-twitch and fast-twitch muscle fibers exhibits interindividual variability and can be influenced by factors such as genetics and training [37].

In this study, we differentiated between the two categories of muscle fibers in our muscle model by adjusting the values of τ_{rise} and τ_{fall} in Equation (10). We set $\tau_{\text{rise}} = 0.1$ and $\tau_{\text{fall}} = 1.0$ for fast-twitch muscle fibers, while for slow-twitch muscle fibers, $\tau_{\text{rise}} = 0.3$ and $\tau_{\text{fall}} = 3.0$. Neural excitation $u = 0.5$ was used for both types of muscle fibers. The temporal variations in the muscle activation level for fast-twitch and slow-twitch muscle fibers are shown in Figure 8.

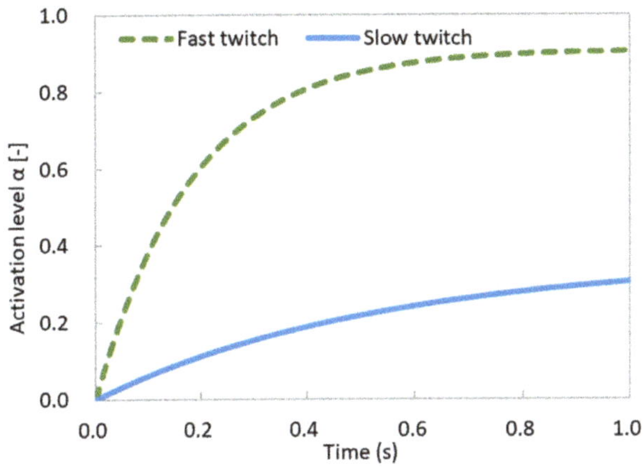

Figure 8. Temporal variations in muscle activation level for fast-twitch and slow-twitch muscle fibers.

Based on Equations (4), (5) and (7), the nominal stress of muscle, including the contributions of both fast-twitch and slow-twitch muscle fibers, is as follows:

$$\begin{aligned} T\left(\tilde{\lambda}_f, \dot{\tilde{\lambda}}_f, \alpha_{SO}, \alpha_{FG}\right) &= T_{SO}\left(\tilde{\lambda}_f, \dot{\tilde{\lambda}}_f, \alpha_{SO}\right) + T_{FG}\left(\tilde{\lambda}_f, \dot{\tilde{\lambda}}_f, \alpha_{FG}\right) \\ &= T_0^M \mu_{SO}\left[f_{PE}\left(\tilde{\lambda}_f\right) + f_L^{CE}\left(\tilde{\lambda}_f\right) f_V^{CE}\left(\tilde{\lambda}_f, \dot{\tilde{\lambda}}_f\right)\alpha_{SO}\right] \\ &+ T_0^M \mu_{FG}\left[f_{PE}\left(\tilde{\lambda}_f\right) + f_L^{CE}\left(\tilde{\lambda}_f\right) f_V^{CE}\left(\tilde{\lambda}_f, \dot{\tilde{\lambda}}_f\right)\alpha_{FG}\right] \end{aligned} \tag{23}$$

where T_{so} and T_{FG} represent the muscle stresses generated by slow and fast-twitch muscle fibers, respectively. Furthermore, μ_{SO} and μ_{FG} denote the percentages of slow-twitch and fast-twitch muscle fibers within the cross-sectional area, respectively. α_{SO} and α_{FG} represent the activation levels of slow-twitch and fast-twitch muscle fibers (Figure 8), respectively.

Alterations in the proportions of fast-twitch fibers play a pivotal role in the age-related decline of muscle function [20,34,35]. As individuals age, there is a proclivity for an augmentation in the proportion of slow-twitch muscle fibers, concomitant with a diminishing trend in the proportion of fast-twitch muscle fibers [38]. In this study, we employed the biceps brachii muscle fiber composition data of young participants (aged 29 ± 5 years), as quantified by Monemi et al., as a baseline (Young in Table 1) [38]. Referring to Hakkinen et al.'s measurements of muscle fiber composition in elderly individuals (61 ± 4 years) [39], we systematically decreased the percentage of fast-twitch muscle fibers by 7%, taking into account the specific context of aging (Elderly I and II in Table 1). Assuming a linear decline in the percentage of fast-twitch muscle fibers during the aging process, we supposed the young case at 30 (±5 years), Elderly I at 45 (±5 years), and Elderly II at 60 (±5 years).

Table 1. Muscle fiber compositions of each case.

Case	Young	Elderly I	Elderly II
Fast-twitch [%]	58	51	44
Slow-twitch [%]	42	49	56

The simulation results showed an increasing trend in the elbow joint flexion angle over time (Figure 9). An increased percentage of fast-twitch muscle fibers resulted in an elevated elbow joint flexion angle throughout the entire time frame. Additionally, at approximately t = 0.1 s, the initiation of forearm elevation was observed. The sequence of forearm initiation unfolded as follows: Young individuals led the way, followed by Elderly I, and finally, Elderly II. A reduced percentage of fast-twitch muscle fibers led to a delay in the onset of forearm elevation. In instances where fast-twitch muscle fibers were scarce, forearm flexion movements were predominantly governed by slow-twitch muscle fibers, which possess a reduced stress generation capacity. It is noted that this conclusion presupposed the maintenance of all other factors in a constant state. According to Mannion et al. [40], the predominant factor influencing high-intensity exercise capacity is the proportion of fast-twitch muscle fibers. A greater proportion of fast-twitch muscle contributes to a superior dynamic exercise performance. Our findings substantiated the pivotal role of muscle fiber composition in the context of forearm flexion dynamics.

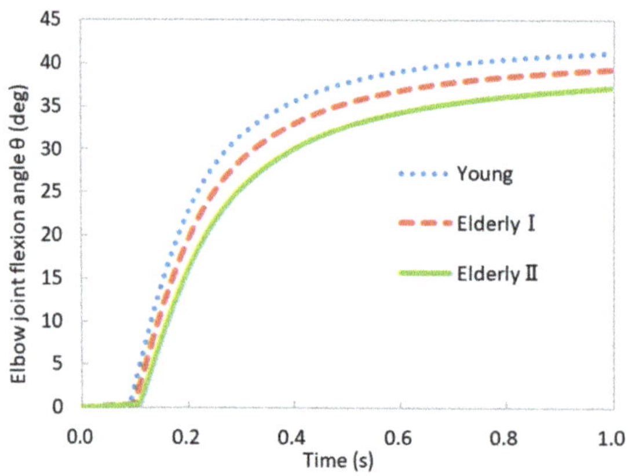

Figure 9. Temporal variations in the elbow joint flexion angle under different muscle fiber compositions.

The maximal degrees of elbow flexion for the Young, Elderly I, and Elderly II cases corresponded to 41.17, 39.28, and 37.19 degrees, respectively (refer to Figure 10). A linear relationship was found between the percentage of fast-twitch muscle fibers and the peak elbow joint flexion angle. As elucidated by Equation (23), there exists a direct linear correspondence between the percentage of fast-twitch muscle fibers and muscle stress. Under the same forearm loading conditions, the greater the proportion of fast-twitch muscle fibers in the biceps brachii, the larger the muscle stress generated, facilitating forearm flexion and resulting in an increased elbow joint flexion angle. The simulation results were consistent with the theoretical model.

We also noted that, with every 10% augmentation in the percentage of fast-twitch muscle fibers, there ensued a corresponding increment of 2.84 degrees in the maximal elbow joint flexion angle. This quantitative analysis introduces a novel methodology for exploring the impact of muscle fiber composition on forearm dynamics. Our findings substantiate the notion that a training program focused on fast-twitch muscle fibers can enhance the forearm flexion ability among older individuals when performing activities under forearm loading conditions. In accordance with Wilson et al. [41], high-intensity, low-volume, and/or high-velocity training programs contribute to an increase in the proportion of fast-twitch muscle fibers. Therefore, engaging in brisk-paced dumbbell bicep curls with lightweight resistance may mitigate the mobility decrease induced by alterations in muscle fiber composition [41,42], aiding in preserving independence and autonomy in the daily lives of elderly individuals.

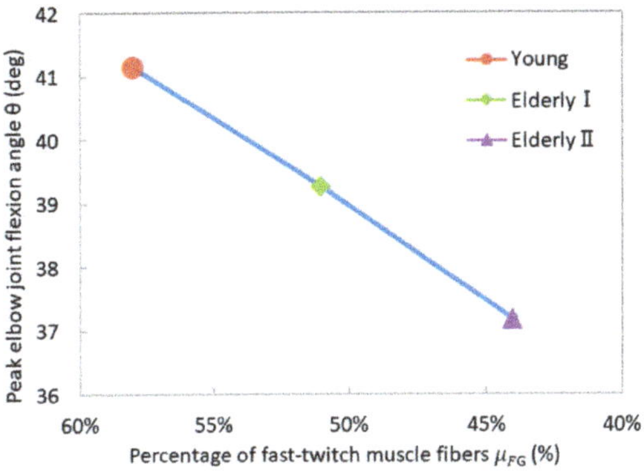

Figure 10. The relationship between the percentage of fast-twitch muscle fibers and peak elbow joint flexion angles.

3.2.2. Biceps Brachii Strength Decline

The aging progression also triggers a conspicuous decline in both muscle mass and strength. This decline becomes particularly evident beyond the age of 40. In comparison to young individuals, those surpassing this age threshold encounter a diminution in muscle strength ranging from 16.6% to 40.9% [43,44]. To elucidate the impact of the decline in the biceps brachii strength on forearm flexion, we introduced a reduction in the maximum muscle stress parameter T_0^M (Equation (23)) from 100% to 70%. The remaining parameters of the simulation remained consistent with those applied to the Young case (refer to Section 3.2.1). The temporal evolution of the elbow joint flexion angle under varying percentages of maximum muscle stress is depicted in Figure 11.

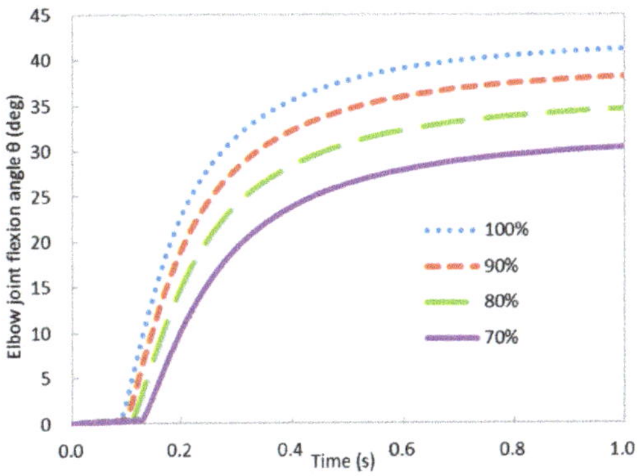

Figure 11. Temporal evolution of the elbow joint flexion angle under varying percentages of maximum muscle stress.

It is noted that an elevated maximum muscle stress T_0^M led to a greater elbow joint flexion angle throughout the entire temporal duration (Figure 11). Additionally, at approximately $t = 0.1$ s, the forearm started to elevate. A reduction in the maximum muscle stress triggered a delayed commencement of forearm elevation. This delay is attributed to the diminished maximal muscle stress, resulting in a smaller actual muscle force at an equivalent level of activation (Equation (23)). This reduction necessitated an extended duration to reach the requisite muscle force for the elevation of the load, ultimately introducing a temporal lag in the initiation of forearm elevation.

The elbow joint flexion angles under different maximum muscle stresses are illustrated in Figure 12. As the maximum muscle stress T_0^M diminished, the peak elbow joint flexion angle also decreased. A nearly linear relationship was observed between the maximum elbow joint flexion angle and the magnitude of the maximum muscle stress. According to Equation (23), the maximum muscle stress parameter acts as a coefficient for generating the muscle force during muscle contraction. Therefore, a greater maximum muscle stress promotes forearm flexion. According to Jung et al. [45], there exists a positive correlation between muscle strength and range of motion. Our simulation results were consistent with this observation.

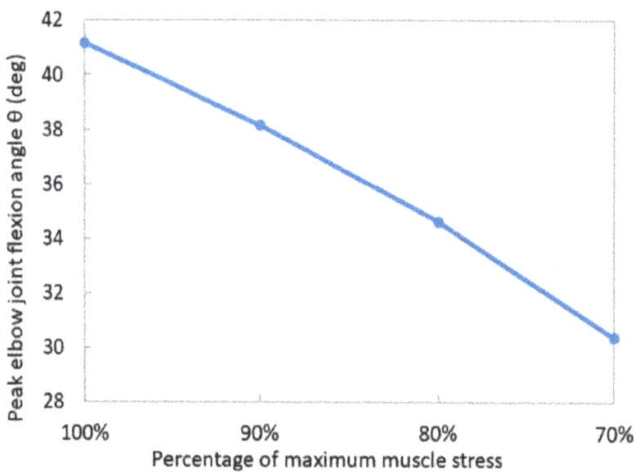

Figure 12. The relationship between the percentage of maximum muscle stress and the peak elbow joint flexion angle.

It was also observed the peak elbow joint flexion angle exhibited a decrement of 3.59 degrees for every 10% reduction in the maximum muscle stress. This quantitative analysis provides a novel perspective for comprehending the impact of diminishing muscle strength on forearm movements. Our study showed that the maximum muscle stress plays an important role in forearm flexion movements. According to Kalapotharakos et al. [46], the continuation of a strength training program is essential for maintaining muscle strength and functional performance in old individuals. Moderate resistance strength training from 2 to 3 days per week can effectively prevent age-related muscle strength decline and improve the quality of life for elderly individuals [47,48].

3.2.3. Neurological Dysfunction

From the generation of neural signals to the initiation of muscle contractions, numerous age-related changes occur in the nervous system. These changes collectively contribute to neurological dysfunction [49–53]. Within the framework of this investigation, we fine-tuned the neural excitation parameter u to emulate the manifestation of neurological dysfunction. It was posited that neural excitation would diminish incrementally from 0.5 to 0.1 in discrete 0.1 intervals, with the aim of replicating the progression of neurological dysfunction. The rest of the simulation conditions were the same as for the Young case (refer to Section 3.2.1). The temporal variations in the forearm flexion angle under different neural excitations are shown in Figure 13.

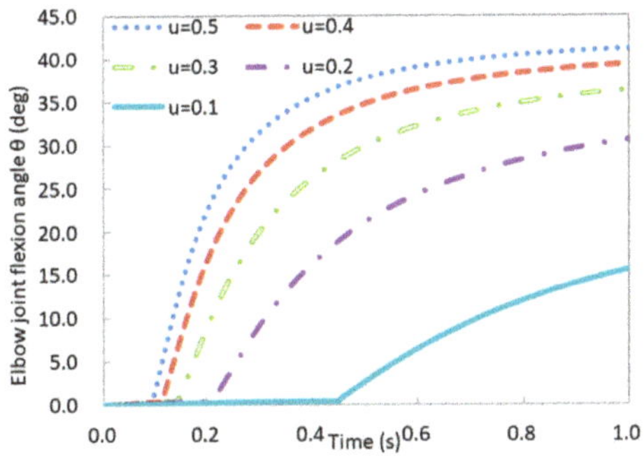

Figure 13. Temporal variations in the elbow joint flexion angle under different neural excitations.

Our observations indicated a positive relationship between the magnitude of neural excitation and the degree of elbow flexion during forearm movement (Figure 13). At approximately 0.1 s, the forearm endowed with the highest neural excitation level $(u = 0.5)$ commenced its elevation. The forearm with the smallest neural excitation $(u = 0.1)$ commenced its elevation at 0.42 s. A greater neural excitation level led to an earlier initiation of forearm elevation. Furthermore, we observed that, in comparison to $u = 0.2$, when $u = 0.1$, there was a significant reduction in the elbow joint flexion angle, accompanied by a noticeable postponement in the timing of forearm elevation. This reduction in neural excitation corresponds to diminished muscle activation levels and muscle stresses (Equations (10) and (23)), resulting in a decline in forearm motion capability. As elucidated by Kwon et al. [54], age-related nervous system changes affect the entire process, from neural signal generation to muscle contraction, further impacting motor performance and muscle force. Our simulation results were consistent with the experimental findings.

The relationship between peak elbow joint flexion angle and neural excitation is illustrated in Figure 14. As the neural excitation decreased, a corresponding reduction occurred in the peak elbow joint flexion angle. This relationship is notably nonlinear, due to the fact that, muscle stress, which has a direct relationship with the peak flexion angle, exhibits a nonlinear association with neural excitation (Equations (10) and (23)). Especially when $u < 0.2$, there was a marked decrease in the peak elbow joint flexion angle. These findings suggest that $u = 0.2$ serves as a critical threshold, below which, the forearm's motion capability undergoes a substantial diminishment. When neural excitation u surpasses the 0.2 threshold, each 10% reduction in neural excitation u corresponds to a concomitant decrease of 1.76 degrees in the peak elbow joint flexion angle. Conversely, when u falls below the threshold of 0.2, each 10% reduction in neural excitation leads to a more pronounced decline of 7.44 degrees in the peak elbow joint flexion angle.

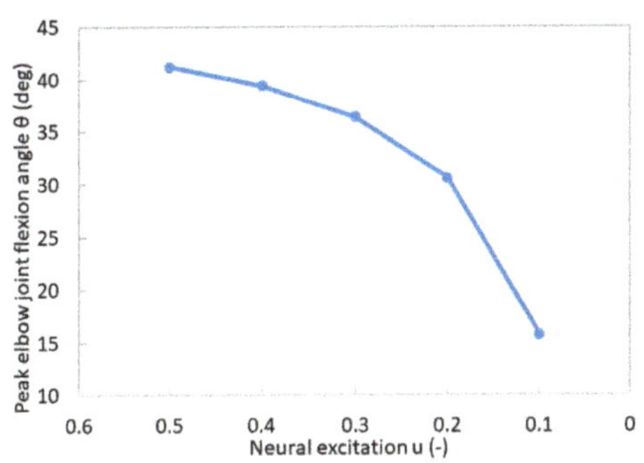

Figure 14. The relationship between peak elbow joint flexion angles and neural excitations.

Clark et al.'s [49] research indicated that age-related strength decline is not only linked to muscle atrophy, but also depends on neurological factors. Our findings can help to explain the impact of neural excitation on forearm movement under loading conditions. Furthermore, our simulation provided valuable information for determining the critical threshold of neural excitation.

3.2.4. Implication of Our Simulations

We succinctly encapsulated the repercussions of a 10% decrement in the investigated factors on the peak flexion angle (Table 2). In instances where the neural excitation value exceeded the threshold ($u > 0.2$), our findings revealed that the most significant influence on forearm flexion kinetics stemmed from the reduction in the biceps brachii strength, resulting in a reduction of 3.59 degrees. Subsequently, alterations in muscle fiber composition contributed to a decrease of 2.84 degrees, while neurological dysfunction exerted the least impact, with a decline of 1.76 degrees. Conversely, when the neural excitation value fell below the threshold ($u < 0.2$), neurological dysfunction emerged as the paramount determinant affecting forearm flexion movements in older individuals, manifesting a substantial reduction of 7.44 degrees.

Table 2. The peak elbow joint flexion angle reduction in elderly subjects under different factors.

	Muscle Fiber Composition Change	**Biceps Brachii Strength Decline**	**Neurological Dysfunction ($u > 0.2$)**	**Neurological Dysfunction ($u < 0.2$)**
Reduced angle (deg)	2.84	3.59	1.76	7.44

When the neural excitation value exceeded the threshold ($u > 0.2$), the decline in the biceps brachii strength became the most significant factor influencing forearm movement, compared to changes in muscle fiber composition. The reason is that the decrease in muscle maximum stress caused by muscle strength decline directly affected the muscle force output (Equation (23)). However, changes in muscle fiber composition indirectly influenced the muscle force and had a smaller impact. When the neural excitation value was under the threshold ($u < 0.2$), the non-linear relationship between neural excitation and the activation level led to a significant decline in muscle stress (Equations (10) and (23)), making it the main factor influencing elbow flexion movement.

According to Clark et al. [49], the aging process is accompanied by a gradual reduction in motor neurons, which impacts the motion capabilities of elderly individuals. When the critical threshold for the number of motor neurons is reached (typically occurring between the ages of 65 and 80), functional disabilities manifest [55]. Our simulation results hold the promise of providing assistance in the development of targeted exercise programs for elderly individuals across different age groups. For elderly individuals under the age of 65, focusing on muscle strength training has proved to be the most effective method for enhancing their motion capabilities, which encompasses implementing progressive strength training or moderate resistance strength training [46]. For those aged 65 and older, exercise programs aimed at improving neurological system functionality become the most effective means for improving their motion capabilities. For instance, developing a training regimen that combines high-resistance training with explosive exercises is an effective approach [56,57].

4. Conclusions

In this study, we developed a simplified forearm finite element model including radius, biceps brachii, and tendons to simulate the forearm flexion motion. Since only the biceps brachii muscle was considered in our study, the synergistic interactions among other tissues were neglected. Therefore, the more complicated motions such as the neck behind-arm flexion extension and bench press movement cannot be reproduced by this model. In this work, we also conducted a parametric study to quantitatively investigate the effects of factors including muscle contraction speed, the proportion of fast-twitch fibers, maximum muscle stress, and neural excitation on the flexion angle with a dumbbell load based on the developed model. In the future, a comprehensive experimental investigation to quantitatively measure these parameters will be necessary for validating the accuracy of our simulation results.

From the simulation results produced by this simplified model, we observed that a slow muscle contraction velocity facilitates the forearm flexion movement, which agreed with the trend of the F-V curve. By analyzing the influence exerted by various factors on forearm motion, we also obtained the subsequent findings:

- A larger percentage of fast-twitch muscle fibers and a greater maximum muscle stress value are benefits for forearm flexion movement;
- The fast-twitch muscle fibers' percentage and maximum muscle stress are linearly correlated with the maximum elbow joint flexion angle;
- The enhancement of neural excitation levels yields advantages in forearm flexion, showcasing a non-linear interplay between neural excitation and the maximum elbow joint flexion angle;
- Moreover, our findings indicated that, when neural excitation levels surpass the threshold, the preeminent factor governing arm flexion movements is the maximal muscle stress. Conversely, in situations where neural excitation levels fall below the threshold, neural excitation takes precedence as the dominant influence on forearm flexion dynamics. Our findings hold significant implications for understanding the mechanisms of forearm motion and guiding rehabilitation training for sarcopenia.

Supplementary Materials: The following supporting information can be downloaded at: https://www.mdpi.com/article/10.3390/bioengineering11010023/s1, Video S1: Animation of the forearm flexion movement simulated by our finite element model.

Author Contributions: Conceptualization, X.C., F.J., C.L. and D.K.; methodology, F.J., X.C., C.L. and D.K.; software, C.L. and D.K.; validation, C.L. and D.K.; formal analysis, D.K. and C.L.; investigation, C.L. and F.J.; resources, X.C. and F.J.; data curation, C.L. and D.K.; writing—original draft preparation, C.L. and F.J.; writing—review and editing, F.J., X.C. and C.L.; visualization, C.L.; supervision, F.J. and X.C.; project administration, F.J.; funding acquisition, F.J. and X.C. All authors have read and agreed to the published version of the manuscript.

Funding: This research received no external funding.

Institutional Review Board Statement: Not applicable.

Informed Consent Statement: Not applicable.

Data Availability Statement: The data that support the findings of this study are available from the corresponding author upon reasonable request.

Conflicts of Interest: The authors declare no conflict of interest.

Appendix A. Validation

To validate the muscle finite element model, a single hexahedral element with a 1 mm side length (Figure A1) was used to simulate the muscle stretching in the passive state and contraction in the active state. The muscle fiber direction was aligned along the Z-axis. The boundary conditions for uniaxial passive stretching and active contraction of the muscle model are illustrated in Figure A1. Additionally, by applying enforced displacement, the upper four nodes underwent the following conditions: a. they were uniformly stretched along the Z-axis at a rate of 0.1 mm/s from 0 to 1 s (passive stretching). b. from 1 to 1.2 s, they experienced uniform contraction at a rate of −1 mm/s (active contraction). In this simulation, we utilized the maximum muscle stress $T_0^M = 0.6688$ Mpa. The neural excitation value was set as $u = 0$ during 0–1 s (passive stretching) and $u = 0.5$ during 1–1.2 s (active contraction), while the rest of the simulation parameters were the same as in Section 2.2.

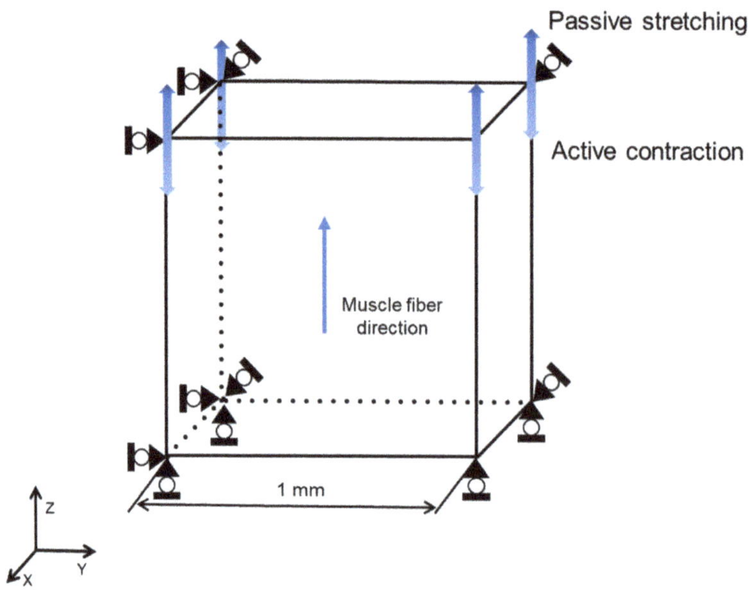

Figure A1. The boundary conditions for the uniaxial passive stretching and active contraction of the muscle model.

We also computed the theoretical value of the second Piola–Kirchhoff stress S_{zz}, as shown in Equation (A1):

$$
\begin{aligned}
S_{zz} = & -\frac{1}{C_{yy}^{-1}}\Big\{cbexp\left(b\left(\tilde{I}_C-3\right)\right)\left(2J^{-\frac{2}{3}}-\frac{2}{3}\tilde{I}_C C_{yy}^{-1}\right) \\
& +T_o^M\left\{-\frac{1}{3}\tilde{\lambda}_f C_{yy}^{-1}\right\}\Big\{2Aaexp\left(a\left(\tilde{\lambda}_f-1\right)^2\right)\left(\tilde{\lambda}_f-1\right) \\
& +\alpha\left[-4\left(\tilde{\lambda}_f-1\right)^2+1\right]\left[-\frac{1}{\mathrm{atan}(5)}\mathrm{atan}\left(-0.5\dot{\tilde{\lambda}}_f\right)+1\right]\Big\}\Big\}C_{zz}^{-1} \\
& +cbexp\left(b\left(\tilde{I}_C-3\right)\right)\left(2J^{-\frac{2}{3}}-\frac{2}{3}\tilde{I}_C C_{zz}^{-1}\right) \\
& +T_o^M\left\{J^{-\frac{2}{3}}\tilde{\lambda}_f^{-1}-\frac{1}{3}\tilde{\lambda}_f C_{zz}^{-1}\right\}\Big\{2Aae^{a\left(\tilde{\lambda}_f-1\right)^2}\left(\tilde{\lambda}_f-1\right) \\
& +\alpha\left[-4\left(\tilde{\lambda}_f-1\right)^2+1\right]\left[-\frac{1}{\mathrm{atan}(5)}\mathrm{atan}\left(-0.5\dot{\tilde{\lambda}}_f\right)+1\right]\Big\}
\end{aligned}
\quad \text{(A1)}
$$

where, under uniaxial passive stretching and active contraction condition, there exist: $C_{yy}^{-1}=\tilde{\lambda}_f$, $C_{zz}^{-1}=\tilde{\lambda}_f^{-2}$, $\tilde{I}_c=\tilde{\lambda}_f^{2}+2\tilde{\lambda}_f^{-1}$, $\dot{\tilde{\lambda}}_f=0.1s^{-1}$ (passive stretching), $\dot{\tilde{\lambda}}_f=-1s^{-1}$ (active contraction). Additionally, according to Equation (10), during passive stretching $\alpha=0$, where during active contraction, $0<\alpha\leq 0.905$.

The simulated results in terms of the second Piola–Kirchhoff stress S_{zz} are compared with the theoretical values in Figure A2. Figure A2 illustrates the relationship between the S_{zz} and the muscle fiber stretch ratio $\tilde{\lambda}_f$ during passive stretching and active contraction. The simulated S_{zz} results matched the theoretical curve throughout the entire process, which validated the finite element discretization.

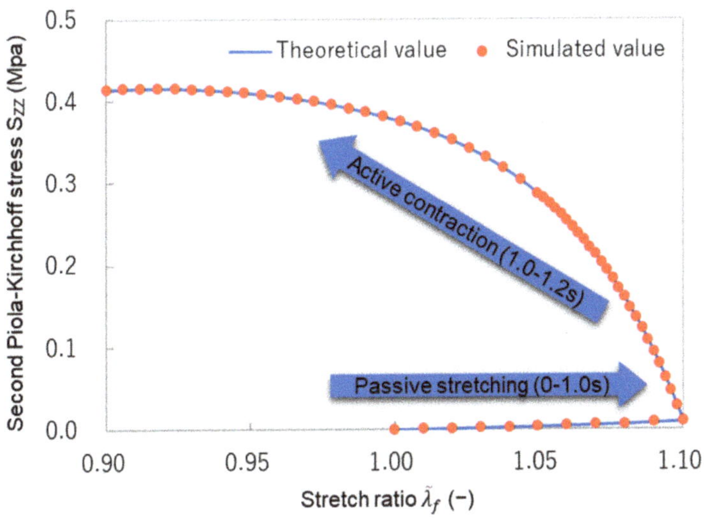

Figure A2. The relationship between the stress ratio $\tilde{\lambda}_f$ and the second Piola–Kirchhoff stress S_{zz} during the muscle model's passive stretching and active contraction.

References

1. Ambrósio, J.; Quental, C.; Pilarczyk, B.; Folgado, J.; Monteiro, J. Multibody biomechanical models of the upper limb. *Procedia IUTAM* **2011**, *2*, 4–17. [CrossRef]
2. Teran, J.; Sifakis, E.; Blemker, S.S.; Ng-Thow-Hing, V.; Lau, C.; Fedkiw, R. Creating and simulating skeletal muscle from the visible human data set. *IEEE Trans. Vis. Comput. Graph.* **2005**, *11*, 317–328. [CrossRef] [PubMed]
3. Dereshgi, H.A.; Serbest, K.; Balik, B.; Sahin, S.N. Stress-strain response of muscle fibers in biceps brachii under dynamic force: An analysis of biceps curl exercise. *Politeknik Dergisi* **2022**, *25*, 1777–1783. [CrossRef]
4. Dereshgi, H.A. The rest-pause biceps curl exercise effect on biceps brachii muscle of women: A study of mechanical responsiveness. *IEEE Access* **2023**, *11*, 116967–116978. [CrossRef]
5. Chen, D.T.; Zeltzer, D. Pump It Up: Computer animation of a biomechanically based model of muscle using the finite element method. In Proceedings of the 19th Annual Conference on Computer Graphics and Interactive Techniques, New York, NY, USA, 1 July 1992.
6. Blemker, S.S.; Pinsky, P.M.; Delp, S.L. A 3D model of muscle reveals the causes of nonuniform strains in the biceps brachii. *J. Biomech.* **2005**, *38*, 657–665. [CrossRef]
7. Hopkins, P.M. Skeletal muscle physiology. *Contin. Educ. Anaesth. Crit. Care Pain* **2006**, *6*, 1–6. [CrossRef]
8. Greig, C.A.; Jones, D.A. Muscle physiology and contraction. *Surgery* **2013**, *31*, 147–154.
9. Zhang, G.; Chen, X.; Ohgi, J.; Miura, T.; Nakamoto, A.; Matsumura, C.; Sugiura, S.; Hisada, T. Biomechanical simulation of thorax deformation using finite element approach. *Biomed. Eng. Online* **2016**, *15*, 18. [CrossRef]
10. Best, T.M.; McElhaney, J.H.; Garrett, W.E.; Myers, B.S. Axial strain measurements in skeletal muscle at various strain rates. *J. Biomech. Eng.* **1995**, *117*, 262–265. [CrossRef]
11. Jiang, F.; Sakuramoto, I.; Nishida, N.; Onomoto, Y.; Ohgi, J.; Chen, X. The mechanical behavior of bovine spinal cord white matter under various strain rate conditions: Tensile testing and visco-hyperelastic constitutive modeling. *Med. Biol. Eng. Comput.* **2023**, *61*, 1381–1394. [CrossRef]
12. Dao, T.T.; Tho, M.C.H.B. A systematic review of continuum modeling of skeletal muscles: Current trends, limitations, and recommendations. *Appl. Bionics. Biomech.* **2018**, *2018*, 7631818. [CrossRef] [PubMed]
13. Wakeling, J.M.; Febrer-Nafría, M.; De Groote, F. A review of the efforts to develop muscle and musculoskeletal models for biomechanics in the last 50 years. *J. Biomech.* **2023**, *155*, 111657. [CrossRef] [PubMed]
14. Kojic, M.; Mijailovic, S.; Zdravkovic, N. Modelling of muscle behaviour by the finite element method using Hill's three-element model. *Int. J. Numer. Methods. Eng.* **1998**, *43*, 941–953. [CrossRef]
15. Tang, C.Y.; Tsui, C.P.; Stojanovic, B.; Kojic, M. Finite element modelling of skeletal muscles coupled with fatigue. *Int. J. Mech. Sci.* **2007**, *49*, 1179–1191. [CrossRef]
16. Johansson, T.; Meier, P.; Blickhan, R. A finite-element model for the mechanical analysis of skeletal muscles. *J. Theor. Biol.* **2000**, *206*, 131–149. [CrossRef] [PubMed]

17. Martins, J.A.C.; Pires, E.B.; Salvado, R.; Dinis, P.B. A numerical model of passive and active behavior of skeletal muscles. *Comput. Methods Appl. Mech. Eng.* **1998**, *151*, 419–433. [CrossRef]
18. Martins, J.A.C.; Pato, M.P.M.; Pires, E.B. A finite element model of skeletal muscles. *Virtual Phys. Prototyp.* **2006**, *1*, 159–170. [CrossRef]
19. Tanimoto, Y.; Watanabe, M.; Sun, W.; Tanimoto, K.; Shishikura, K.; Sugiura, Y.; Kusabiraki, T.; Kono, K. Association of sarcopenia with functional decline in community-dwelling elderly subjects in Japan. *Geriatr Gerontol Int.* **2013**, *13*, 958–963. [CrossRef]
20. Marcell, T.J. Sarcopenia: Causes, consequences, and preventions. *J. Gerontol. A Biol. Sci. Med. Sci.* **2003**, *58*, M911–M916. [CrossRef]
21. Yang, J.; Jiang, F.; Yang, M.; Chen, Z. Sarcopenia and nervous system disorders. *J. Neurol.* **2022**, *269*, 5787–5797. [CrossRef]
22. Netter, F.H. *Atlas of Human Anatomy*, 4th ed.; Elsevier Saunders: Philadelphia, PA, USA, 2006; pp. 431–435.
23. Zeng, W.; Hume, D.R.; Lu, Y.; Fitzpatrick, C.K.; Babcock, C.; Myers, C.A.; Rullkoetter, P.J.; Shelburne, K.B. Modeling of active skeletal muscles: A 3D continuum approach incorporating multiple muscle interactions. *Front. Bioeng. Biotechnol.* **2023**, *11*, 1153692. [CrossRef] [PubMed]
24. Humphrey, J.D.; Yin, F.C.P. On constitutive relations and finite deformations of passive cardiac tissue: I. A pseudostrain-energy function. *J. Biomech. Eng.* **1987**, *109*, 298–304. [CrossRef] [PubMed]
25. Pandy, M.G.; Zajac, F.E.; Sim, E.; Levine, W.S. An optimal control model for maximum-height human jumping. *J. Biomech.* **1990**, *23*, 1185–1198. [CrossRef] [PubMed]
26. Bosisio, M.R.; Talmant, M.; Skalli, W.; Laugier, P.; Mitton, D. Apparent Young's modulus of human radius using inverse finite-element method. *J. Biomech.* **2007**, *40*, 2022–2028. [CrossRef] [PubMed]
27. Wakabayashi, I.; Itoi, E.; Sano, H.; Shibuya, Y.; Sashi, R.; Minagawa, H.; Kobayashi, M. Mechanical environment of the supraspinatus tendon: A two-dimensional finite element model analysis. *J. Shoulder. Elbow. Surg.* **2003**, *12*, 612–617. [CrossRef] [PubMed]
28. Zienkiewicz, O.C.; Taylor, R.L.; David, D.F. *The Finite Element Method for Solid and Structural Mechanics*, 7th ed.; Butterworth-Heinemann: Oxford, UK, 2013; pp. 450–463.
29. Morrey, B.F. *The Elbow and Its Disorders*, 4th ed.; Saunders: Philadelphia, PA, USA, 2008; pp. 620–625.
30. Yang, J.; Lee, J.; Lee, B.; Kim, S.; Shin, D.; Lee, Y.; Lee, J.; Han, D.; Choi, S. The effects of elbow joint angle changes on elbow flexor and extensor muscle strength and activation. *J. Phys. Ther. Sci.* **2014**, *26*, 1079–1082. [CrossRef] [PubMed]
31. Chow, J.W.; Darling, W.G. The maximum shortening velocity of muscle should be scaled with activation. *J. Appl. Physiol.* **1999**, *86*, 1025–1031. [CrossRef]
32. Gülch, R.W. Force-velocity relations in human skeletal muscle. *Int. J. Sports Med.* **1994**, *15*, S2–S10. [CrossRef]
33. Alcazar, J.; Csapo, R.; Ara, I.; Alegre, L.M. On the shape of the force-velocity relationship in skeletal muscles: The linear, the hyperbolic, and the double-hyperbolic. *Front. Physiol.* **2019**, *10*, 769. [CrossRef]
34. Nilwik, R.; Snijders, T.; Leenders, M.; Groen, B.B.; van Kranenburg, J.; Verdijk, L.B.; Van Loon, L.J.C. The decline in skeletal muscle mass with aging is mainly attributed to a reduction in type II muscle fiber size. *Exp. Gerontol.* **2013**, *48*, 492–498. [CrossRef]
35. Walston, J.D. Sarcopenia in older adults. *Curr. Opin. Rheumatol.* **2012**, *24*, 623–627. [CrossRef] [PubMed]
36. Eberstein, A.; Goodgold, J. Slow and fast twitch fibers in human skeletal muscle. *Am. J. Physiol.* **1968**, *215*, 535–541. [CrossRef] [PubMed]
37. Simoneau, J.A.; Bouchard, C. Genetic determinism of fiber type proportion in human skeletal muscle. *FASEB J.* **1995**, *9*, 1091–1095. [CrossRef] [PubMed]
38. Monemi, M.; Eriksson, P.O.; Kadi, F.; Butler-Browne, G.S.; Thornell, L.E. Opposite changes in myosin heavy chain composition of human masseter and biceps brachii muscles during aging. *J. Muscle Res. Cell Motil.* **1999**, *20*, 351–361. [CrossRef] [PubMed]
39. Hakkinen, K.; Newton, R.U.; Gordon, S.E.; Mccormick, M.; Volek, J.S.; Nindl, B.C.; Gotshalk, L.A.; Campbell, W.W.; Evans, W.J.; Hakkinen, A.; et al. Changes in muscle morphology, electromyographic activity, and force production characteristics during progressive strength training in young and older men. *J. Gerontol. A Biol. Sci. Med. Sci.* **1998**, *53*, B415–B423. [CrossRef]
40. Mannion, A.F.; Jakeman, P.M.; Willan, P.L. Skeletal muscle buffer value, fibre type distribution and high intensity exercise performance in man. *Exp. Physiol.* **1995**, *80*, 89–101. [CrossRef]
41. Wilson, J.M.; Loenneke, J.P.; Jo, E.; Wilson, G.J.; Zourdos, M.C.; Kim, J.S. The effects of endurance, strength, and power training on muscle fiber type shifting. *J. Strength Cond. Res.* **2012**, *26*, 1724–1729. [CrossRef]
42. Simoneau, J.A.; Lortie, G.; Boulay, M.R.; Marcotte, M.; Thibault, M.C.; Bonchard, C. Human skeletal muscle fiber type alteration with high-intensity intermittent training. *Eur. J. Appl. Physiol.* **1985**, *54*, 250–253. [CrossRef]
43. Keller, K.; Engelhardt, M. Strength and muscle mass loss with aging process. Age and strength loss. *Muscles Ligaments Tendons J.* **2013**, *3*, 346–350. [CrossRef]
44. Frontera, W.R.; Hughes, V.A.; Fielding, R.A.; Fiatarone, M.A.; Evans, W.J.; Roubenoff, R. Aging of skeletal muscle: A 12-yr longitudinal study. *J. Appl. Physiol.* **2000**, *88*, 1321–1326. [CrossRef]
45. Jung, H.; Yamasaki, M. Association of lower extremity range of motion and muscle strength with physical performance of community-dwelling older women. *J. Physiol. Anthropol.* **2016**, *35*, 30. [CrossRef] [PubMed]
46. Kalapotharakos, V.I.; Smilios, I.; Parlavatzas, A.; Tokmakidis, S.P. The effect of moderate resistance strength training and detraining on muscle strength and power in older men. *J. Geriatr. Phys. Ther.* **2007**, *30*, 109–113. [CrossRef] [PubMed]

47. Seguin, R.; Nelson, M.E. The benefits of strength training for older adults. *Am. J. Prev. Med.* **2003**, *25*, 141–149. [CrossRef] [PubMed]
48. Ratamess, N.A.; Alvar, B.A.; Evetoch, T.E.; Housh, T.J.; Ben Kibler, W.; Kraemer, W.J.; Triplett, N.T. Progression models in resistance training for healthy adults. *Med. Sci. Sports. Exerc.* **2009**, *41*, 687–708.
49. Clark, D.J.; Fielding, R.A. Neuromuscular contributions to age-related weakness. *J. Gerontol. A Biol. Sci. Med. Sci.* **2012**, *67*, 41–47. [CrossRef] [PubMed]
50. Jang, Y.C.; Van Remmen, H. Age-associated alterations of the neuromuscular junction. *Exp. Gerontol.* **2011**, *46*, 193–198. [CrossRef] [PubMed]
51. Clark, L.A.; Manini, T.M.; Wages, N.P.; Simon, J.E.; Russ, D.W.; Clark, B.C. Reduced neural excitability and activation contribute to clinically meaningful weakness in older adults. *J. Gerontol. A Biol. Sci.* **2021**, *76*, 692–702. [CrossRef]
52. Delbono, O. Neural control of aging skeletal muscle. *Aging Cell* **2003**, *2*, 21–29.
53. Jensen, G.L. Inflammation: Roles in aging and sarcopenia. *JPEN J. Parenter. Enteral. Nutr.* **2008**, *32*, 656–659. [CrossRef]
54. Kwon, Y.N.; Yoon, S.S. Sarcopenia: Neurological point of view. *J. Bone. Metab.* **2017**, *24*, 83–89. [CrossRef]
55. McNeil, C.J.; Doherty, T.J.; Stashuk, D.W.; Rice, C.L. Motor unit number estimates in the tibialis anterior muscle of young, old, and very old men. *Muscle Nerve* **2005**, *31*, 461–467. [CrossRef] [PubMed]
56. Häkkinen, K.; Kallinen, M.; Linnamo, V.; Pastinen, U.M.; Newton, R.U.; Kraemer, W.J. Neuromuscular adaptations during bilateral versus unilateral strength training in middle-aged and elderly men and women. *Acta Physiol. Scand.* **1996**, *158*, 77–88. [CrossRef] [PubMed]
57. Häkkinen, K.; Kallinen, M.; Izquierdo, M.; Jokelainen, K.; Lassila, H.; Mälkiä, E.; Kraemer, W.J.; Newton, R.U.; Alen, M. Changes in agonist-antagonist EMG, muscle CSA, and force during strength training in middle-aged and older people. *J. Appl. Physiol.* **1998**, *84*, 1341–1349. [CrossRef] [PubMed]

bioengineering

MDPI

Article

Elastic Resistance and Shoulder Movement Patterns: An Analysis of Reaching Tasks Based on Proprioception

Gyuseok Shim [1], Duwon Yang [1,†], Woorim Cho [2,†], Jihyeon Kim [3], Hyangshin Ryu [3,*], Woong Choi [4,*] and Jaehyo Kim [1,*]

1 Department of Human Ecology & Technology, BrainKorea21 FOUR, Handong Global University, Pohang 37554, Republic of Korea; gyuseoksa@handong.ac.kr (G.S.); doonebest0730@gmail.com (D.Y.)
2 Department of Information and Communications Engineering, Tokyo Institute of Technology, Yokohama 226-8503, Japan; cho.w.ab@m.titech.ac.jp
3 Department of Digital Healthcare, Human Integrated Solution, Goyang 10464, Republic of Korea; jihyeon@hisolution.co.kr
4 College of ICT Construction & Welfare Convergence, Kangnam University, Yongin 16979, Republic of Korea
* Correspondence: rhs@hisolution.co.kr (H.R.); wchoi@kangnam.ac.kr (W.C.); jhkim@handong.edu (J.K.)
† These authors contributed equally to this work.

Abstract: This study departs from the conventional research on horizontal plane reach movements by examining human motor control strategies in vertical plane elastic load reach movements conducted without visual feedback. Here, participants performed shoulder presses with elastic resistances at low, moderate, and high intensities without access to visual information about their hand position, relying exclusively on proprioceptive feedback and synchronizing their movements with a metronome set at a 3 s interval. The results revealed consistent performance symmetry across different intensities in terms of the reach speed (p = 0.254–0.736), return speed (p = 0.205–0.882), and movement distance (p = 0.480–0.919). This discovery underscores the human capacity to uphold bilateral symmetry in movement execution when relying solely on proprioception. Furthermore, this study observed an asymmetric velocity profile where the reach duration remained consistent irrespective of the load (1.15 s), whereas the return duration increased with higher loads (1.39 s–1.45 s). These findings suggest that, in the absence of visual feedback, the asymmetric velocity profile does not result from the execution of the action but rather represents a deliberate deceleration post-reach aimed at achieving the target position as generated by the brain's internal model. These findings hold significant implications for interpreting rehabilitation approaches under settings devoid of visual feedback.

Keywords: elastic resistance; shoulder press; proprioception; reaching; OpenPose; skewness; exercise intensity; symmetry

1. Introduction

In everyday life, humans execute numerous reaching movements, employing a combination of the brain's internal model [1], visual information [2], and the intricate interplay of the musculoskeletal system [3] to achieve precise targeting. Notably, among all body joints, the shoulder joint offers the highest degree of freedom for these movements [4]. The control of the shoulder joint during reaching movements is primarily influenced by two key factors: muscle fatigue [5] and visual feedback [6]. Muscle fatigue can significantly diminish the force-generating capacity of the shoulder's surrounding muscles, posing a challenge to maintaining movement performance. Within this context, visual feedback assumes a pivotal role. It refers to the sensory information received through the eyes, which aids in coordinating and adjusting movements based on visual cues [7]. However, when visual feedback is unavailable, reliance shifts to proprioception. Proprioception, or the proprioceptive sense, recognizes body position and the necessary force adjustments without relying on visual inputs [8,9]. While proprioception is crucial for movement control, it inherently lacks the precision offered by visual feedback [10]. When visual feedback is unavailable and elastic resistance is introduced as an external force, an essential component of proprioception, known as movement feedback, experiences enhancement [11]. This enhancement results in an increased level of accuracy in reaching movements. Elastic bands provide a resistance that intensifies as the distance from the neutral position increases, thereby furnishing finely tuned feedback for joint position and muscle force control [12]. This directly contributes to the enhancement of proprioception.

Past studies have predominantly examined the influence of load on reaching movements within a two-dimensional horizontal plane with visual feedback [13,14]. Human movements typically follow straight trajectories from the initial point to the target, characterized by symmetric, bell-shaped velocity profiles [15], as elucidated by the minimum variance model [16] and the minimum torque-change model [17]. When an elastic load is applied, the minimum variance model predicts asymmetrical velocity profiles due to the influence of the elastic force, whereas the minimum torque-change model anticipates symmetrical velocity profiles regardless of the magnitude of the external force. Nevertheless, human movements encompass not only horizontal but also vertical components. Thus, for a comprehensive understanding of human reaching movement control, it becomes imperative to analyze reaching movements across various planes, considering the presence or absence of visual feedback.

The primary objective of this study was to examine the strategies governing movement control during reaching motions within a vertical plane, particularly when visual feedback was absent and elastic resistance was introduced. In this context, participants engaged in shoulder presses utilizing elastic bands, emphasizing the compensatory role played by somatosensory feedback and the impact of muscle fatigue when experiencing elastic resistance. Generally, when individuals rely solely on somatosensory feedback, an expected outcome is an asymmetry in the movement speed between the dominant and non-dominant arms, attributable to differences in sensory reliance [18]. Furthermore, exercises that primarily employ somatosensory feedback are anticipated to prioritize the minimization of muscle force fluctuations over the reaching accuracy, likely resulting in symmetrical velocity profiles [19]. This approach can advance our comprehension of proprioception development in diverse reaching movement contexts and offers a more intuitive framework for movement analysis.

2. Materials and Methods

2.1. Subjects

Thirty healthy participants, with an average age of 22.8 $\pm$ 1.97 years and no physical impairments, were selected for this experiment. All participants were provided with comprehensive written and verbal explanations detailing the experiment's purpose, background, precautions, and procedures. Subsequently, written informed consent was obtained from each participant. This study received approval from the Institutional Review Board of Handong Global University (Approval No. 2022-HGUA020) on 25 September 2023. Table 1 provides a summary of the participants' information. The participants were recruited through the use of advertisements. During the initial screening process, questionnaires were employed to evaluate all participants for the presence of any physical injuries. Only those individuals without injuries were considered eligible for participation in the experiment. The inclusion criterion for participation in the study was either no prior experience in resistance exercises or less than two months of experience. Exclusion criteria included a maximum muscle strength lower than 2.63 kgf for each arm and the presence of physical or mental disabilities.

Table 1. Information on the participants.

	Male (n = 17)	Female (n = 13)	Total (n = 30)
Age (years)	24.0 ± 4.2	26.2 ± 4.9	24.9 ± 4.6
Dominant hand	Right (n = 17)	Right (n = 12) Left (n = 1)	Right (n = 29) Left (n = 1)
Body length (cm)	40.9 ± 2.3	36.6 ± 2.1	40.2 ± 2.4
Left arm length (cm)	56.3 ± 2.2	49.0 ± 2.4	54.7 ± 3.0
Right arm length (cm)	56.6 ± 2.8	49.1 ± 2.5	54.8 ± 3.2
Maximal strength	18.3 ± 3.19	8.1 ± 2.5	13.9 ± 5.8

2.2. Experimental Setup

In this experiment, participants performed a band shoulder press. The bands used were TheraBand elastic bands (TheraBand, Performance Health, Akron, OH, USA) with seven different resistance levels ranging from the yellow-colored band with minimum tension (1.36 kgf, 100% of elongation) to the gold-colored band with maximum tension (6.44 kgf, 100% of elongation). As the elastic bands stretched, the resistance increased. The maximum joint range of motion (ROM) of the participants was measured to ensure a consistent maximum band tension in the experiment. Half of the measured length from the arm to the body was set as the length of the elastic band. This helped ensure that the elastic load did not exceed 100% during exercise.

To analyze the participants' movements, we captured videos using an RGB camera (STREAMCAM, Logitech, Lausanne, Switzerland). The camera supported a resolution of 1080 p and recorded 60 frames per second (fps). The LogiCapture software 2.08.12 (Logitech, Lausanne, Switzerland) was used to record videos at 60 fps. The camera was positioned on a tripod at a height of 1 m from the ground and a distance of 2.2 m away from the participants in the frontal view.

To validate the accuracy of the joint positions estimated by OpenPose (version 1.6.0) from the camera data, inertial measurement units (IMUs) were attached to both forearms in front of the elbows of the participants. The IMUs consisted of a transmitter (EBIMU24GV5, E2BOX, Hanam-si, Gyeonggi-do, Republic of Korea) and a receiver (EBIMU24GV5, E2BOX, Hanam-si, Gyeonggi-do, Republic of Korea) capable of recording quaternion, gyro, and acceleration data. The IMUs were sampled at 60 fps to match the camera data. The receiver was attached to the ground and placed approximately 50 cm in front of the participants to ensure that it did not interfere with their movements (Figure 1).

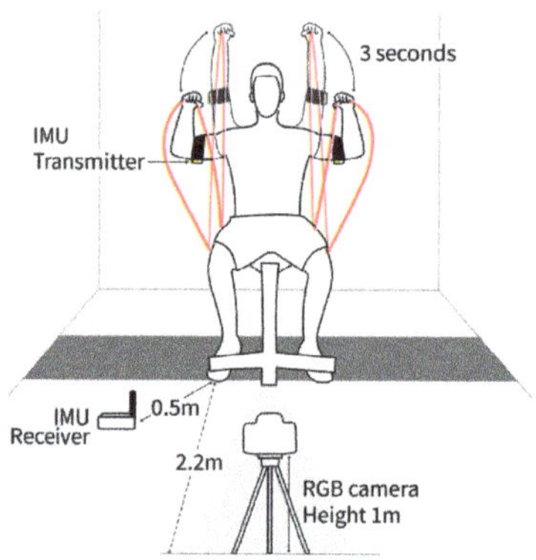

Figure 1. Schematic of the experimental environment. The RGB camera was positioned 2.2 m from the participants and at a height of 1.1 m from the ground. Each participant repeatedly performed lifting and lowering actions in sync with a metronome that rang at 3 s intervals.

To minimize the influence of psychological factors and individual variations in exercise repetition speed, a metronome with a tempo set at 20 beats per minute was employed [20]. Per the metronome's auditory cues, participants raised and lowered the elastic band in synchrony with each sound. The metronome function was programmed using MATLAB R2021b and transmitted through the speakers of the measurement equipment, a Precision 7760 laptop (Dell Technologies Inc, Round Rock, TX, USA).

2.3. *Experimental Procedure*

2.3.1. 1–Repetition Maximum Measurement Session

Initially, a session was conducted to measure the 1–repetition maximum (1 RM) to set the weights according to different exercise intensities. First, an explanation of the shoulder press posture was provided to the participants. A familiarization session followed this to ensure accurate performance in terms of the movements. Female participants performed the exercises without employing an elastic band, whereas male participants utilized a yellow band, and each group completed the exercise regimen five times. This methodological choice was based on the hypothesis that the lower maximum muscular strength typically observed in females might impede their ability to attain accurate posture when guided by the lightest resistance band. By contrast, considering that the maximum muscular strength in males is estimated to surpass the weight of the lightest band by more than five-fold, using a yellow band was deemed suitable for this group. Subsequently, starting with the yellow band, the participants incrementally performed a single shoulder press for each stage. The posture was considered correct when the elbow level exceeded the height of the nose when the arms were fully extended. A successful lift was recorded if the participant performed the shoulder press within a sufficient range of motion; otherwise, it was considered a failure. Upon successfully lifting the weight, the participants rested for 2 min before attempting to lift the next weight in the following order: yellow, red, blue, green, black, gray, and then gold. The measurement was repeated after successful attempts with the gold band, starting with the lighter bands. The weight in the previous successful attempt was considered 1 RM if the participant could no longer perform a single repetition or failed to achieve the standard range of motion.

2.3.2. Intensity-Specific Exercise Sessions

After a 3-day rest period, intensity-specific exercise sessions (low, high, and moderate) were conducted. The intensity criteria were as follows:

- Low intensity: bands with a weight less than or equal to 40% of 1 RM [21].
- Moderate intensity: bands with a weight greater than or equal to 50% of 1 RM but less than high-intensity bands.
- High intensity: bands with a weight greater than or equal to 80% of 1 RM [22].

The experiment was conducted in the following order: low, high, and moderate intensity. Eston et al. reported, using the Borg-15 scale, that individuals perceived weight as "low" in intensity when it corresponded to 40% of their 1 RM (one-repetition maximum). Furthermore, Morishita, S. documented that a weight perceived as "high" in intensity aligned with over 80% of the 1 RM. Because a paucity of research explicitly defines the percentage of 1 RM associated with the "moderate" intensity level, an intermediate weight falling between the "low" and "high" categories was established for this categorization. This was repeated for a maximum of 15 times [22] or until the participant could no longer lift.

If the elbow did not touch the height of chin or the movement did not match the beats per minute, the number of repetitions was recorded, and the participant was asked to rest for a certain period. After each session, a 5 min rest period was allowed, during which participants assessed their exercise intensity using the Borg 15-point RPE scale. After 5 min, the participants were asked about muscle fatigue. If fatigue was experienced, an additional 2 min rest period was allowed to minimize the impact of muscle fatigue.

2.3.3. Openpose Validation Session

Eight randomly selected participants were chosen to validate the OpenPose data following the intensity-specific exercise sessions. The selected subjects wore IMU sensors in front of their elbows and performed 15 repetitions with a yellow band.

2.4. Data Analysis

2.4.1. Data Processing

The recorded videos were processed using the OpenPose to estimate the joint positions. The exercise data of the participants were represented as individual positional data using the Body_25 format. Upon conversion of the data to the Body_25 format, matrices representing pixel data x_i, y_i for joints in the human body were obtained. The vertical positions of the endpoints of the right and left hands were denoted as y_4 and y_7, respectively.

A first-order low-pass filter with a cutoff frequency of 0.5 Hz was applied to remove outliers and high-frequency noise from the data of the participants. The transformed data were recorded in terms of pixels. Notably, individual body lengths or situational factors can influence the analysis of the data in pixel coordinates. Therefore, the z-score technique was employed to normalize the OpenPose data for each participant. Each normalized joint position was obtained using the following:

$$x_i = \frac{x_i - \mu}{\sigma} \tag{1}$$

Here, x_i refers to the joint position data, while μ and σ denote the mean and standard deviation of the joint position data during one trial, respectively.

2.4.2. Openpose and IMU Comparison

To validate the precision of the OpenPose technology, a comparison was conducted between the shoulder angle measurements obtained from both the IMU and OpenPose. The OpenPose approach involved the computation of the shoulder angle utilizing vector mathematics.

$$\text{vector}_1 = \left(P_{2x} - P_{1x}, P_{2y} - P_{1y}\right)$$
$$\text{vector}_2 = \left(P_{3x} - P_{1x}, P_{3y} - P_{1y}\right)$$
$$\theta = \cos^{-1}\left(\frac{\text{vector}_1 \cdot \text{vector}_2}{|\text{vector}_1| \cdot |\text{vector}_2|}\right)$$

$$P_{1x}, P_{1y} = x_{2\text{ or }5}, y_{2\text{ or }5} / P_{2x}, P_{2y} = x_{9\text{ or }12}, y_{9\text{ or }12} / P_{3x}, P_{3y} = x_{3\text{ or }6}, y_{3\text{ or }6}$$

This process facilitated accurate estimation of joint positions and the computation of joint angles by utilizing OpenPose's advanced pose estimation algorithms. By contrast, the IMUs yielded a distinct yet complementary angle estimation. The quaternions recorded by the IMUs were meticulously converted into Euler angles, representing roll, pitch, and yaw. When the IMUs were placed on the participants during the band shoulder press exercise, the roll angle corresponded to the shoulder angle in the frontal plane. This specific angle was then compared to the angle derived from OpenPose.

- RMSE (Root Mean Square Error): To understand the error between the two measurement techniques, the root mean square error method was employed. Here, y_{PP} represents the estimated angle of the shoulder from Openpose, and y_{IMU} is the angle estimated from the IMU. n denotes the length of data for each measurement.

$$\text{RMSE} = \sqrt{\frac{1}{n}\sum_{i=1}^{n}\left(y_{PP} - y_{IMU}\right)^2}$$

- Correlation coefficient (CC): To analyze the correlation, the CC for the angle of the shoulder measured using both the IMU and OpenPose was calculated. A CC value of

0.8 or above indicated a strong correlation between the two measurement methods. The coefficient was calculated using the following formula:

$$CC = \frac{\sum_{i=1}^{n}(y_{PP} - \overline{y}_{PP})(y_{IMU} - \overline{y}_{IMU})}{\sqrt{\sum_{i=1}^{n}(y_{PP} - \overline{y}_{PP})^2}\sqrt{\sum_{i=1}^{n}(y_{IMU} - \overline{y}_{IMU})^2}}. \quad (2)$$

Here, y_{PP} is the angle of the shoulder obtained from OpenPose, y_{IMU} is the angle obtained from the IMU, and $\overline{y}_{PP}$ and $\overline{y}_{IMU}$ are the mean angles of the shoulder calculated from each respective source.

2.4.3. Skewness

The skewness of the velocity profile indicates whether the speed distribution is symmetric or biased in one direction. If the skewness is close to zero, the speed distribution is symmetric. If it is not zero, the distribution is biased in one direction. The skewness was calculated using the density function of the gamma distribution [23].

$$\mu = \frac{\sum_{i=1}^{180} t_i \cdot v(t_i) \cdot \Delta t}{\sum_{i=1}^{180} v(t_i) \cdot \Delta t}. \quad (3)$$

$$\sigma^2 = \frac{\sum_{i=1}^{180} (t_i - \mu)^2 \cdot v(t_i) \cdot \Delta t}{\sum_{n=1}^{180} v(t_i) \cdot \Delta t}. \quad (4)$$

$$S = \frac{\sum_{i=1}^{180} (t_i - \mu)^3 \cdot v(t_i) \cdot \Delta t}{\sigma^3 \sum_{n=1}^{180} v(t_i) \cdot \Delta t}. \quad (5)$$

In this formula, μ is the expectation value of the velocity profile, σ^2 is the variance of the velocity profile, $v(t_i)$ is the velocity profile, and Δt is the measuring interval, i.e., 1/60 of a second. The skewness was calculated for the velocity profile within the 0–3 s interval, and the calculation was repeated every 6 s from the neutral position to the maximum elastic load.

2.5. Statistical Analysis

IBM SPSS Statistics 21 (IBM Corp., New York, NY, USA) was employed for data analysis using the two-way repeated analysis of variance (ANOVA) technique. In this analysis, the first factor was "hand", representing the dominant hand (DH) and non-dominant hand (NDH), and the second factor was "intensity", categorized into three levels: low (I1), moderate (I2), and high intensity (I3). This analysis determined the main effects of each factor and the interactions between the two factors. Statistical significance was set at <0.05. In cases where the main effects or interaction effects were statistically significant, post-hoc tests were conducted to determine where significant differences occurred. Bonferroni correction was applied to mitigate errors resulting from multiple comparisons. Additionally, the mean (M), standard error (SE), and standard deviation of the data were computed. Furthermore, Mauchly's sphericity test assessed the assumption of sphericity for the ANOVA results obtained from repeated measurements.

3. Results

3.1. Comparison of Bilateral Performance in Lifting and Lowering Speeds at Various Intensities

In Section 3.1, our primary interest lies in assessing the symmetry between the DH and NDH. The study focused on lifting and lowering movements and aimed to investigate whether hand dominance would impact performance when participants interacted with a resistance of varying intensity levels. This inquiry was particularly relevant in proprioceptive feedback, where visual cues were absent, and the primary emphasis relied on the body's internal sensory feedback mechanisms. Our analysis utilized a two-way repeated-measures ANOVA to discern any significant disparities in performance between DH and NDH across low, moderate, and high intensity levels (Figure 2).

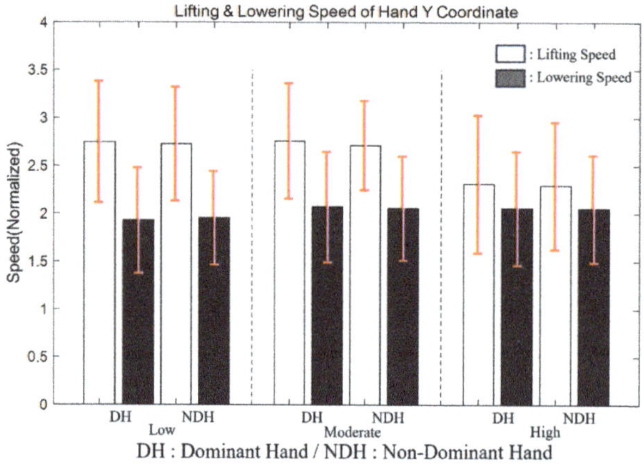

Figure 2. Boxplot for the lifting and lowering speeds at each intensity level and hand dominance.

The boxplot comparison in Figure 2 illustrates normalized speeds for both lifting and lowering at each intensity level, categorized by hand dominance. The results of the two-way repeated-measures ANOVA indicated no significant interaction effect on the lifting speed of the hand's y-coordinate ($F(2,58) = 0.854$, $p = 0.431$, partial $\eta^2 = 0.029$, as detailed in Supplementary Table S1). Specifically, no discernible performance differences were observed between DH and NDH across the intensity levels. At low intensity (I1), DH and NDH demonstrated equivalent lifting speeds (DH: M = 2.747, SE = 0.636; NDH: M = 2.727, SE = 0.595; $p = 0.490$), and this pattern persisted across moderate (I2) and high intensities (I3) with minimal variance. Likewise, the lowering speeds exhibited a similar trend, with no significant interaction effect between hand dominance and intensity ($F(2,58) = 1.159$, $p = 0.321$, partial $\eta^2 = 0.038$, as detailed in Supplementary Table S2). This finding indicates that the process of returning from the vertical target point to the starting position remained consistent between DH and NDH at all tested intensities. For instance, at low intensity, both hands displayed comparable results (DH: M = 1.928, SE = 0.552; NDH: M = 1.955, SE = 0.490; $p = 0.205$), a pattern that was also valid at moderate and high intensities. In summary, the lifting and lowering speeds between DH and NDH were statistically indistinguishable under various loading conditions. This suggests that hand dominance does not significantly impact the speed of arm movement coordination in tasks performed without visual feedback.

3.2. *Comparison of Lifting Speed, Lowering Speed, and Range of Motion at Various Intensities*

This section expands beyond the bilateral symmetry focus discussed in Section 3.1. It delves into how the body reacts to differing levels of imposed load. By classifying intensity into three distinct levels—low, moderate, and high—we can pinpoint noteworthy variations in performance, especially in lifting speed, which exhibit significant differences at higher intensities. Figure 3 displays a boxplot analysis structured to elucidate the effects of exercise intensity on three kinematic parameters: lifting speed, lowering speed, and range of motion.

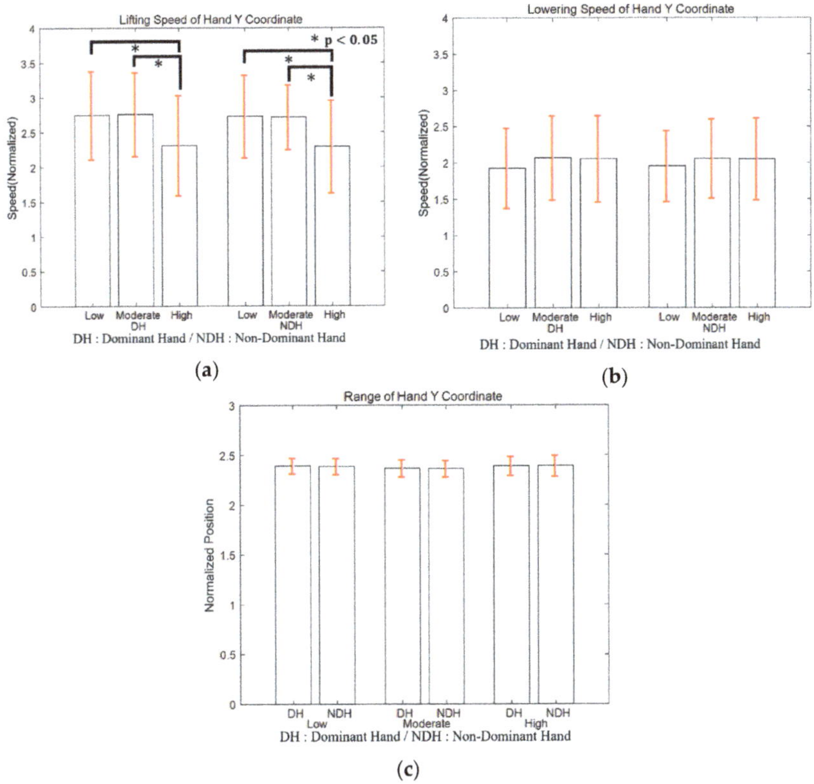

Figure 3. Boxplot for the (**a**) lifting speed, (**b**) lowering speed, and (**c**) range of motion at each intensity level.

(a) Lifting Speed: The analysis revealed a noteworthy reduction in lifting speed at high intensity (I3), with the DH exhibiting a mean speed of 2.311 (SE = 0.720) and the NDH displaying a mean speed of 2.293 (SE = 0.666). This represents a significant decrease from the lifting speeds observed at low intensity (I1), where DH had a mean speed of 2.747 (SE = 0.636), and NDH had a mean speed of 2.727 (SE = 0.595). Both DH and NDH demonstrated statistically significant differences (DH: $p = 0.001$; NDH: $p = 0.001$) when comparing the high-intensity to low-intensity conditions.

A similar pattern of significant reduction in lifting speed was observed when comparing high intensity to moderate intensity (I2). DH had a mean speed of 2.758 (SE = 0.604), and NDH had a mean speed of 2.714 (SE = 0.467), with both DH and NDH again showing statistically significant differences (DH: $p < 0.001$; NDH: $p < 0.001$). However, it is worth noting that the transition from low to moderate intensity did not yield significant differences in lifting speed (DH: $p = 1.00$; NDH: $p = 1.00$). This suggests that the impact of exercise intensity on lifting speed becomes more pronounced at the higher end of the intensity spectrum.

(b) Lowering Speed: In contrast to the findings related to lifting speed, no significant differences were observed in the lowering speed across the various intensity levels. This consistent pattern was observed for both the DH, with a mean speed of 1.928 (SE = 0.552) at low intensity, and NDH, with a mean speed of 1.955 (SE = 0.490). These results suggest that the presence of elastic resistance does not significantly influence control during the lowering phase. Statistical analysis supported this observation, with no significant differences found for DH ($p = 0.544$ at moderate intensity and $p = 0.303$ at high intensity) or NDH

($p = 0.066$ at moderate intensity and $p = 0.181$ at high intensity) when comparing different intensity levels.

(c) Range of Motion: The range of motion remained consistent across all intensities, with low intensity (I1) demonstrating a mean value for DH at 2.394 (SE = 0.078) and for NDH at 2.388 (SE = 0.081). This consistency persisted through moderate intensity (I2) (DH: M = 2.367, SE = 0.086; NDH: M = 2.363, SE = 0.083) and high intensity (I3) (DH: M = 2.391, SE = 0.096; NDH: M = 2.393, SE = 0.105), with no statistically significant differences (DH: $p = 0.150$; NDH: $p = 0.160$ between low and moderate, and DH: $p > 0.99$; NDH: $p > 0.99$ between moderate and high).

In summary, these observations highlight that, except for a noticeable reduction in lifting speed at the highest intensity, the participants' performance in terms of both speed and range of motion remained relatively unaffected by the intensity of the exercise.

3.3. Changes in the Velocity Profile with Varying Intensities

Among the kinematic data previously categorized into low, moderate, and high intensities, we specifically compare the velocity profiles under low- and high-intensity conditions. Figure 4 depicts the velocity profile of the lifting speed by intensity level.

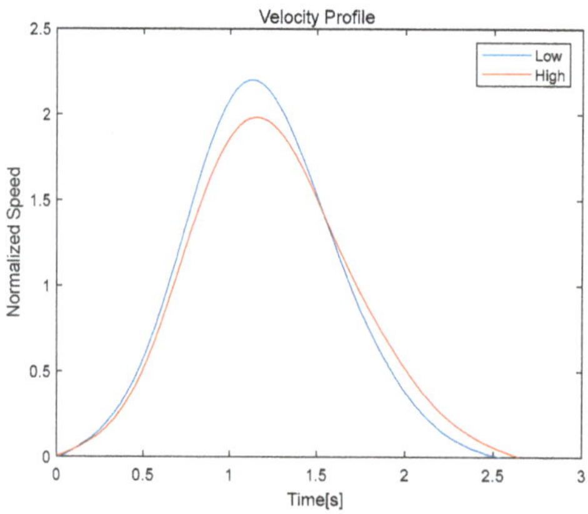

Figure 4. Modulation in velocity profiles with a shift in exercise intensity from a low to high level.

In Table 2, indicators representing the characteristics of velocity profiles for each intensity level are organized and recorded.

Table 2. Skewness, peak velocity, and the time to peak velocity during reaching.

Intensity	Skewness	Peak Velocity	Time to Peak Velocity	Exercise Duration
Low	0.294	2.200	1.122	2.514
High	0.351	1.982	1.151	2.601

The low-intensity condition exhibited a velocity profile with a skewness of 0.294, indicating a relatively symmetrical distribution of speeds with a peak velocity of 2.200 reached within 1.122 s after movement initiation. This profile was captured during the phase of motion, where participants stretched upwards in response to a metronome cue over a 3 s interval. Notably, the exercise duration for the low-intensity condition averaged 2.514 s.

By contrast, the high-intensity trials displayed a velocity profile with a skewness of 0.351, reflecting a slightly more asymmetrical distribution of speeds. The peak velocity observed was lower at 1.982, and the time to reach this peak was slightly longer, at 1.151 s. The exercise duration for these trials was, on average, marginally longer at 2.601 s.

Comparing these two profiles underscores the impact of intensity on the dynamics of movement execution. Specifically, the increase in skewness and the decrease in peak velocity at higher intensities may suggest a shift in strategy to accommodate the greater resistance, potentially implicating the recruitment of different muscle groups or changes in neuromuscular control.

3.4. Comparative Analysis of Shoulder Angles Using OpenPose and IMU

To determine the positional accuracy of OpenPose in kinematic assessments, we conducted a comparison with the established IMU-based measurements of upper arm inclination angles during repetitive exercises. Figure 5 illustrates this comparison across 15 exercise repetitions, visually representing the agreement between the two methods.

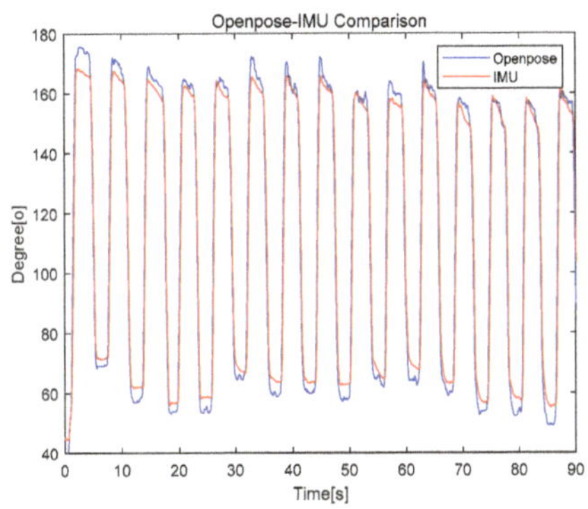

Figure 5. Alignment of shoulder angle measurements obtained from OpenPose and IMU during a series of upper arm movements.

In Table 3 we present a comparison of the results obtained from OpenPose and IMU, utilizing the root mean square error (RMSE) and the CC as key metrics for evaluation. Remarkably, the CC values, indicative of the degree of correlation between the two measurement techniques, consistently remained at a high level of 0.99 across all conditions. This remarkable level of correlation underscores an excellent agreement between the OpenPose and IMU methods, suggesting that OpenPose is a dependable tool for the real-time capture of upper arm kinematics.

Table 3. Comparison Result of Openpose and IMU.

	1	**2**	**3**	**4**	**5**	**6**	**7**	**8**
RMSE	8.65	9.03	9.25	11.85	11.30	9.59	11.68	9.84
CC	0.99	0.99	0.99	0.99	0.99	0.99	0.99	0.99

The RMSE values, which ranged from 8.65 to 11.85, demonstrate a relatively narrow margin of error between the readings obtained from OpenPose and IMU across the participants. This consistent RMSE range indicates that OpenPose can estimate the upper arm shoulder angle with an accuracy similar to that of the IMU. Furthermore, the consistent maintenance of relatively low RMSE values strengthens the assertion that both methodologies closely align when estimating kinematic data.

4. Discussion

The findings of this study make a substantial contribution to our comprehension of motor control in situations lacking visual feedback, particularly in the presence of elastic loads. The notable preservation of symmetry in reaching movements, regardless of hand dominance, represents a remarkable aspect that calls into question the traditional understanding of proprioception's role in motor coordination.

4.1. Symmetry under Elastic Load

Our experiment has substantiated that symmetry in reaching movements persists even when an elastic load is applied without visual information. Conventionally, bilateral coordination in movements with visual feedback has been acknowledged for its symmetry, attributed to the substantial influence of visual cues on trajectory generation and adjustment [24]. However, our study has unveiled that even without visual feedback, humans can uphold movement symmetry through proprioception. This finding suggests that internal motor control mechanisms are pivotal in preserving symmetry rather than relying solely on external visual feedback. The physical positioning and load detected under elastic resistance are communicated to both arms through commands generated in the primary motor cortex (M1). Arm dominance introduces disparities in the sensory information that each arm targets.

Previous research has indicated that the DH prioritizes visual targets, whereas the NDH prioritizes proprioceptive targets [25]. Consequently, in high-intensity exercises where muscle fatigue is a factor, it is anticipated that control by the NDH would become more prominent, potentially leading to asymmetric movements. However, our results demonstrate that even without visual targets, proprioception does not bestow dominance upon the NDH; instead, reaching control strives to engage both arms symmetrically, utilizing somatosensory feedback. This discovery, in contrast to prior theories, underscores the pivotal role of proprioception in upholding bilateral symmetry.

4.2. Elastic Load and Velocity Profile during Reaching

Our findings revealed that in the absence of visual feedback and when external forces were applied, the velocity profile during reaching movements exhibited a forward skew, indicative of an asymmetric form. This was observed through increased skewness and movement time, whereas the time required to reach peak velocity and the range of motion remained unchanged. These results imply that even without visual feedback, individuals adjust their speed to attain a position virtually generated by the brain's internal model.

If we had observed that the velocity profile remained unaffected by external forces, as predicted by the minimum torque-change model, it could have suggested that humans prioritize muscle control generated by the brain's internal model regardless of visual feedback. However, the results are per the minimum variance model, which posits that smaller target sizes result in speed control with an asymmetric velocity profile. This model is typically applied in situations involving visual feedback. However, our findings demonstrate its applicability even without visual feedback, underscoring the prioritization of reaching accuracy. Furthermore, as corroborated by our statistical analysis, the absence of significant differences in the movement range across different intensities suggests that the brain's internal model prioritizes reaching accuracy over mitigating muscle fatigue induced by increased load.

4.3. Openpose Validation by Comparing with IMU

Two primary methodologies are commonly employed in biomechanical motion tracking: motion capture using OpenPose and the Inertial Measurement Unit (IMU) approach. In our study, the accuracy of OpenPose in estimating the upper arm shoulder angle was compared with that of the IMU. The Root Mean Square Error (RMSE) values, ranging from 8.65 to 11.85, demonstrate a relatively narrow margin of error between OpenPose and IMU measurements across participants. This consistency in RMSE values suggests that OpenPose can estimate the upper arm shoulder angle with an accuracy comparable to the IMU.

In the analysis of arm and forearm movements, OpenPose data exhibited fewer joint tracking errors under static conditions, while IMU data showed reduced errors during dynamic movements. Furthermore, the angles derived from video recordings using OpenPose displayed a robust positive correlation with those obtained through inertial sensors, with a correlation coefficient (CC) greater than 0.95. This strong correlation not only confirms the reliability of OpenPose in capturing accurate kinematic data but also strengthens the assertion that OpenPose offers valuable measurements for biomechanical motion tracking. These findings suggest that even with a single 2D camera, OpenPose provides reliable data that closely align with the measurements obtained from more complex IMU systems.

4.4. Limitations and Future Work

One of the primary limitations of our study was the overrepresentation of right-handed participants. This demographic bias could potentially limit the generalizability of our findings. Coordination dynamics vary between left-handed and right-handed individuals due to inherent neurological and biomechanical differences associated with handedness. Future research would benefit from a more balanced inclusion of left-handed individuals, which could offer a broader perspective on how handedness influences coordination in response to different force fields and proprioceptive demands.

Our study's focus on proprioceptive feedback in movement coordination under elastic load aligns with the increasing emphasis on proprioception in rehabilitation. Research, such as that published Smith et al. [26], has underscored proprioceptive impairments in various populations and the potential benefits of proprioceptive training in enhancing motor function. Similarly, findings by Johnson and Lee [27] emphasize the significance of proprioception in neurological rehabilitation. These studies resonate with our observations, suggesting that exercises centered on proprioception, particularly in environments devoid of visual feedback, can play a crucial role in rehabilitation programs.

From a practical perspective, our findings indicate that rehabilitation exercises utilizing elastic resistance in a vertical plane can be effectively conducted with reduced reliance on visual feedback. This approach may be especially advantageous for patients recovering from injuries or conditions that impair their visual perception. By leveraging proprioceptive cues, therapists can tailor rehabilitation programs to enhance movement accuracy and control, thus compensating for reduced or absent visual inputs. This underscores the potential of proprioceptive training in improving motor control and facilitating recovery in visually impaired populations.

5. Conclusions

The findings of this study offer valuable insights into human motor control strategies during vertical plane elastic load reach movements, particularly when visual feedback is absent. The bilateral symmetry in performance across different intensities highlights the human capacity for precise proprioceptive-based movement control. Despite variations in the load intensity, participants consistently demonstrated symmetric reaching movements, indicating a robust internal model of movement execution within the brain.

However, an asymmetrical velocity profile, characterized by varying return durations at higher loads, suggests an adaptive strategy for controlled deceleration. This adaptation underscores the brain's ability to adjust motor outputs in response to changing mechanical demands, ensuring accurate target achievement.

These results hold implications for the understanding of motor control in diverse sensory conditions and could inform rehabilitation practices where proprioception plays a critical role in the absence of visual cues.

Supplementary Materials: The following supporting information can be downloaded at: https://www.mdpi.com/article/10.3390/bioengineering11010001/s1, Table S1: Summary of Statistical Analysis for Lifting Speed of the Hand Y Coordinate. Table S2: Summary of Statistical Analysis for Lowering Speed of the Hand Y Coordinate. Table S3: Summary of Statistical Analysis for Range of the Hand Y Coordinate.

Author Contributions: Conceptualization, G.S., H.R. and J.K. (Jaehyo Kim); methodology, G.S., D.Y., W.C. (Woong Choi) and J.K. (Jaehyo Kim); software, G.S., D.Y. and J.K. (Jihyeon Kim); validation, G.S., D.Y., W.C. (Woorim Cho), W.C (Woong Choi) and J.K. (Jaehyo Kim); formal analysis, G.S. and H.R.; investigation, G.S. and J.K. (Jihyeon Kim); resources, G.S., W.C. (Woong Choi) and H.R.; data curation, G.S., D.Y., H.R. and J.K. (Jaehyo Kim); writing—original draft preparation, G.S., D.Y. and W.C. (Woorim Cho); writing—review and editing, H.R., W.C. (Woong Choi) and J.K. (Jaehyo Kim); visualization, G.S.; supervision, H.R., W.C. (Woong Choi) and J.K. (Jaehyo Kim); project administration, H.R., W.C. (Woong Choi) and J.K. (Jaehyo Kim); funding acquisition, W.C. (Woong Choi) and J.K. (Jaehyo Kim). All authors have read and agreed to the published version of the manuscript.

Funding: This study was supported by the Translational R&D Program on Smart Rehabilitation Exercises, National Rehabilitation Center, Ministry of Health and Welfare, Korea (#TRSRE-MD02); National Research Foundation of Korea (NRF) Grant Number 2022R1A2C1092178; and National Research Foundation (NRF), Republic of Korea, under project BK21 FOUR (No. 5199990314060).

Institutional Review Board Statement: This study was conducted per the Declaration of Helsinki and approved by the Handong Global University Institutional Review Board (protocol code 2022-HGUA020, approval date: 25 September 2023).

Informed Consent Statement: Informed consent was obtained from all participants involved in the study. Written informed consent was obtained from all participants for the publication of this paper.

Data Availability Statement: Data available on request due to privacy concerns. The data presented in this study are available on request from the corresponding author. The data are not publicly available because our experimental data consist of video recordings featuring participants' faces, and several participants have refused to expose their faces.

Conflicts of Interest: The authors declare no conflict of interest.

References

1. Lonini, L.; Dipietro, L.; Zollo, L.; Guglielmelli, E.; Krebs, H.I. An internal model for acquisition and retention of motor learning during arm reaching. *Neural Comput.* **2009**, *21*, 2009–2027. [CrossRef] [PubMed]
2. Berthier, N.E.; Clifton, R.K.; Gullapalli, V.; McCall, D.D.; Robin, D.J. Visual information and object size in the control of reaching. *J. Mot. Behav.* **1996**, *28*, 187–197. [CrossRef] [PubMed]
3. Sy, H.V.N.; Nambu, I.; Wada, Y. The adjustment of muscle synergy recruitment by controlling muscle contraction during the reaching movement. In Proceedings of the 2016 IEEE International Conference on Systems, Man, and Cybernetics (SMC), Budapest, Hungary, 9–12 October 2016; IEEE: New York, NY, USA, 2016.
4. Haering, D.; Raison, M.; Begon, M. Measurement and description of three-dimensional shoulder range of motion with degrees of freedom interactions. *J. Biomech. Eng.* **2014**, *136*, 084502. [CrossRef] [PubMed]
5. Lee, H.M.; Liau, J.J.; Cheng, C.K.; Tan, C.M.; Shih, J.T. Evaluation of shoulder proprioception following muscle fatigue. *Clin. Biomech.* **2003**, *18*, 843–847. [CrossRef] [PubMed]
6. Dube, M.-O.; Roy, J.-S. Effect of fatigue and the absence of visual feedback on shoulder motor control in an healthy population during a reaching task. *Gait Posture* **2019**, *74*, 135–141. [CrossRef] [PubMed]
7. Saunders, J.A.; Knill, D.C. Humans use continuous visual feedback from the hand to control fast reaching movements. *Exp. Brain Res.* **2003**, *152*, 341–352. [CrossRef] [PubMed]
8. Proske, U.; Gandevia, S.C. The proprioceptive senses: Their roles in signaling body shape, body position and movement, and muscle force. *Physiol. Rev.* **2012**, *92*, 1651–1697. [CrossRef]
9. Van Beers, R.J.; Sittig, A.C.; Denier van der Gon, J.J. The precision of proprioceptive position sense. *Exp. Brain Res.* **1998**, *122*, 367–377. [CrossRef]
10. Gosselin-Kessiby, N.; Kalaska, J.F.; Messier, J. Evidence for a proprioception-based rapid on-line error correction mechanism for hand orientation during reaching movements in blind subjects. *J. Neurosci.* **2009**, *29*, 3485–3496. [CrossRef]
11. Anderson, D.I. The discrimination, acquisition, and retention of aiming movements made with and without elastic resistance. *Hum. Factors* **1999**, *41*, 129–138. [CrossRef]
12. Bahrick, H.P.; Bennett, W.F.; Fitts, P.M. Accuracy of positioning responses as a function of spring loading in a control. *J. Exp. Psychol.* **1955**, *49*, 437. [CrossRef] [PubMed]
13. Muceli, S.; Boye, A.T.; d'Avella, A.; Farina, D. Identifying representative synergy matrices for describing muscular activation patterns during multidirectional reaching in the horizontal plane. *J. Neurophysiol.* **2010**, *103*, 1532–1542. [CrossRef] [PubMed]
14. Koshland, G.F.; Galloway, J.C.; Nevoret-Bell, C.J. Control of the wrist in three-joint arm movements to multiple directions in the horizontal plane. *J. Neurophysiol.* **2000**, *83*, 3188–3195. [CrossRef] [PubMed]

15. Rosenbaum, D.A.; Engelbrecht, S.E.; Bushe, M.M.; Loukopoulos, L.D. A model for reaching control. *Acta Psychol.* **1993**, *82*, 237–250. [CrossRef] [PubMed]
16. Harris, C.M.; Wolpert, D.M. Signal-dependent noise determines motor planning. *Nature* **1998**, *394*, 780–784. [CrossRef] [PubMed]
17. Kawato, M.; Maeda, Y.; Uno, Y.; Suzuki, R. Trajectory formation of arm movement by cascade neural network model based on minimum torque-change criterion. *Biol. Cybern.* **1990**, *62*, 275–288. [CrossRef] [PubMed]
18. Goble, D.J.; Brown, S.H. The biological and behavioral basis of upper limb asymmetries in sensorimotor performance. *Neurosci. Biobehav. Rev.* **2008**, *32*, 598–610. [CrossRef] [PubMed]
19. Novak, K.E.; Miller, L.E.; Houk, J.C. The use of overlapping submovements in the control of rapid hand movements. *Exp. Brain Res.* **2002**, *144*, 351–364. [CrossRef]
20. Gearhart, R.F., Jr.; Goss, F.L.; Lagally, K.M.; Jakicic, J.M.; Gallagher, J.; Robertson, R.J. Standardized scaling procedures for rating perceived exertion during resistance exercise. *J. Strength Cond. Res.* **2001**, *15*, 320–325.
21. Eston, R.; Evans, H.J.L. The validity of submaximal ratings of perceived exertion to predict one repetition maximum. *J. Sports Sci. Med.* **2009**, *8*, 567.
22. Morishita, S.; Tsubaki, A.; Takabayashi, T.; Fu, J.B. Relationship between the rating of perceived exertion scale and the load intensity of resistance training. *Strength Cond. J.* **2018**, *40*, 94–109. [CrossRef] [PubMed]
23. Abramowitz, M.; Stegun, I.A. *Handbook of Mathematical Functions with Formulas, Graphs, and Mathematical Tables*, 9th ed.; Series 55; National Bureau of Standards Applied Mathematics: Springfield, VA, USA, 1972.
24. Abujaber, S.; Pozzi, F.; Zeni, J., Jr. Influence of weight bearing visual feedback on movement symmetry during sit to stand task. *Clin. Biomech.* **2017**, *47*, 110–116. [CrossRef] [PubMed]
25. Sarlegna, F.R.; Sainburg, R.L. The roles of vision and proprioception in the planning of reaching movements. In *Progress in Motor Control: A Multidisciplinary Perspective*; Springer: Boston, MA, USA, 2009; pp. 317–335.
26. Rand, D. Proprioception deficits in chronic stroke—Upper extremity function and daily living. *PLoS ONE* **2018**, *13*, e0195043. [CrossRef] [PubMed]
27. Etoom, M.; Altaim, T.A.; Alawneh, A.; Aljuhini, Y.; Alanazi, F.S.; Gaowgzeh, R.A.M.; Alanazi, A.O.; Neamatallah, Z.; Alfawaz, S.; Abdullahi, A. Single-textured insole for the less affected leg in freezing of gait: A hypothesis. *Front. Neurol.* **2022**, *13*, 892492. [CrossRef]

bioengineering

MDPI

Article

Spinal Cord Epidural Stimulation Improves Lower Spine Sitting Posture Following Severe Cervical Spinal Cord Injury

Kundan Joshi [1,2], Enrico Rejc [1,3,4], Beatrice Ugiliweneza [1,3], Susan J. Harkema [1,3,5] and Claudia A. Angeli [1,2,5,*]

1 Kentucky Spinal Cord Injury Research Center, University of Louisville, Louisville, KY 40202, USA; kundan.joshi@louisville.edu (K.J.); enrico.rejc@louisville.edu (E.R.); beatrice.ugiliweneza@louisville.edu (B.U.); susan.harkema@louisville.edu (S.J.H.)
2 Department of Bioengineering, University of Louisville, Louisville, KY 40292, USA
3 Department of Neurological Surgery, University of Louisville, Louisville, KY 40202, USA
4 Department of Medicine, University of Udine, 33100 Udine, Italy
5 Frazier Rehabilitation Institute, University of Louisville Health, Louisville, KY 40202, USA
* Correspondence: claudia.angeli@louisville.edu; Tel.: +1-502-582-7443

Abstract: Cervical spinal cord injury (SCI) leads to impaired trunk motor control, negatively impacting the performance of activities of daily living in the affected individuals. Improved trunk control with better sitting posture has been previously observed due to neuromuscular electrical stimulation and transcutaneous spinal stimulation, while improved postural stability has been observed with spinal cord epidural stimulation (scES). Hence, we studied how trunk-specific scES impacts sitting independence and posture. Fourteen individuals with chronic, severe cervical SCI with an implanted neurostimulator performed a 5-min tall-sit task without and with trunk-specific scES. Spine posture was assessed by placing markers on five spine levels and evaluating vertical spine inclination angles. Duration of trunk manual assistance was used to assess independence along with the number of independence changes and average independence score across those changes. With scES, the sacrum-L1 inclination and number of independence changes tended to decrease by 1.64 ± 3.16° (p = 0.07; Cohen's d = 0.53) and 9.86 ± 16.8 (p = 0.047; Cohen's d = 0.59), respectively. Additionally, for the participants who had poor sitting independence without scES, level of independence tended to increase by 12.91% [0%, 31.52%] (p = 0.38; Cohen's d = 0.96) when scES was present. Hence, trunk-specific scES promoted improvements in lower spine posture and lower levels of trunk assistance.

Keywords: epidural stimulation; sitting posture; independence

1. Introduction

Spinal cord injury (SCI) is generally associated with impaired sensorimotor control below the level of injury. Consequently, injuries at the cervical level affect the ability to recruit hip and trunk musculature to maintain postural stability, which further limits upper extremity function during activities of daily living [1,2]. Sitting postural stability is also influenced by posture kinematics [3,4]. Upright posture in sitting is accomplished by activation of muscles to counteract the movement of the center of gravity of the trunk [3,5]. This ability is severely impacted by injuries above the C4 level, and it is also affected to varying degrees by injuries in the lower cervical and upper thoracic levels [6]. As a result, individuals with thoracic level SCI employ compensatory strategies such as using the upper limbs and non-postural muscles to maintain upright sitting posture [7]. If erect posture cannot be achieved, individuals adopt a more kyphotic posture that increases static sitting stability whilst also increasing the risk of low back conditions [1,6,8]. Better sitting posture is thus crucial to re-gaining trunk stability, which is one of the top rehabilitation goals of individuals with SCI [9].

Recovery of the ability to maintain sitting upright posture has been achieved to varying degrees with the reactivation of hip and trunk musculature via different electrical stimulation modalities [10–15]. Neuromuscular electrical stimulation (NMES) applied to the hip and trunk muscles of individuals with SCI led to improvements in pelvic tilt and shoulder height in static sitting [10,11]. Furthermore, it also led to the anterior shift of maximum interface pressure from the posterior sacral region of sacral sitters. This potentially reduced the risks of pressure ulcers for sacral sitters, while upright sitters demonstrated low interface pressure in the sacral region [12]. Closed-loop control systems have also been developed to maintain erect posture in static and dynamic sitting by stimulating abdominal muscles when the trunk is flexed over a pre-set threshold [1,16,17]. A combination of NMES with mat-based exercises also led to higher independence in reaching tasks [18]. In contrast to NMES that directly stimulates the agonist muscle responsible for the movement, transcutaneous spinal cord stimulation re-engages spinal neurocircuitry at different sites of the spinal cord that, in-turn, innervates the required muscles [13–15]. Consequently, stimulation of T11 and L1 regions in adults with SCI led to better static sitting posture characterized by decreased trunk angle and trunk curvature [14]. Stimulation at the same spinal levels in children with SCI also led to improved lower trunk angles in comparison to baseline relaxed sitting, and volitional effort to maintain erect posture without stimulation while postural control did not improve even with decreased lower trunk inclination induced by a passive anterior pelvic tilt [15]. Another neuromodulation modality, spinal cord epidural stimulation (scES), has also been used to re-engage spinal circuitry in individuals with motor complete SCI [19]. Previous studies have established that the lumbar spinal cord has the potential to evoke coordinated motor outputs similar to synergistic locomotor activity [20,21]. Optimization of scES parameters has led to the recovery of activation patterns for weight-bearing standing and locomotion [22,23]. However, the effects of scES on sitting posture or level of independence have not been studied. Increased trunk control and reach distances have been observed in individuals with thoracic SCI [24]. Decreased lumbar curvature was observed when scES was applied targeting the erector spinae and quadratus lumborum muscles during repeated trunk flexion/extension in reaching and retrieving tasks and during four-point kneeling movement [25]. Thus, scES has the potential to improve posture of individuals with SCI in static sitting which in turn could enable them to perform activities of daily living (ADLs) with increased independence.

Effects of epidural stimulation in stand, step, and reaching activities have been studied, while its effects on sitting posture and independence has not been explored [22–24]. This study aims to analyze the effects of trunk-specific scES on sitting posture and trunk control of individuals with chronic severe cervical SCI. We hypothesize that trunk-specific scES will improve spine curvature and level of independence compared to no stimulation.

2. Materials and Methods

2.1. Experimental Protocol

Fourteen individuals with chronic severe cervical SCI (Age: 37.8 ± 10.9 yrs.; time post-injury: 13.1 ± 10 yrs.; injury levels: C4–C6; American Spinal Injury Association Impairment Scale (AIS): A–C; body mass index (BMI) 16.7–27.9) were implanted with a scES unit (Table 1, Appendix A). Based on the BMI, eight participants were classified as normal, while three were classified as overweight and three as underweight. All the participants had sedentary lifestyles. Among them, eight participants used power wheelchairs; four used manual wheelchairs; and two used manual wheelchairs with SmartDrive. Caregivers were required on a 24-h basis for seven participants, and on a periodic basis for six participants, while one participant was independent. Seven participants required one assistant and a transfer board to perform transfers, while six participants required two assistants. The participant who did not require caregivers performed independent transfers using the transfer board. As previously reported, implantation consisted of a 16-electrode array implanted at the L1–S1 spinal cord level connected to an Intellis neurostimulator (Medtronic, Minneapolis, MN, USA) internalized in the lower back [26]. All participants provided written informed consent as described in the study protocol approved by the University of Louisville's Institutional Review Board. The study was registered in clinical trials.gov prior to participant enrollment (NCT03364660). The participants had not undergone any training to improve sitting posture before enrollment. At the time of assessment, the participants were at different stages of a randomized controlled trial with 5 out of the 14 participants having received an intervention comprising trunk exercises.

Table 1. Participant Demographics.

ID	Gender	Age	Time Since Injury	Neuro Level	AIS	BMI	Mobility	Lifestyle	Caregiver	Transfers
A64	M	55.7	38.6	C4	A	21.6	Power wheelchair	Sedentary	24 h	Two-person
A97	M	38.6	15.4	C4	A	16.7	Power wheelchair	Sedentary	24 h	Two-person
A127	F	40.6	13.1	C4	A	23.9	Manual wheelchair	Sedentary	Periodic	One person Transfer board
A128	M	38.6	8.7	C4	A	23.7	Manual wheelchair	Sedentary	Periodic	One person Transfer board
A119	F	26.4	11.5	C5	A	17.6	Power wheelchair	Sedentary	Periodic	Two-person
A133	M	34.6	13.1	C5	A	27.9	Power wheelchair	Sedentary	Periodic	One person Transfer board
B38	M	21.9	3.3	C4	B	26.8	Power wheelchair	Sedentary	Periodic	Two-person
B40	M	36.0	4.7	C4	B	20.3	Power wheelchair	Sedentary	24 h	Two-person
B42	M	58.7	7.5	C4	B	26.8	Power wheelchair	Sedentary	24 h	Two-person
B212	F	47.9	29.7	C4	B	24.8	Manual wheelchair	Sedentary	Periodic	One person Transfer board
B213	F	25.1	5.4	C4	B	19.5	Power wheelchair	Sedentary	24 h	One person Transfer board
B194	F	37.8	18.2	C5	B	17.9	Manual wheelchair + SmartDrive	Sedentary	Independent	Independent Transfer board
C193	F	41.1	8.9	C4	C	24.4	Manual wheelchair + SmartDrive	Sedentary	Periodic	One person Transfer board
C231	F	26.8	5.7	C6	C	23.5	Manual wheelchair	Sedentary	24 h	One person Transfer board

Note: AIS—American Spinal Injury Association Impairment Scale, BMI—Body Mass Index.

A full-body motion capture marker set (modified Helen Hayes model—Helen Hayes Hospital, West Haverstraw, NY, USA) and eight Kestrel motion capture cameras (Motion Analysis Corporation, Santa Rosa, CA, USA) were used to capture kinematics. Markers were placed on five spine levels—the C3/C4 marker was placed behind the neck, and the sacral marker was placed on the mid-point of the posterior superior iliac spines. The other three spine markers were placed on estimated locations on T10, T3/T4, and L1 spine levels such that the five markers divided the spine into four equidistant segments. Marker placements were carried out by experienced research staff. Participants were seated on a standard experiment mat to perform the designated activity.

Data were acquired at 100 Hz using Cortex software Version 6.2.3.1732 (Motion Analysis Corporation, Santa Rosa, CA, USA). The participants were instructed to sit as tall and stable as possible without upper limb support for 5 min. They were asked to call out the start of the activity which was initially performed without scES and then repeated with optimal trunk-specific scES. The stimulation configuration was optimized for each participant in order to enable sitting postural control. Due to the customization, configurations contained either a single cohort to facilitate maintenance of static sitting posture, as well as trunk extension and leaning, or multiple cohorts running simultaneously with specific functionalities (Appendix B). Since the implantation occurs at the L1–S1 spinal region that innervates primarily lower extremity muscle fibers, the electrode configurations are rostrally arranged such that the stimulation can be directed at the superior from the lumbar region towards the trunk and abdominal muscles.

Research staff provided assistance as needed to maintain safety or upright sitting during the assessments by supporting lower to midback to maintain posture (maximum assistance) or to prevent a backward fall (minimum to moderate assistance) or by supporting the sternum in case they were falling forward (Figure 1). The support was removed if the participant could regain sitting balance. Participants were also allowed to place their hands on the mat or their legs in case of loss of balance. A manual pulse was used to record changes in the level of external assistance provided to accomplish the task.

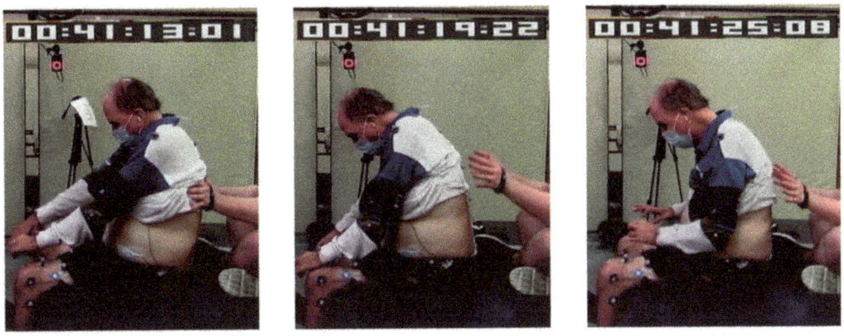

(a) (b) (c)

Figure 1. A participant requiring various levels of assistance to complete the task: (**a**) posterior trunk assistance from research staff, (**b**) anterior assistance by placing hands on legs, and (**c**) no external assistance.

2.2. Data Analysis

Marker identification in the kinematic data was performed in the Cortex software Version 6.2.3.1732 (Motion Analysis Corporation, Santa Rosa, CA, USA). In case of motion capture frames missing any marker data when blocked from view by research staff providing assistance, linear and polynomial interpolation techniques were used to remove missing gaps. Ortho Trak software Version 6.6.4 (Motion Analysis Corporation, Santa Rosa, CA, USA) was then used to generate 3D locations of the markers. A custom MATLAB code written in MATLAB Version R2017b (MathWorks, Natick, MA, USA) was used to isolate planar locations of the markers at the five spine levels (Sacrum, L1, T10, T3/T4, and C3/C4) in the sagittal plane (Figure 2a). Vertical inclination angles of the four spine segments were also calculated as below:

$$\theta_{S-L1} = \tan^{-1}\left(\frac{X_{L1} - X_S}{Z_{L1} - Z_S}\right) \quad (1)$$

$$\theta_{L1-T10} = \tan^{-1}\left(\frac{X_{T10} - X_{L1}}{Z_{T10} - Z_{L1}}\right) \quad (2)$$

$$\theta_{T10-T3T4} = \tan^{-1}\left(\frac{X_{T3/T4} - X_{T10}}{Z_{T3/T4} - Z_{T10}}\right) \quad (3)$$

$$\theta_{T3T4-C3C4} = \tan^{-1}\left(\frac{X_{C3/C4} - X_{T3/T4}}{Z_{C3/C4} - Z_{T3/T4}}\right) \quad (4)$$

where X_{marker} & Z_{marker} are the horizontal and vertical coordinates of the specified marker, respectively; $\theta_{inferior\ marker-superior\ marker}$ is the inclination angle of the spine segment joining the specified inferior and superior spine markers. To quantify curvature of the spine, a least-squares circle was fitted onto the sagittal plane coordinates of the five markers, and a radius of the fit circle (radius of curvature) was obtained (Figure 2b). The method used to determine the radius of the fit circle was by the minimization of the equation of the circle after substituting the equation with the available five marker locations. Consider if the equation of the circle was:

$$(x-k)^2 + (y-m)^2 = r^2 \quad (5)$$

where (k, m) is the center of the circle, and r, the radius, the following equation expressed in the sagittal (XZ) plane was minimized to obtain best-fit values for k, m, and $r_{curvature}$:

$$F(k,\ m,\ r_{curvature}) = \sum\left[\left(X_{marker} - k\right)^2 + \left(Z_{marker} - m\right)^2 - r_{curvature}{}^2\right]^2 \quad (6)$$

where $F(k,\ m,\ r_{curvature})$ is the function to be minimized with respect to k, m, and $r_{curvature}$.

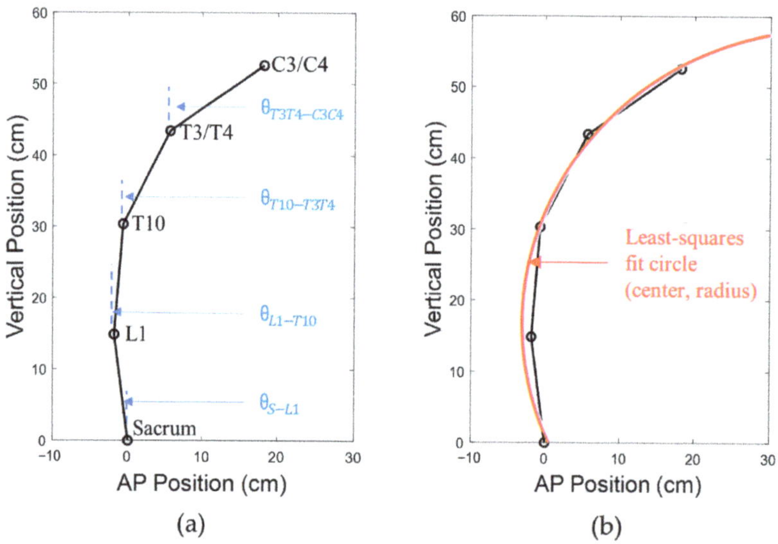

Figure 2. Calculation of (**a**) vertical spine inclination angles for the spine segments, and (**b**) least-squares fit circle to obtain radius of curvature.

From the manual pulse data, events were separated where the participants were fully independent (labeled as "independent"). Likewise, the label "assisted" was assigned when they were externally supported by research staff due to loss of postural stability ("assisted trunk") or if they placed their hands on their legs/the mat ("assisted hand/hands"). The duration of these events was summed up to obtain the fraction of the total 5 min duration where the participants were independent or needed to be assisted. The number of independence changes was also calculated from the events. For each event due to a change in independence, a custom independence score was used to rate the level of assistance needed. The ratings were from 0 (fully independent) to 6 (fully assisted on the trunk and both hands down). An average score was obtained by summing individual independence scores for all the events and dividing the sum by the number of events.

2.3. Statistical Comparisons

Prior to statistical analysis, normality was evaluated using visual examination of variable distribution supplemented by evaluation of skewness and kurtosis. Acceptable normality was defined as having a distribution visually with normal and skewness between −2 and 2 and kurtosis between −7 and 7 [27]. Variables that satisfied these criteria were summarized with mean and standard deviation (SD) and analyzed by paired t-tests. Those that did not were summarized with interquartile range (25th and 75th percentiles) and analyzed by the signed rank test. The significance level was set to 5%. To quantify the observed changes, Cohen's d effect sizes (ES = mean/SD) were used for normally distributed outcomes [28]. For non-normally distributed variables, a non-parametric equivalence to Cohen's d was calculated as the median divided by the median absolute deviation (MAD), i.e., ES = median/MAD. Sawilowsky's extension to Cohen's criteria was used to classify the obtained effect sizes as very small (<0.2), small (0.2–0.49), median (0.5–0.79), large (0.8–1.19), very large (1.2–1.99), and huge (>2.0). The threshold of 0.5 was used for meaningfulness as it was found to be the minimally important difference in health-related quality of life [29,30].

3. Results

3.1. Posture Outcomes

There were no statistically significant differences observed for all four spine inclination angles as well as the radius of curvature when scES OFF and scES ON conditions were compared (Figure 3; Table 2). However, there was a medium-effect size change of 1.64 ± 3.16° (p = 0.07; Cohen's d = 0.52) in the sacrum to the L1 inclination angle between scES OFF and ON conditions (Figure 3a). There was also a medium-effect-size increase of 1.9 ± 3.35° (p = 0.054; Cohen's d = 0.57) in the L1 to T10 inclination angle when scES was applied (Figure 3b). There were no statistically significant changes observed in the anterior-posterior or vertical coordinate of all the spine markers between scES OFF and scES ON with all effect sizes being small or very small. Even though statistically significant differences were not found, the S.D. of the anterior-posterior and vertical coordinates of all the spine markers were lower in the scES ON condition compared to the scES OFF condition (Figure 3c).

Table 2. Inferential statistics for posture and independence outcomes.

Parameter	scES OFF	scES ON	Change	p-Value	Effect Size	Classification
$\theta_{S\text{-}L1}$ (°)	−7.6 ± 8.02	−5.96 ± 7.68	1.64 ± 3.16	0.07	0.52 **	Medium
$\theta_{L1\text{-}T10}$ (°)	2.46 ± 6.67	4.36 ± 5.78	1.9 ± 3.35	0.054	0.57 **	Medium
$\theta_{T10\text{-}T3T4}$ (°)	24.32 ± 10.76	25.46 ± 8.9	1.14 ± 4.6	0.37	0.25	Small
$\theta_{T3T4\text{-}C3C4}$ (°)	51.16 ± 10.48	52.15 ± 10.34	1 ± 6.06	0.55	0.16	Very small
$r_{curvature}$ (cm)	42.72 ± 6.26	43.15 ± 6.79	0.42 ± 4.41	0.72	0.1	Very small
% Independent	98.5 [22.81, 100]	100 [71.74, 100]	0.12 [0, 12.65]	0.18	0.12	Small
% Assisted	1.5 [0, 77.19]	0 [0, 28.26]	−0.12 [−12.65, 0]	0.18	0.12	Small
No. of Independence Changes	13.29 ± 22.1	3.43 ± 8.46	−9.86 ± 16.8	**0.047** *	0.59 **	Medium
Independence Score	0.93 [0, 2.33]	0 [0, 2]	−0.17 [−0.67, 0]	0.34	0.43	Small

Note: Statistics are mentioned in the formats—mean ± SD or median [IQR] depending on the validity of assumption of normality. * implies p-value < 0.05. ** implies Cohen's d ≥ 0.5.

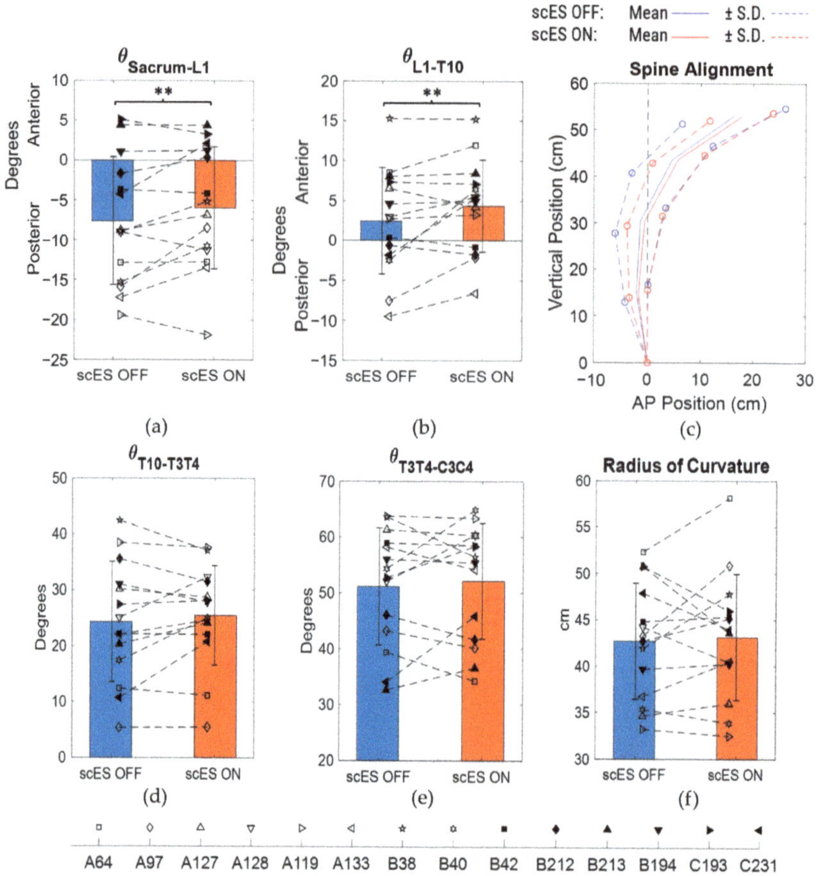

Figure 3. Comparison of spine inclination angles, spine posture, and radius of curvature between scES OFF and scES ON conditions: (**a**) sacrum to L1 angle, (**b**) L1 to T10 angle, (**c**) mean ± S.D. of spine marker coordinates, with sacrum as reference origin, (**d**) T10 to T3/T4 angle, (**e**) T3/T4 to C3/C4 angle, and (**f**) radius of curvature obtained from least-squares fit circle. Note: ** implies p-value not significant but Cohen's d $\geq$ 0.5.

3.2. Level of Independence

In the scES OFF condition, the participants performed the task independently for a median [IQR] duration of 98.5% [22.81%, 100%] of the total time and needed assisted for 1.5% [0%, 77.19%] (Table 2; Figure 4a). In the scES ON condition, they were independent for 100% [71.74%, 100%] and assisted for 0% [0%, 28.26%]. The 0.12% [0%, 12.65%] change in duration of independence (p = 0.18; Cohen's d = 0.12) between the scES OFF and scES ON conditions was not statistically significant. However, there was a statistically significant mean decrease of −9.86 ± 16.8 in the number of independence changes (p = 0.047; Cohen's d = 0.59). On the other hand, the −0.17 [−0.67, 0] change in median [IQR] independence score was not statistically significant (p = 0.34; Cohen's d = 0.43) (Figure 4b,c).

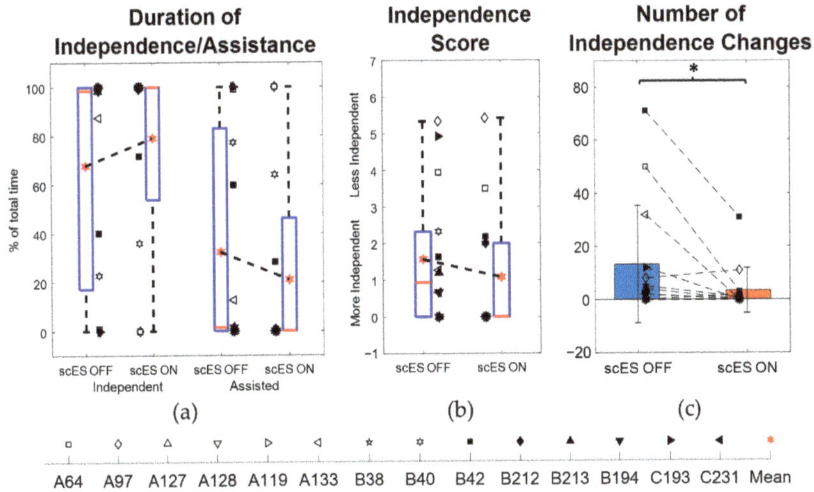

Figure 4. Comparison of independence outcomes between scES OFF and scES ON conditions: (**a**) percentage duration of independence and needing assistance, (**b**) independence score, and (**c**) number of independence changes. Note: * implies p-value < 0.05.

3.3. Subset Analysis

Based on the number of independence changes, a subset analysis was performed on N = 6 participants (A64, A97, A133, B40, B42, C193) by excluding the other 8 participants who showed a relatively better sitting postural control with scES OFF, as they were independent for more than 98% of the total time performing the task and had fewer than 4 independence changes in both scES OFF and scES ON conditions. There were no statistically significant changes observed in the spine inclination angles and the radius of curvature of the trunk (Table 3). However, compared to the scES OFF condition, there were medium-effect size changes of 2.25 ± 3.54° (p = 0.18; Cohen's d = 0.63) in the sacrum to L1 inclination angle and of 1.62 ± 3.21° (p = 0.27; Cohen's d = 0.5) in the T10 to T3/T4 inclination angle in the scES ON condition (Figure 5a,d). In addition, there was a large-effect size change of 3.2 ± 3.72° (p = 0.09; Cohen's d = 0.86) in the L1 to T10 inclination angle (Figure 5b). There were no statistically significant changes observed in the anterior-posterior or vertical coordinate of all the spine markers between scES OFF and scES ON with effect sizes being small or very small. Interestingly, the S.D. of the anterior-posterior and vertical coordinates of all the spine markers were lower in the scES ON condition compared to the scES OFF condition (Figure 5c).

When comparing the level of independence and assistance, there were no statistically significant changes observed between the scES OFF and scES ON condition. However, a large-effect-size increase of 12.91% [0%, 31.52%] in median [IQR] duration of independence was observed (p = 0.38, Cohen's d = 0.96). In addition, there was a statistically significant decrease of 22 ± 20.48 in the mean (SD) number of independence changes (p = 0.047, Cohen's d = 1.07), along with a medium-effect-size change of 0.39 [−1.27, 0.08] in median [IQR] independence scores (p = 0.69, Cohen's d = 0.57) from scES OFF to scES ON conditions. There was also a medium-effect-size change of 0% [−15.6%, 0%] in the median [IQR] duration of assistance with one hand on the mat (p = 0.5, Cohen's d = 0.63) and a large-effect-size change of −4% [−8.87%, 0%] in duration of assistance on the trunk by research staff and one hand on the mat (p = 0.25, Cohen's d = 1).

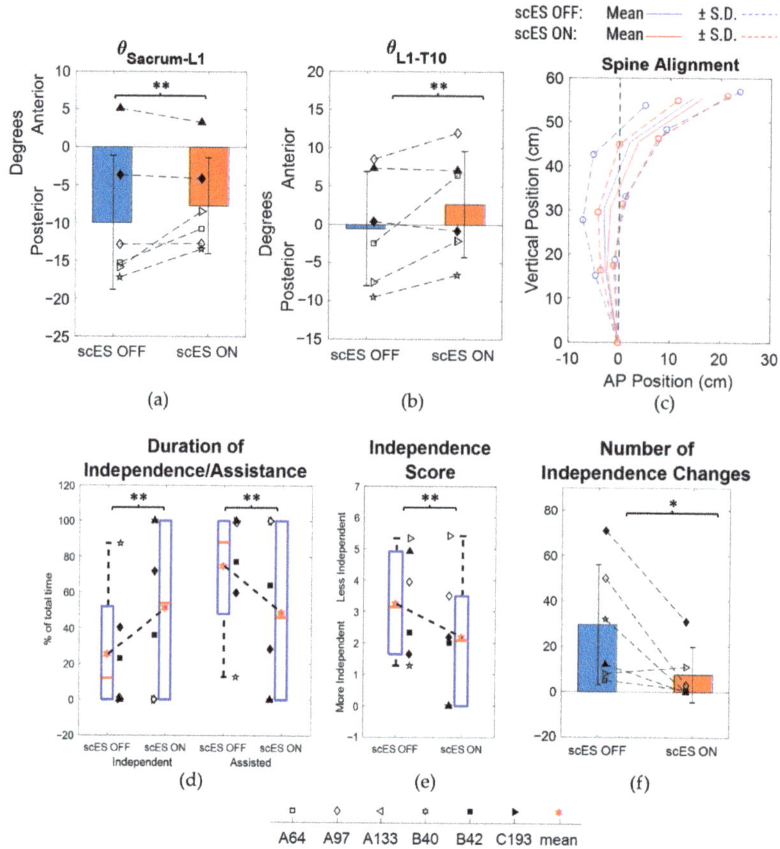

Figure 5. Comparison of spine inclination angles, spine posture, and radius of curvature between scES OFF and scES ON conditions for the subset (N = 6): (**a**) sacrum to L1 angle, (**b**) L1 to T10 angle, (**c**) mean ± S.D. of spine marker coordinates, with sacrum as reference origin, (**d**) T10 to T3/T4 angle, (**e**) T3/T4 to C3/C4 angle, and (**f**) radius of curvature obtained from least-squares fit circle. Note: * implies p-value < 0.05; ** implies p-value not significant but Cohen's d ≥ 0.5.

Table 3. Inferential statistics of the subset (N = 6) for posture and independence outcomes.

Parameter	scES OFF	scES ON	Change	p-Value	Effect Size	Classification
$\theta_{S\text{-}L1}$ (°)	−9.97 ± 8.84	−7.73 ± 6.36	2.25 ± 3.54	0.18	0.63 **	Medium
$\theta_{L1\text{-}T10}$ (°)	−0.55 ± 7.46	2.65 ± 6.95	3.2 ± 3.72	0.09	0.86 **	Large
$\theta_{T10\text{-}T3T4}$ (°)	17.78 ± 7.92	19.4 ± 8.99	1.62 ± 3.21	0.27	0.5 **	Medium
$\theta_{T3T4\text{-}C3C4}$ (°)	51.13 ± 8.05	51.7 ± 11.9	0.58 ± 6.21	0.83	0.09	Very small
$r_{curvature}$ (cm)	43.86 ± 6.97	45.77 ± 8.36	1.9 ± 4.67	0.37	0.41	Small
% Independent	11.88 [0, 40.23]	53.87 [0, 100]	12.91 [0, 31.52]	0.38	0.96 **	Large
% Assisted	88.12 [59.77, 100]	46.13 [0, 100]	−12.91 [−31.52, 0]	0.38	0.96 **	Large
% Assisted (1 Hand Only)	0 [0, 15.6]	0 [0, 0]	0 [−15.6, 0]	0.5	0.63 **	Medium
% Assisted (2 Hands)	5.94 [0, 17.44]	0 [0, 5.97]	0 [−11.47, 0]	1	0.23	Small
% Assisted (Trunk Only)	22.89 [1.33, 53.59]	1.18 [0, 20.58]	−1.21 [−21.75, 0]	0.38	0.19	Very Small
% Assisted (Trunk + 1 Hand)	4 [0, 14.73]	0 [0, 0]	−4 [−8.87, 0]	0.25	1 **	Large

Table 3. *Cont.*

Parameter	scES OFF	scES ON	Change	p-Value	Effect Size	Classification
% Assisted (Trunk + 2 Hands)	8.87 [0, 31.4]	0.61 [0, 1.7]	−0.38 [−15.75, 1.7]	1	0.06	Very Small
No. of Independence Changes	29.67 ± 26.52	7.67 ± 12.16	−22 ± 20.48	**0.047** *	1.07 **	Large
Independence Score	3.14 [1.64, 4.92]	2.09 [0, 3.5]	−0.39 [−1.27, 0.08]	0.69	0.57 **	Medium

Note: Statistics are mentioned in the formats—mean ± SD or median [IQR] depending on the validity of assumption of normality. * implies p-value < 0.05. ** implies Cohen's d ≥ 0.5.

Among the participants in the subset analysis, one participant (C193) was assisted fully during the scES OFF condition and was fully independent during scES ON condition. During the 1st minute of the 5-min task, the assistance on the trunk enabled her to obtain upright posture in the scES OFF condition (Figure 6a), but her trunk tilted progressively anteriorly until the last minute (Figure 6c). In contrast, with scES, she started in an anteriorly tilted trunk posture to begin but corrected it progressively until she was fully upright especially in the lower back without needing any assistance (Figure 6b,c).

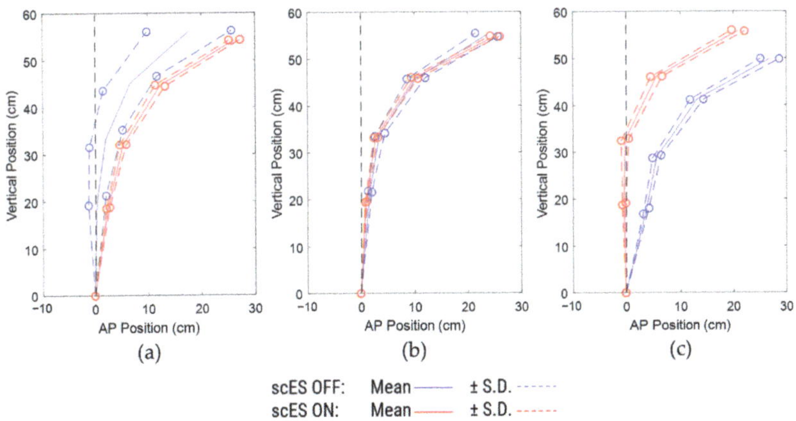

Figure 6. Comparison of spine posture for different 1-min periods for participant C193: (**a**) 1st minute, (**b**) 3rd minute, and (**c**) 5th minute.

4. Discussion

The participants of this study were able to obtain more erect sitting posture in the lower spine with the aid of scES targeted at trunk stability compared to sitting without stimulation. The effects of scES on upper spine posture as well as overall curvature of the spine, however, were not statistically significant. In the presence of scES, the participants had decreased frequency in independence changes, indicating that stimulation enabled them to hold a certain independence level for longer periods. When a subset of participants was analyzed by excluding those participants with almost full independence and no more than four independence changes, sitting posture of the lower spine improved with stimulation along with obtaining a higher level of trunk independence, lower frequency of independence changes, and better independence scores. Results from one participant in the subset indicated that scES substituted the need of external trunk assistance throughout the 5-min task, and sitting posture progressed from an anterior trunk tilt in the first minute to an erect lower spine in the last minute. This target was unachievable for the participant without stimulation even with full assistance provided by research staff.

4.1. Posture and Independence with scES

Epidural stimulation optimized for trunk stability targets abdominal muscle groups responsible for trunk flexion and extension. This neuromodulation approach provides excitability to the muscles in the lower abdomen, and with the assistance of innervation from the residual circuitry, causes a resultant motor output [19–21]. For the tall-sit activity in our study, the excitation to the rectus abdominus and paraspinal muscles enabled the participants to modulate motor output and improve postural stability, independence, and maintain upright lower spine evidenced by a decrease in spine inclination of the Sacrum to L1 segment. The improved ability of the participants to hold an assistance or independence level with stimulation was reflected in the trend of the decreased spread of the anterior-posterior coordinates of spine markers from scES OFF to scES ON conditions. Analogous to these results, a previous study conducted with functional electrical stimulation of the trunk and hip extensors led to improved static shoulder height, pelvic tilt, and trunk lean in a fraction of participants [10]. Improved lower trunk extension, trunk curvature, and angle were observed along with increased activity in L3 level-erector spinae and oblique muscles as a result of transcutaneous stimulation of T11 and L1 spinal regions [13]. Upright posture of the L5 to S1, and pelvic to T8 segments, were observed due to transcutaneous stimulation of the T11 and L1 regions of children with SCI [15]. While achieving erect posture helps to maintain sitting stability, being able to perform the task without external assistance is also important.

Not many studies have investigated the effects of stimulation on the level of independence; instead, the individuals with SCI were asked to perform certain tasks until they lost control or independence [11,13,24]. In one study, upon application of functional electrical stimulation on the quadriceps and gastrocnemius muscles, individuals with SCI were able to perform mat-based reaching and retrieving tasks with more independence scores in the Spinal Cord Independence Measure-III (SCIM-III) scale [18]. In our study, the median [IQR] level of independence was 98.5% [22.81%, 100%] without stimulation and 100% [71.74%, 100%] with stimulation. Because a fraction of participants (8/14) showed good independence without stimulation, the changes were statistically not significant. Hence, when we performed a subset analysis for the rest of the participants, there were improvements seen in the level of independence, number of independence changes, and independence score when scES was applied (Figure 5d–f, Table 3). The pattern of assistance provided also changed with decreases in the duration of one hand needing support with or without trunk support with stimulation (Table 3). It is likely that without stimulation, participants needed to put a hand on the mat to maintain stability more often than when stimulation was present. Even though there were no significant changes in spine marker coordinate locations in the presence of stimulation, the lower spine tended to be more erect (Figure 5c). Without stimulation, the lower spine tended to be more inclined even when more assistance was provided to aid in posture. This result reflected the strategy of the participants focusing on gaining independence and then on maintaining posture, a strategy that was highlighted in one participant (C193). In particular, without stimulation, she was fully assisted, but even with assistance, her posture progressively became anteriorly tilted. With stimulation, she did not need any external assistance, and her lower spine posture progressively became more erect from an initial anterior tilt (Figure 6a–c). These opposing responses indicate that epidural stimulation has the potential to substitute external assistance with an immediate effect. Continuous stimulation allows the individual to modulate neuromuscular activation resulting in spinal posture improvements along with improved independence. The transition from an anteriorly tilted to an erect posture also highlights the differences due to the intended duration of the task. Previous studies asked the participants to maintain static sitting bouts for as few as 10 s to a maximum of 1 min [13,15]. While smaller intended durations may maximize immediate improvements due to stimulation, the desirable effect would be steady improvements that last for a longer period. The ability to maintain better posture for a longer duration helps to perform other functional tasks that start from unsupported sitting such as trunk movements or reaching for objects [31].

Better sitting posture would also conceivably decrease the likelihood of pressure ulcers that arise from poor postures such as sacral sitting [6,8,12]. Given the participants' sedentary lifestyles with around half of them requiring power wheelchairs, 24-h caretakers, and two persons to transfer, epidural stimulation has the potential to increase the range of potential achievable seated tasks that the participants could perform (Table 1). When taken together, these improved outcomes can help achieve better quality of life for individuals with SCI.

4.2. Physiological Response to scES

As previously reported, the epidural stimulator was implanted between L1 and S1 spinal cord levels, a section typically responsible for innervating hip muscle fibers [19–23]. On the other hand, nerve and muscle fibers responsible for trunk functions are present in the thoracic spinal cord. Consequently, trunk specific scES configurations are generally rostral with cathodes lining up the first row of the implanted electrode array and allowing for tonic stimulation to be projected from the lumbar region towards the pelvis and the trunk muscles (Appendix B). Tonic stimulation in combination with residual descending supraspinal drive across the lesion enables the participant to maintain static balance, independence, and posture [19,23,24]. This approach leads to a focal pattern of motor unit recruitment to maintain posture, analogous to the autonomous regulation of posture in uninjured population [24,32]. This coordinated activation pattern as a result of L1 level epidural stimulation was most likely responsible for improving lower spine posture, and the ability to hold a level of independence/assistance, as well as drastically improving the level of independence for the participants who did not have a high level of pre-existing trunk independence without stimulation.

The potential of epidural stimulation to improve seated posture and independence had not been investigated previously. Our results highlight the need for further research on neurophysiological changes leading to changes in seated posture in various functional tasks brought about by epidural stimulation, in a manner similar to generation of locomotor patterns with stimulation of the lumbosacral spinal cord [20–22]. Comparatively more pronounced improvements in posture were observed in past studies that used transcutaneous spinal cord stimulation for neuromodulation [13]. However, the increased ease of using the trunk-specific scES configuration in home and community environments implies the need for further studies to link stimulation with posture improvements in seated tasks, as well as improvements in execution of activities of daily living. All the participants in the study had sedentary lifestyles with 5 out of 14 participants having undergone an intervention program comprising trunk exercises at the time of assessment of spine posture (Appendix A). The improvements seen in lower spine posture regardless of different stages of intervention suggests that trunk-specific scES could be a beneficial tool for them to increase their level of activity overall and potentially increase independence during activities of daily living (Table 1).

4.3. Limitations

There was a lack of validated assessments of sitting posture as well as limited past literature. Hence, comparative analysis of the results of our study with past studies was not intuitive. The participants' characteristics in the current study ranged in age, gender, level of injury, time since injury, and AIS scores and sitting ability prior to implantation. All these add to the variability in our sample population.

5. Conclusions

The effect-size analysis of sitting posture suggested that epidural stimulation targeted at gaining trunk stability led to improved upright lower spine control in the individuals with SCI enrolled in the present study. Given the variations in participant demographics, their injury levels, and initial trunk control, the primary hypothesis of improvements in overall trunk curvature was not achieved. The stimulation did lead to improved independence in performing the static sitting for individuals who did not already have good independence without stimulation, while also significantly reducing the frequency of changes in independence levels of all participants to maintain balance and posture. These results validate our second hypothesis that trunk-specific stimulation leads to improved independence in those with more severe motor control impairments. Further research should focus on standardization of the assessment of sitting posture. Future work can also entail how stimulation substitutes external assistance needed to maintain posture and if/how it stabilizes with time. The long-term effects of stimulation can also be manifested in rehabilitation programs aimed at improving trunk control and posture, which would in turn lead to better quality of life for the individuals with SCI.

Author Contributions: Following were the contributions of the authors of this manuscript: Conceptualization, S.J.H., and C.A.A.; methodology, C.A.A., E.R., and S.J.H.; software, K.J.; validation, K.J.; formal analysis, B.U., and K.J.; investigation, S.J.H., E.R., and C.A.A..; resources, S.J.H.; data curation, K.J., B.U., and C.A.A.; writing—original draft preparation, K.J.; writing—review and editing, K.J, E.R., B.U., S.J.H., and C.A.A.; visualization, K.J.; supervision, C.A.A.; project administration, S.J.H., E.R., and C.A.A.; funding acquisition, S.J.H. All authors have read and agreed to the published version of the manuscript.

Funding: This research was funded by the Christopher and Dana Reeve Foundation, grant number ES_BI-2017, the University of Louisville Hospital, and Medtronic Plc.

Institutional Review Board Statement: The study was conducted in accordance with the Declaration of Helsinki and approved by the Institutional Review Board of the University of Louisville (protocol 16-0179 and approved on 10/19/2017).

Informed Consent Statement: Informed consent was obtained from all subjects involved in the study.

Data Availability Statement: The data presented in this study are available on request from the corresponding author. The data are not publicly available due to lack of available repository.

Acknowledgments: We are indebted to our research participants for their courage, dedication, motivation, and perseverance that made these research findings possible. Maxwell Boakye performed surgical implantation and provided medical oversight. Glen Hirsch, Darryl Kaelin, and Sarah Wagers provided medical oversight. Yukishia Austin, Lynn Robbins, and Kristen Johnson provided medical management. We would like to thank Yangsheng Chen and Sharon Zdunowski for engineering leadership and Taylor Blades for project management. Justin Vogt, Katie Pfost, Katelyn Brockman, Brittany Logdson, Dylan Pfost, Eric Davis, Curtis Standafer, and Darrius Lopez lead research interventions and provided support of research participants.

Conflicts of Interest: The authors declare no conflict of interest.

Appendix A. Additional Demographics

Table A1. Participant Spine Characteristics.

PID	Spine Characteristics	Trunk-Specific Intervention?
A64	- Mildly desiccated intervertebral discs throughout lumbar spine with small posterior bulges at L3–S1. - No significant stenosis.	No
A97	- S-shaped scoliosis, dextroscoliotic in the thoracic spine with levoscoliotic compensation at the cervical-thoracic junction. Additional levoscoliotic compensation in lumbar spine. - No significant spinal stenosis or foraminal narrowing in thoracic spine. - Partial fusion of the lower sacroiliac joints bilaterally. - Generalized osteoporosis involving the sacrum and iliac bones.	No
A127	- Counterclockwise rotary scoliosis of C2 relative to C1. Alignment returning to normal at C5 through the thoracic inlet. - Minimal disc bulge at L5–S1.	Yes–80 sessions

Table A1. *Cont.*

PID	Spine Characteristics	Trunk-Specific Intervention?
A128	- L5-S1 intervertebral disc mildly desiccated and associated with a minimal bulge that results in no significant stenosis.	No
A119	- Cervical lordosis mildly reversed at C3 and C4. - Lumbar spine alignment is near anatomic with minimal retrolisthesis of L5 relative to S1 and hyper-lordosis of the L5–S1 level.	No
A133	- Trace retrolisthesis of C3 on C4 with posterior disc bulge and ligamentum flavum buckling contributing to moderate spinal stenosis at the C3–4 level. - Lumbar lordosis is mildly reversed at the L1–L2 level. - L5 is minimally subluxed posteriorly relative to S1. - The L5-S1 disc is desiccated and mildly narrowed, with a posterior central protrusion.	No
B38	- Cervical lordosis is straightened from C1 through T1. - Mild broad dextroscoliosis is centered at about T8.	Yes–160 sessions
B40	- Cervical lordosis is focally reversed at C4–5. - Dextroscoliosis is moderate to marked in the thoracic spine with the apex at T5–6. - L5 is minimally posteriorly subluxed relative to S1.	No
B42	- Mild endplate irregularities at the inferior endplate of T8 and the superior endplate of T11. - Minimal central to anterior compression at T12. - Sharp osteophyte at the T6–7 level that results in moderate spinal stenosis. - Lumbar spine is mildly hyper-lordotic at the lumbosacral junction. - There is minimal retrolisthesis of L5 relative to L6 with an associated bulge.	No
B212	- Cervical lordosis is mildly focally reversed at C5–6. - Small posterior disc bulges are at T2–3 and T3–4. A minimal inferior extrusion at T3–4 results in no significant stenosis.	Yes–80 sessions
B213	- Cervical lordosis is straightened from C1 through C6 with minimal angulated reversal of lordosis at C7–T1.	Yes–80 sessions
B194	- Mild dextroscoliosis in the dependent thoracic spine, centered at T5–T6. Small posterior central protrusions are at T1–T2 and T6–T7. Disc bulges eccentric to the left at T3–4 and T4–5. None resulting in significant stenosis. - Small posterior bulges at L3–4 and L4–5	Yes–80 sessions
C193	- Cervical lordosis is straightened and mildly lordotic from C1 through C6. - Mildly accentuated kyphosis at T11–12 and T12–L1. - Intervertebral discs are partially desiccated from T8-9 through L1. - Mild endplate irregularities at the inferior endplates of T9–T11 and the superior endplates of T11–L1.	No
C231	- Cervical lordosis is smoothly reversed with the reversal centered at approximately C4.	No

Appendix B. scES Electrode Configurations for Trunk Stability

Electrode configurations for trunk stability contain either a single cohort (for 4 out of 14 participants) that enables all aspects of sitting postural control such as trunk extension and leaning in addition to the maintenance of static sitting posture, or multiple cohorts (for 10 participants) that run simultaneously with specific functionality of each cohort (Table A2). Additional cohorts can be added to target weaker muscle groups or balance agonists and antagonists. For example, if a cohort meant for extension leads to trunk hyperextension, another cohort is added to increase the strength of abdominal muscles. Similarly, a cohort can be added to aid the participant's weaker side during lateral leaning activities. Cohorts that decrease muscle activity in the lower extremities or aid in cardiovascular functions also help participants achieve better sitting posture for longer periods. All these variations lead to specific optimization of the stimulation parameters unique to the participants. However, a common arrangement of cathodes (0-/5-/11-) and anodes (2+/7+/13+) is seen as part of a cohort for most of the participants (Figure A1). This arrangement allows for the stimulation to be projected upward from the lumbar region towards the trunk.

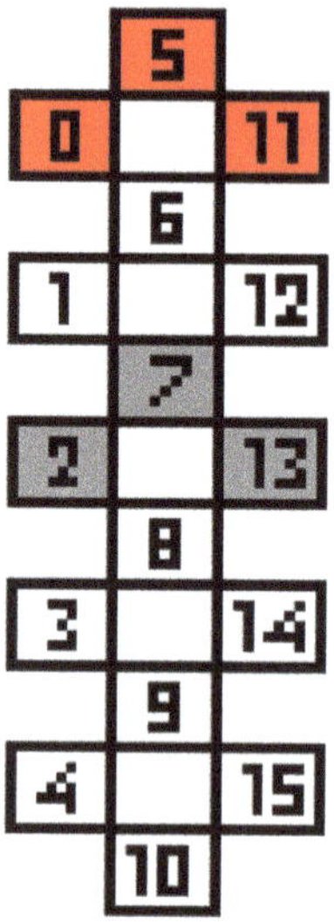

Figure A1. An arrangement of cathodes (in red) and anodes (in grey) commonly seen within the scES configurations based on Table A1. 8/14 participants had 0-/5-/11- as a part of the cathode arrangement, and 9/14 participants had 2+/7+/13+ as a part of the anode arrangement for at least one cohort. 6 participants had both in a single cohort.

Table A2. List of optimized scES configurations for each participant.

PID	Configuration	Frequency	Pulse Width	Amplitude
A64	C1: (0-/5-/11-//1+/2+/7+/8+/12+/13+)	21.67 Hz	800 µs	11.2 mA
	C2: (0-/5-/11-//2+/3+/8+/9+/13+/14+)	21.67 Hz	800 µs	13.5 mA
A97	C1: (0-/5-//2+/7+)	20 Hz	650 µs	6.9 mA
	C2: (6-//0+/1+/2+/3+/4+/5+/7+/8+/9+/10+/11+/12+/13+/14+/15+)	100 Hz	500 µs	5.5 mA
A127	C1: (5-/11-//0+/1+/6+/7+/12+)	35 Hz	650 µs	18.8 mA
A128	C1: (5-//0+/11+)	16.67 Hz	1000 µs	25.5 mA
	C2: (8-//0+/1+/2+/3+/4+/5+/6+/7+/9+/10+/11+/12+/13+/14+/15+)	100 Hz	500 µs	10 mA
A119	C1: (0-/5-/11-//2+/7+/8+/13+)	37.5 Hz	600 µs	12.1 mA
	C2: (3-/8-/14-//1+/2+/4+/7+/9+/10+/12+/13+/15+)	150 Hz	300 µs	10 mA
A133	C1: (0-/1-/5-/11-/12-//2+/3+/8+/13+/14+)	25 Hz	600 µs	12. 9 mA
	C2: (0-/11-//7+/8+/9+/10+)	16.67 Hz	600 µs	5 mA
B38	C1: (0-/5-/11-//2+/3+/7+/8+/13+/14+)	30 Hz	950 µs	15.3 mA
B40	C1: (5-//0+/11+)	30 Hz	850 µs	3.5 mA
	C2:(7-//0+/1+/2+/3+/4+/6+/8+/9+/10+/11+/12+/13+/14+/15+)	90 Hz	450 µs	8 mA
	C3: (0-//6+/12+)	22.5 Hz	700 µs	4.4 mA
B42	C1: (1-/6-/12-//2+/3+/7+/8+/13+/14+)	32 Hz	650 µs	12.9 mA

Table A2. *Cont.*

PID	Configuration	Frequency	Pulse Width	Amplitude
B212	C1: (5-/11-//0+/6+/12+)	21.67 Hz	900 μs	8.2 mA
	C2: (1-/7-/12-//0+/2+/3+/4+/6+/8+/9+/10+/11+/13+/14+/15+)	130 Hz	300 μs	6.2 mA
B213	C1: (0-/5-/11-//1+/6+/12+)	16.67 Hz	1000 μs	17 mA
B194	C1: (0-/5-/6-/11-/12-//1+/2+/7+/13+)	28 Hz	700 μs	7.8 mA
	C2: (0-/1-/2-//5+/6+/7+)	140 Hz	300 μs	2 mA
C193	C1: (0-/5-/11-//1+/2+/6+/7+/12+/13+)	25 Hz	800 μs	10.1 mA
	C2: (0-/1-/5-/6-/11-/12-//2+/3+/13+/14+)	25 Hz	700 μs	11.5 mA
C231	C1: (0-/5-/11-//2+/7+/8+/9+/13+)	19.17 Hz	700 μs	6.1 mA
	C3: (10-//2+/3+/4+/7+/8+/9+/13+/14+/15+)	9.58 Hz	300 μs	3.1 mA

References

1. Murphy, J.O.; Audu, M.L.; Lombardo, L.M.; Foglyano, K.M.; Triolo, R.J. Feasibility of closed-loop controller for righting seated posture after spinal cord injury. *J. Rehabil. Res. Dev.* **2014**, *51*, 747–760. [CrossRef] [PubMed]
2. Hagen, E.; Eide, G.E.; Rekand, T.; Gilhus, N.; Gronning, M. A 50-year follow-up of the incidence of traumatic spinal cord injuries in Western Norway. *Spinal Cord* **2010**, *48*, 313–318. [CrossRef] [PubMed]
3. Lanzetta, D.; Cattaneo, D.; Pellegatta, D.; Cardini, R. Trunk control in unstable sitting posture during functional activities in healthy subjects and patients with multiple sclerosis. *Arch. Phys. Med. Rehabil.* **2004**, *85*, 279–283. [CrossRef] [PubMed]
4. Granata, K.; Wilson, S. Trunk posture and spinal stability. *Clin. Biomech.* **2001**, *16*, 650–659. [CrossRef]
5. Lissy, D.; Kukke, S. Preliminary performance of a surgically implanted neuroprosthesis for standing and transfers—Where do we stand? *Development* **2001**, *38*, 609–617.
6. Minkel, J.L. Seating and mobility considerations for people with spinal cord injury. *Phys. Ther.* **2000**, *80*, 701–709. [CrossRef]
7. Seelen, H.A.M.; Potten, Y.J.M.; Huson, A.; Spaans, F.; Reulen, J.P.H. Impaired balance control in paraplegic subjects. *J. Electromyogr. Kinesiol.* **1997**, *7*, 149–160. [CrossRef] [PubMed]
8. Hobson, D.A.; Tooms, R.E. Seated lumbar/pelvic alignment: A comparison between spinal cord-injured and noninjured groups. *Spine* **1992**, *17*, 293–298. [CrossRef] [PubMed]
9. Anderson, K.D. Targeting recovery: Priorities of the spinal cord-injured population. *J. Neurotrauma* **2004**, *21*, 1371–1383. [CrossRef]
10. Triolo, R.J.; Bailey, S.N.; Miller, M.E.; Lombardo, L.M.; Audu, M.L. Effects of stimulating hip and trunk muscles on seated stability, posture, and reach after spinal cord injury. *Arch. Phys. Med. Rehabil.* **2013**, *94*, 1766–1775. [CrossRef] [PubMed]
11. Bergmann, M.; Zahharova, A.; Reinvee, M.; Asser, T.; Gapeyeva, H.; Vahtrik, D. The effect of functional electrical stimulation and therapeutic exercises on trunk muscle tone and dynamic sitting balance in persons with chronic spinal cord injury: A crossover trial. *Medicina* **2019**, *55*, 619. [CrossRef]
12. Wu, G.A.; Lombardo, L.; Triolo, R.J.; Bogie, K.M. The effects of combined trunk and gluteal neuromuscular electrical stimulation on posture and tissue health in spinal cord injury. *PM&R* **2013**, *5*, 688–696.
13. Rath, M.; Vette, A.H.; Ramasubramaniam, S.; Li, K.; Burdick, J.; Edgerton, V.R.; Gerasimenko, Y.P.; Sayenko, D.G. Trunk stability enabled by noninvasive spinal electrical stimulation after spinal cord injury. *J. Neurotrauma* **2018**, *35*, 2540–2553. [CrossRef]
14. Gerasimenko, Y.; Gorodnichev, R.; Moshonkina, T.; Sayenko, D.; Gad, P.; Edgerton, V.R. Transcutaneous electrical spinal-cord stimulation in humans. *Ann. Phys. Rehabil. Med.* **2015**, *58*, 225–231. [CrossRef] [PubMed]
15. Keller, A.; Singh, G.; Sommerfeld, J.H.; King, M.; Parikh, P.; Ugiliweneza, B.; D'Amico, J.; Gerasimenko, Y.; Behrman, A.L. Noninvasive spinal stimulation safely enables upright posture in children with spinal cord injury. *Nat. Commun.* **2021**, *12*, 5850. [CrossRef] [PubMed]
16. Audu, M.L.; Lombardo, L.M.; Schnellenberger, J.R.; Foglyano, K.M.; Miller, M.E.; Triolo, R.J. A neuroprosthesis for control of seated balance after spinal cord injury. *J. Neuroeng. Rehabil.* **2015**, *12*, 8. [CrossRef]
17. Friederich, A.R.; Bao, X.; Triolo, R.J.; Audu, M.L. Feedback control of upright seating with functional neuromuscular stimulation during a reaching task after spinal cord injury: A feasibility study. *J. Neuroeng. Rehabil.* **2022**, *19*, 139. [CrossRef]
18. Rahimi, M.; Torkaman, G.; Ghabaee, M.; Ghasem-Zadeh, A. Advanced weight-bearing mat exercises combined with functional electrical stimulation to improve the ability of wheelchair-dependent people with spinal cord injury to transfer and attain independence in activities of daily living: A randomized controlled trial. *Spinal Cord* **2020**, *58*, 78–85. [PubMed]
19. Harkema, S.; Gerasimenko, Y.; Hodes, J.; Burdick, J.; Angeli, C.; Chen, Y.; Ferreira, C.; Willhite, A.; Rejc, E.; Grossman, R.G. Effect of epidural stimulation of the lumbosacral spinal cord on voluntary movement, standing, and assisted stepping after motor complete paraplegia: A case study. *Lancet* **2011**, *377*, 1938–1947. [CrossRef] [PubMed]
20. Minassian, K.; McKay, W.B.; Binder, H.; Hofstoetter, U.S. Targeting Lumbar Spinal Neural Circuitry by Epidural Stimulation to Restore Motor Function After Spinal Cord Injury. *Neurotherapeutics* **2016**, *13*, 284–294. [CrossRef]

21. Dimitrijevic, M.R.; Gerasimenko, Y.; Pinter, M.M. Evidence for a spinal central pattern generator in humans. *Ann. N. Y. Acad. Sci.* **1998**, *860*, 360–376. [CrossRef]
22. Rejc, E.; Angeli, C.; Harkema, S. Effects of lumbosacral spinal cord epidural stimulation for standing after chronic complete paralysis in humans. *PLoS ONE* **2015**, *10*, e0133998. [CrossRef] [PubMed]
23. Angeli, C.A.; Boakye, M.; Morton, R.A.; Vogt, J.; Benton, K.; Chen, Y.; Ferreira, C.K.; Harkema, S.J. Recovery of over-ground walking after chronic motor complete spinal cord injury. *N. Engl. J. Med.* **2018**, *379*, 1244–1250. [CrossRef]
24. Gill, M.; Linde, M.; Fautsch, K.; Hale, R.; Lopez, C.; Veith, D.; Calvert, J.; Beck, L.; Garlanger, K.; Edgerton, R. Epidural electrical stimulation of the lumbosacral spinal cord improves trunk stability during seated reaching in two humans with severe thoracic spinal cord injury. *Front. Syst. Neurosci.* **2020**, *14*, 79. [CrossRef]
25. Rowald, A.; Komi, S.; Demesmaeker, R.; Baaklini, E.; Hernandez-Charpak, S.D.; Paoles, E.; Montanaro, H.; Cassara, A.; Becce, F.; Lloyd, B. Activity-dependent spinal cord neuromodulation rapidly restores trunk and leg motor functions after complete paralysis. *Nat. Med.* **2022**, *28*, 260–271. [CrossRef]
26. Angeli, C.A.; Edgerton, V.R.; Gerasimenko, Y.P.; Harkema, S.J. Altering spinal cord excitability enables voluntary movements after chronic complete paralysis in humans. *Brain* **2014**, *137*, 1394–1409. [CrossRef] [PubMed]
27. Hair, J.F., Jr.; Black William, C.; Babin Barry, J.; Anderson Rolph, E. Multivariate data analysis. In *Upper Saddle River*, 7th ed.; Prentice Hall: Hoboken, NJ, USA, 2009.
28. Cohen, J. The effect size. In *Statistical Power Analysis for the Behavioral Sciences*; Lawrence Erlbaum Associates: Hillsdale, NJ, USA, 1988; pp. 77–83.
29. Farivar, S.S.; Liu, H.; Hays, R.D. Half standard deviation estimate of the minimally important difference in HRQOL scores? *Expert Rev. Pharmacoecon. Outcomes Res.* **2004**, *4*, 515–523. [CrossRef]
30. Hansen, T.; Slagsvold, B. The age and subjective well-being paradox revisited: A multidimensional perspective. *Nor. Epidemiol.* **2012**, *22*, 187–195.
31. Boswell-Ruys, C.L.; Harvey, L.A.; Barker, J.J.; Ben, M.; Middleton, J.W.; Lord, S.R. Training unsupported sitting in people with chronic spinal cord injuries: A randomized controlled trial. *Spinal Cord* **2010**, *48*, 138–143. [CrossRef]
32. Carini, F.; Mazzola, M.; Fici, C.; Palmeri, S.; Messina, M.; Damiani, P.; Tomasello, G. Posture and posturology, anatomical and physiological profiles: Overview and current state of art. *Acta Biomed.* **2017**, *88*, 11–16. [CrossRef]

bioengineering

MDPI

Article

Muscular and Kinematic Responses to Unexpected Translational Balance Perturbation: A Pilot Study in Healthy Young Adults

Cheuk Ying Tong [1,†], Ringo Tang-Long Zhu [1,2,†], Yan To Ling [1,3], Eduardo Mendonça Scheeren [4], Freddy Man Hin Lam [5], Hong Fu [6,*] and Christina Zong-Hao Ma [1,2,*]

1 Department of Biomedical Engineering, The Hong Kong Polytechnic University, Hong Kong SAR 999077, China; cheuk-ying.tong@connect.polyu.hk (C.Y.T.); ringo-tanglong.zhu@connect.polyu.hk (R.T.-L.Z.); jane.yt.ling@connect.polyu.hk (Y.T.L.)
2 Research Institute for Smart Ageing, The Hong Kong Polytechnic University, Hong Kong SAR 999077, China
3 Centre for Developmental Neurobiology, King's College London, London SE1 1UL, UK
4 Graduate Program in Health Technology, Pontifícia Universidade Católica do Paraná, Curitiba 80215-901, Brazil; eduardo.scheeren@pucpr.br
5 Department of Rehabilitation Sciences, The Hong Kong Polytechnic University, Hong Kong SAR 999077, China; freddy-mh.lam@polyu.edu.hk
6 Department of Mathematics and Information Technology, The Education University of Hong Kong, Hong Kong SAR 999077, China
* Correspondence: hfu@eduhk.hk (H.F.); czh.ma@polyu.edu.hk (C.Z.-H.M.); Tel.: +852-2766-7671 (C.Z.-H.M.); Fax: +852-2334-2429 (C.Z.-H.M.)
† These authors contributed equally to this work.

Abstract: Falls and fall-related injuries are significant public health problems in older adults. While balance-controlling strategies have been extensively researched, there is still a lack of understanding regarding how fast the lower-limb muscles contract and coordinate in response to a sudden loss of standing balance. Therefore, this pilot study aims to investigate the speed and timing patterns of multiple joint/muscles' activities among the different challenges in standing balance. Twelve healthy young subjects were recruited, and they received unexpected translational balance perturbations with randomized intensities and directions. Electromyographical (EMG) and mechanomyographical (MMG) signals of eight dominant-leg's muscles, dominant-leg's three-dimensional (3D) hip/knee/ankle joint angles, and 3D postural sways were concurrently collected. Two-way ANOVAs were used to examine the difference in timing and speed of the collected signals among muscles/joint motions and among perturbation intensities. This study has found that (1) agonist muscles resisting the induced postural sway tended to activate more rapidly than the antagonist muscles, and ankle muscles contributed the most with the fastest rate of response; (2) voluntary corrective lower-limb joint motions and postural sways could occur as early as the perturbation-induced passive ones; (3) muscles reacted more rapidly under a larger perturbation intensity, while the joint motions or postural sways did not. These findings expand the current knowledge on standing-balance-controlling mechanisms and may potentially provide more insights for developing future fall-prevention strategies in daily life.

Keywords: translational balance perturbation; moving platform; muscle activation; muscle co-contraction; onset latency; time to peak; electromyography (EMG); mechanomyography (MMG)

1. Introduction

Falls are one of the major public health problems in the world. Approximately one in three older adults fall worldwide [1], and 28.7% of older adults fall in the United States annually [2]. Every year, there are around 684,000 fatal falls, and it is the second leading cause of unintentional injury death [1,3]. For the non-fatal injuries, about one in ten older adults experiences a fall-related injury annually [4]. Falls cause physical and mental impacts on older adults and can further heavily burden society [1]. Balance and gait disorder is the major cause of falls excepting accidents [5]. The appropriate and timely postural adjustments and lower-limb muscle activities are vital to maintain postural balance. The in-depth investigation into these strategies for how a person reacts to sudden balance perturbations can facilitate our understanding of the underlying mechanisms of falls. This could also provide more insights and inspire the future development of fall-prevention strategies.

Humans have different patterns of lower-limb joint motions in response to varied intensities of balance perturbations. Previous studies have identified three fundamental strategies to maintain the static standing balance, i.e., the ankle strategy, hip strategy, and stepping strategy [6]. The ankle strategy is reached mainly by the dorsiflexion and plantarflexion of ankle joint, with minimal movement of the other proximal joints [7]. This strategy is dominantly employed when no external perturbation exists [8]. The hip strategy is used when the ankle strategy is not enough to keep the center of mass (COM) within the base of support (BOS) [7]. If the ankle and hip muscles cannot contract sufficiently to compensate for the large balance perturbations, the stepping strategy would be employed [9]. Sometimes a "mixed strategy" can also be used to maintain balance with typical characteristics of using the combined above-mentioned strategies depending on the specific situation [10].

An investigation of the rapidity and appropriate sequence of movements in the hip, knee, and ankle joints is crucial for understanding the balance-controlling strategy, especially during unexpected and intense balance perturbations. Previous studies have primarily focused on the peak responses of postural sways and joint angles in maintaining standing balance [11–13], and only a few studies have analyzed the onset sequence of various lower-limb joint motions in response to balance perturbations in the sagittal plane [14]. When specifically looking at the lower-limb responses following the translational perturbations induced by a suddenly forward-moving platform, the lower-limb joints commonly react with the sequence of ankle dorsiflexion, knee flexion, and finally hip flexion [14]. However, research on the timing and speed of lower-limb joint responses to balance perturbations in the frontal plane remains inadequate. Therefore, a study of the temporal parameters, such as onset latency and time to peak, of whole-body postural sways as well as lower-limb joint motions in response to the balance perturbations with various intensities and directions is warranted.

In addition to examining the lower-limb joint motions, analyzing the lower-limb muscle activities can provide greater insights into the underlying balance-controlling strategies. Irrespective of the balance-controlling strategy utilized, the acceleration of any body segment resulting from a perturbation must be generated by the contraction of the corresponding skeletal muscles. Most previous studies investigated the signals of only one or a couple of lower-limb muscles for maintaining balance [15–21]. Specifically, most previous studies on static balance control mainly investigated the EMG signals of the ankle dorsiflexor and plantarflexor [6,15–17]. During the walking task with unexpectedly induced slipping, the previous literature has reported that older adults who failed to maintain balance tended to have delayed EMG onset in the knee flexors/extensors of the slipping legs [18,19]. Some other studies also reported that the large rate of EMG rise in the ankle plantarflexor and knee flexor of the stance leg was important for preventing tripping [20] and that in the hip abductors/adductors was important for protective stepping [21] in older people. However, until now, there has been insufficient evidence on how fast the major hip, knee, and ankle muscles can react to the balance perturbations with varying intensities and directions.

Meanwhile, one of our recent works investigated the rapid responses of eight dominant-leg muscles following the sudden loss of balance induced by waist-pull perturbations, by quantifying the EMG-onset latency, time to peak EMG amplitude, and rate of EMG rise of the captioned muscles [22]. It mainly identified that the agonist muscles exhibited quicker activation than the antagonist muscles, and ankle muscles tended to activate faster than the remaining six muscles (i.e., hip flexor/extensor, hip abductor/adductor, and knee flexor/extensor) in response to the waist-pull balance perturbation in young adults [22]. However, it has remained unclear whether young adults would adopt similar strategies in response to the moving-platform balance perturbation, which mimics a more real-life situation of standing in the buses/trains/boats and merits further study.

Apart from the joint reactions and muscle electrical activities, the response of other events along the motor output pathway during balance control has been less explored. The generation of a joint motion goes through activation in neuromuscular junctions, muscle mechanical activities (shortening and lateral vibrations), and force propagation to tendons [23]. However, it is unknown whether the timing of muscle mechanical activities plays a role in the recovery from balance perturbations of varying intensities and directions. Mechanomyography (MMG) can detect such mechanical activities of a contracting muscle by recording the lateral vibrations that are perpendicular to the muscle fiber direction on the skin surface [24]. Previous research has reported that the onset of the MMG signal was later than that of the EMG signal during the isometric contraction [24]. For dynamic situations, MMG signals have been investigated in the tasks of maintaining walking balance [25,26] and standing balance [22]. The MMG peak timing was found to be later than the EMG peak timing for the ankle plantarflexor during a gait cycle [25]; however, the onset and peak timing of MMG signals were found generally earlier than that of EMG signals following the sudden perturbations induced by waist pulls, which might be affected by the noise of passive body-segment movements induced by perturbations [22]. Therefore, this study made further attempts to explore the timing and coordination patterns of major lower-limb muscles' mechanical activities during balance control.

To bridge the above research gaps, this study aimed to explore how healthy young adults respond to the moving-platform-induced balance perturbations with multiple directions and intensities from the perspectives of postural sways, lower-limb joint motions, and lower-limb muscle activities. The objectives of this study were to examine the differences in speed (onset latency, time to peak, and/or rate of rise) and peak responses of (1) the forward/backward, medial/lateral, and upward/downward COM displacements; (2) the eight lower-limb joint motions (i.e., hip flexion/extension, hip abduction/adduction, knee flexion/extension, and ankle dorsiflexion/plantarflexion); and (3) the eight dominant-leg muscles' electrical and mechanical activities (i.e., hip flexor/extensor, hip abductor/adductor, knee flexor/extensor, and ankle dorsiflexor/plantarflexor) under the different perturbation intensities. Such comprehensive analysis of kinematics and muscle activities under the sudden loss of balance that simulates daily scenarios is expected to uncover the more in-depth mechanisms underlying standing-balance control. We hypothesized that (1) agonist muscles resisting the induced postural sway would have faster activation than antagonist muscles; (2) involuntary/passive joint motions and postural sways induced by the unexpected perturbation would occur earlier than voluntary/active ones for balance recovery; and (3) higher intensities of unexpected perturbations would induce faster muscle activities, joint motions, and postural sways.

2. Materials and Methods

2.1. Study Design and Subjects

This is an observational/cross-sectional and exploratory study. A total of 12 young healthy adults aged between 18 to 24 were recruited through the method of convenience sampling. Ethical approval was granted by the Institutional Review Board (IRB) of The Hong Kong Polytechnic University (HSEARS20201230002). The subjects satisfied the following inclusion criteria [27]:

- No high-intensity sports within 24 h before the experiment;
- No known neurological or musculoskeletal deficits;
- No history of balance disorders, walking disorders, or dizziness;
- No history of lower-limb injuries within a week;

- No sight or hearing disorders;
- No medication intake that could affect muscle activities.

2.2. Equipment

2.2.1. Moving-Platform Perturbation System

A moving-platform perturbation system was developed to induce the unexpected balance perturbations (see Figure 1). It consisted of (1) an aluminum alloy frame, (2) four servo motors (130-07725AS4, Wenzhou Guomai Electronics Ltd., Wenzhou, China), (3) a customized circular wooden platform (diameter: 80.0 cm; thickness: 3.5 cm), (4) four braided polyethylene wires (diameter: 1.2 mm), (5) a set of rails, and (6) a safety harness system (PG-360, Physio Gait Dynamic Unweighting System, Healthcare International Ltd., Langley, WA, USA). An Arduino UNO board (Arduino Uno Rev3, The Arduino Team, Somerville, America) and a customized Arduino program were used to control the servo motors and deliver the unexpected balance perturbations via the wires. Each of the four wires connected the edge of the platform with a motor, and the motor would pull the platform to slide along the rails so as to induce the horizontal balance perturbation in one of the four directions with regard to the subject's body (anterior, posterior, left, and right). Figure 2 shows the flow of generating one perturbation. Firstly, the system delivered a sudden pull to the wooden platform with a randomized direction and intensity. Then, the platform would remain stationary for 8 s. Finally, the system pulled the wooden platform to return to its original position. The direction, intensity, and starting time of each perturbation were randomized.

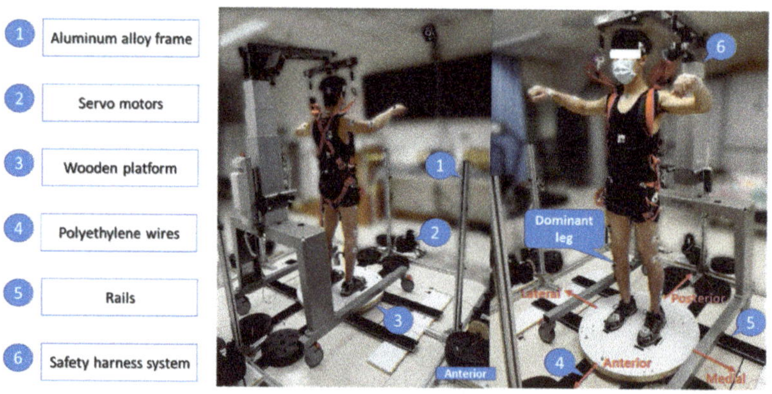

Figure 1. The moving-platform perturbation system with a subject.

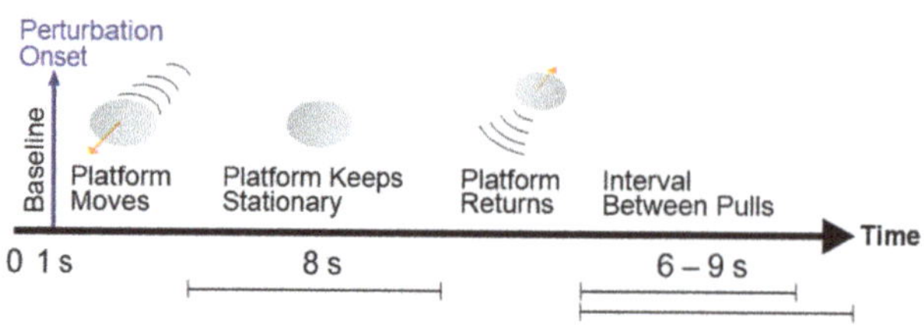

Figure 2. The flow of a pulling perturbation.

2.2.2. Data Sampling Equipment

A three-dimensional capture and analysis system, i.e., the Vicon system (Nexus 2.11, Vicon Motion Systems Ltd., Yarnton, UK), with eight cameras, was applied to capture the whole-body kinematics. The sampling rate was 250 Hz. A total of 39 reflective markers were adhered to the subject's body based on the full-body plug-in-gait dynamic model, including twelve on the bilateral lower limbs (bilateral thigh, lateral condyle of femur, shank, lateral malleolus, heel, and 2nd metatarsal head), four on the pelvis (bilateral anterior superior iliac spine [ASIS], and bilateral posterior superior iliac spine), five on the torso (sternal notch, xiphoid process of the sternum, spinous process of the 7th cervical vertebra, spinous process of 10th thoracic vertebra, and right scapula), fourteen on the bilateral upper limbs (bilateral acromion, upper arm, lateral epicondyle of humerus, forearm, radial styloid process, ulnar styloid process, and 3rd metacarpal head), and four on the head (bilateral temples and bilateral back head) [28]. To ensure the reflective markers were firmly fixed on the subject's body surface, tight clothes and shorts were provided for subjects to wear during the experiment.

Eight major lower-limb muscles' activities were collected by an eight-channel Trigno Wireless Biofeedback System (SP-W02D-1110, Delsys Inc., Natick, MA, USA). Each Delsys Trigno Avanti sensor (mass: 14 g; dimension: 37 mm × 27 mm × 13 mm) consisted of an EMG sensor (double-differential silver bar electrodes; inter-electrode distance: 10 mm; each electrode size: 5 mm × 1 mm; analogue Butterworth filter bandwidth: 20–450 Hz) and a 3-axis accelerometer (range: ±16 g; resolution: 10 bits) to serve as the MMG sensor [29]. The sampling rates of the EMG and MMG were 2000 Hz and 250 Hz, respectively. According to the Surface ElectroMyoGraphy for the Non-Invasive Assessment of Muscles (SENIAM) recommendation [30], the subject's skin was shaved to remove the hair, and alcohol wipes were used to clean the skin surface. After the alcohol vaporized and when the skin was dry, the eight EMG and MMG sensors were placed over the investigated eight lower-limb muscles, respectively (see Table 1), and firmly fixed using double-sided adhesives (Adhesive Interfaces for Trigno Sensors, Delsys, Boston, MA, USA) and pressure-sensitive tapes (Haishi Hainuo Group, Qingdao, China). The Trigno Wireless Biofeedback System was commercially synchronized with the Vicon system. Infrared light bulbs were connected to the moving-platform perturbation system, and the flash of infrared light indicating each perturbation could be detected by the Vicon system. In this way, the three systems were synchronized during data collection.

Table 1. Eight investigated muscles and the corresponding EMG/MMG sensor placement.

Muscle	EMG/MMG Sensor Placement
Ankle dorsiflexor: tibialis anterior (TA)	• One-third of the way from the tip of the fibula to the tip of the medial malleolus [30];
Ankle plantarflexor: medial gastrocnemius (MG)	• On the most prominent bulge of the muscle [30];
Knee extensor: rectus femoris (RF)	• Halfway from the superior boarder of the patella to the ASIS [30];
Knee flexor: semitendinosus (ST)	• Halfway from the medial epicondyle of the tibia to the ischial tuberosity [30];
Hip flexor: sartorius (SA)	• At 8 cm distal from the ASIS along the line between the ASIS and the median of the tibial tuberosity [31];
Hip extensor: gluteus maximus (GMax)	• Halfway from the greater trochanter to the sacral vertebrae [30];
Hip abductor: gluteus medius (GMed)	• Halfway from the greater trochanter to the highest point of iliac crest [30];
Hip adductor: adductor maximus (AM)	• Halfway from the medial femoral epicondyle to the pubic tubercle [32].

2.3. Protocol

2.3.1. Subjective Assessment

Each subject firstly accomplished the demographic data collection and the subjective assessments. Body mass and height were measured using a standard scale (DETECTO 3P704, Webb City, MI, USA), and other anthropometrics such as leg length were measured using a tape measure and a caliper. The International Physical Activity Questionnaire—Short version (IPAQ-S) [33] and the Falls Efficacy Scale—International (FES-I) short version [22,34–36] were used to evaluate the physical and mental factors that might affect the balance performance in each subject, respectively. A larger value calculated from the IPAQ-S reflects a higher level of physical activity in the past 1 week, and a higher score of the FES-I short version (7 items; full score: 28 points) reflects greater concerns over falling [33,34]. The Mini-Balance Evaluation System Test (Mini-BEST) was also performed to evaluate the subject's balance capacity in four categories: anticipatory postural control, reactive postural control, sensory organization, and dynamic gait [37]. A higher score of the Mini-BEST (14 items; full score: 28 points) indicates better balance capacity. Finally, the subject's dominant leg was ascertained using the balance recovery test, ball-kick test, and step-up test [38]. The leg used most frequently in nine total trials (3 trials $\times$ 3 tests) was considered the dominant leg [38].

2.3.2. Instrumented Data Collection

Before the perturbation experiment, the reflective markers and the EMG and MMG sensors were attached to subjects, and instructions and explanation of the experimental protocol were given. To simulate the daily situation, the subject was asked to wear his/her usual shoes during the whole perturbation experiment. The subject was instructed to stand naturally with two feet shoulder-width apart in the middle of the platform and knees fully extended; subjects were instructed that when the platform moved, he/she should try his/her best to maintain balance without stepping or return to the original foot position as soon as possible if stepped. The subject held a light bar in front of the body at the waist level, and the reflective markers was not blocked during data collection in this way [11]. Dark-colored tapes were adhered below the subject's shoes to mark the original foot position on the wooden platform.

Each subject received a total of 48 unexpected balance perturbations induced by the moving platform (4 directions $\times$ 4 intensities $\times$ 3 repetitions), and the kinematic, EMG, and MMG data of the subject's responses were collected. These balance perturbations were randomly allocated into four perturbation trials during the experiment, and there was a 5 min rest between the two trials to avoid the effects of fatigue. For each perturbation, the starting time, direction (anterior, posterior, medial, or lateral), or intensity (highest, high, low, or lowest) was random. The direction of a balance perturbation was defined as the moving direction of the platform in reference to the subject's dominant leg. For example, for a subject with the right leg as the dominant leg, pulling the platform toward the left was regarded as a "medial" perturbation, while pulling toward the right was a "lateral" perturbation (see Figure 1). Different intensities of balance perturbations were induced by the different displacements and velocities of the moving platform. Based on previous works and our pilot studies, the displacements under the "highest" intensity for the perturbations in anterior, posterior, medial, and lateral directions were set as 4%, 2.67%, 5.33%, and 5.33% of the subject's height, respectively [22,39–41]. The displacements under the "high", "low", and "lowest" intensities corresponded to 3/4, 2/4, and 1/4 of that under the "highest" intensity, respectively. The pulling duration of each perturbation was measured from the flash time of the infrared light (see Table S1 in Supplementary Material). The displacement, velocity, and acceleration of each perturbation were measured based on the trajectory of the reflective marker fixed on the moving platform (see Figure S1 in Supplementary Material). By examining these parameters, the moving-platform perturbation system showed good reliability in delivering three repetitive balance perturbations with the same direction and intensity (see Table S1 in Supplementary Material). Videos were taken during the entire perturbation experiment to evaluate the subject's stepping strategy following the unexpected perturbations.

2.4. Data Processing

The kinematic data, i.e., the whole body's center of mass (COM) and the hip, knee, and ankle angles, were firstly processed by the plug-in-gait dynamic model of the Vicon system and then zeroed to the baseline, i.e., mean signal value over the 1000 ms interval before each perturbation via a customized MATLAB program (MATLAB 2019b, The MathWorks, Inc., Natick, MA, USA). The COM displacement was further subtracted from the displacement of the platform to obtain the COM displacement relative to the base of support (BOS).

For the muscle activity data, the raw EMG data were firstly zeroed to the mean signal value over the whole perturbation trial, then full-wave rectified, and low-pass filtered by a bi-directional 4th-order Butterworth filter (cut-off frequency: 4 Hz) to obtain the EMG signal envelopes [22]. To extract MMG data, the z-axis accelerometry signals were firstly filtered through an adaptive filter in an attempt to eliminate the noise caused by limb motion by removing the trajectory of the reflective marker that was close to the MMG sensor. Next, the signals were further band-pass filtered by a 4th-order Butterworth filter (5–50 Hz) [25,26], full-wave rectified, and low-pass filtered by a bi-directional 4th-order Butterworth filter (cut-off frequency: 4 Hz) to obtain the MMG signal envelopes [42]. The EMG and MMG signal envelopes were further divided by the 1000 ms baseline mean values before the whole perturbation trial for normalization.

The onset latency, time to peak amplitude, peak amplitude, and/or rate of rise were analyzed for the kinematic, EMG, and MMG data (see Figure 3). The onset and peak points were identified within 2 s after the start of each perturbation. The onset point of a signal was determined as the first time point when the corresponding amplitude exceeded five times of standard deviation (SD) plus the mean of baseline (mean + 5 SD) [43,44]. The mean of baseline was calculated from the 1000 ms signal values before the start of each perturbation. The onset latency indicated the delayed time between the start of each perturbation and the onset point of a signal. The time to peak indicated the delayed time between the start of each perturbation and the peak point of a signal. The rate of rise indicated the slope of signal rise over the 50 ms interval after onset. For each parameter (i.e., onset latency, time to peak, peak value, or rate of rise), each subject's mean of the three values in three repetitive perturbation trials with the same direction and same intensity was used for the statistical analysis.

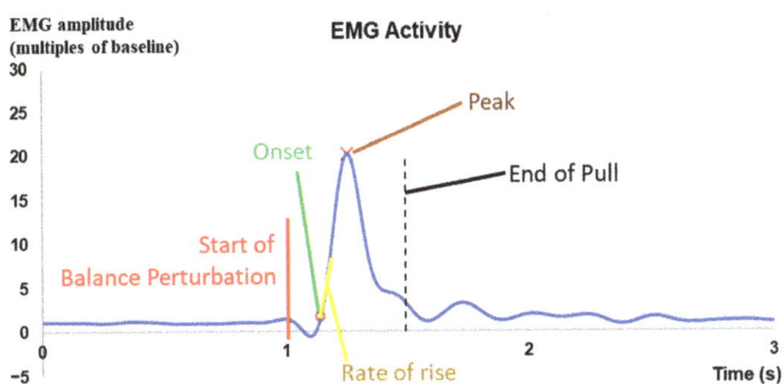

Figure 3. An example of EMG signal showing the examined parameters for one balance-perturbation trial.

2.5. Statistical Analyses

The IBM SPSS version 25 was used for statistical analyses, and the significance level was set as 0.05. For each of the four perturbation directions, two-way analysis of variance and post hoc pairwise comparisons with Bonferroni corrections were applied to analyze the effects of the below two factors on the onset latency, time to peak, peak amplitude, or rate of rise of the investigated signals:

1. EMG signal difference among the eight different muscles and among the four different perturbation intensities (muscle × perturbation intensity);
2. MMG signal difference among the eight different muscles and among the four different perturbation intensities (muscle × perturbation intensity);
3. Joint angle difference among the eight different joint motions and among the four different perturbation intensities (joint motion × perturbation intensity);
4. COM trajectory difference among the six different postural sway directions and among the four different perturbation intensities (postural sway direction × perturbation intensity).

3. Results

The demographic data and the subjective assessment results of 12 subjects are shown in Table 2. All subjects had the right leg as the dominant leg. No fall or disastrous event took place during experiments. All subjects reported that the safety harness system provided adequate protection while not restricting their motions.

Table 2. Demographic data and subjective assessments (mean ± SD) of twelve subjects.

	Male (n = 6)	Female (n = 6)	Total (n = 12)
Age (year)	21.2 ± 1.2	21.5 ± 0.5	21.3 ± 0.9
Height (cm)	174.8 ± 5.8	166.1 ± 4.9	170.4 ± 6.9
Body Mass (kg)	59.2 ± 8.9	56.8 ± 3.6	58.0 ± 6.6
BMI (kg/m^2)	19.3 ± 2.2	20.6 ± 1.0	20.0 ± 1.7
Dominant Leg	Right (n = 6)	Right (n = 6)	Right (n = 12)
Leg Length (cm)	88.8 ± 4.6	85.0 ± 3.2	86.9 ± 4.3
IPAQ-S (Kcal/week)	2017.3 ± 1253.3	1238.2 ± 883.6	1627.8 ± 1111.0
FES-I Short Version	10.8 ± 3.4	10.0 ± 2.8	10.4 ± 3.0
Mini-BEST Score	27.0 ± 0	27.5 ± 0.5	27.3 ± 0.5

Note: BMI, body mass index; IPAQ-S, International Physical Activity Scale—Short Version; FES-I, Fall Efficacy Scale—International; Mini-BEST, Mini-Balance Evaluation System Test.

Under the lowest, low, and high perturbation intensities, all young subjects were able to maintain balance without stepping or lifting their feet (0/432). Under the highest intensity of perturbations, eight subjects stepped for a total of 14 times following the anterior perturbations (14/36), no subject stepped following the posterior perturbation (0/36), one subject took a step with the non-dominant leg following the medial perturbation (1/36), and one subject took a step with the dominant leg following the lateral perturbation (1/36). Among the stepping responses following anterior perturbations, six subjects took two steps to maintain balance (7/14), three took one step with the dominant leg (4/14), and three took one step with the non-dominant leg (3/14).

3.1. COM Displacements

Figure 4 plots the mean whole-body COM displacement relative to the BOS of twelve subjects following unexpected balance perturbations in each of the four directions and four intensities (n = 12). A red dotted line specifies the start of the balance perturbation (t = 1 s). The mean and standard error (mean ± SE, n = 12) values of onset latencies, time to peak, and peak values are also plotted against the different directions of COM displacement in Figure 5.

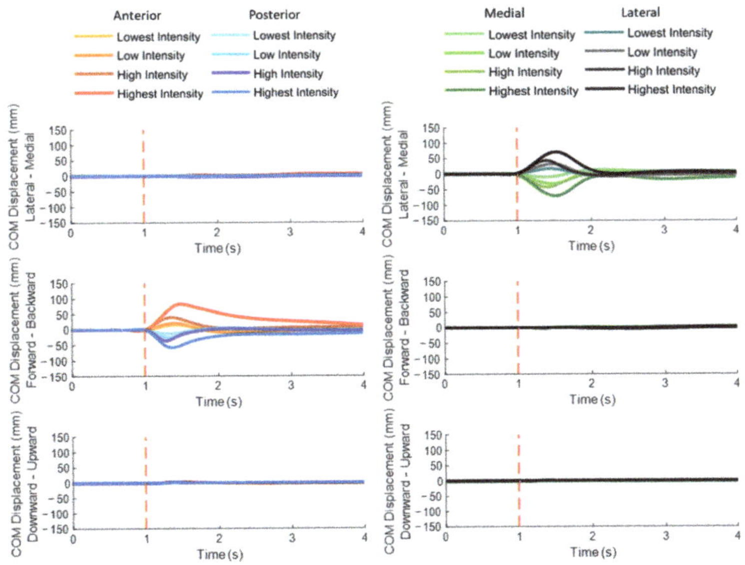

Figure 4. The mean whole-body COM displacements of twelve subjects following the unexpected perturbations with four directions and four intensities ($n = 12$). (Note: **COM**, center of mass; **red dotted line** specifies the start of the balance perturbation).

For each of the four perturbation directions, the initial COM displacement was found in the direction opposite to the perturbation, followed by the COM displacement toward the perturbation significantly ($p < 0.05$). Perturbation intensity showed significant effect on the peak COM displacement ($p < 0.05$) but not on the timing of COM displacement.

The unexpected perturbation also induced the early response of COM displacement in the vertical direction. Following anterior perturbations, the COM displacement had significantly earlier onset and significantly shorter time to peak in the upward direction than in downward/forward/medial/lateral directions ($p < 0.05$). Following posterior perturbations, the significantly shorter time to peak COM displacement was observed in the downward direction compared to the upward/backward/medial/lateral directions ($p < 0.05$). Following medial perturbations, the COM displacement in the upward direction had significantly earlier onset and significantly shorter time to peak than in downward/forward/backward direction ($p < 0.05$). Following lateral perturbations, the COM displacement had significantly earlier onset and significantly shorter time to peak in the upward direction than in downward/lateral/forward/backward direction ($p < 0.05$).

3.2. Dominant-Leg Joint Motions

Figure 6 plots the mean dominant-leg joint angle changes of the twelve subjects following unexpected translational balance perturbations ($n = 12$). Figure 7 shows the mean and standard error (mean ± SE, $n = 12$) values of onset latencies, time to peak, and peak values of the dominant-leg joint angles.

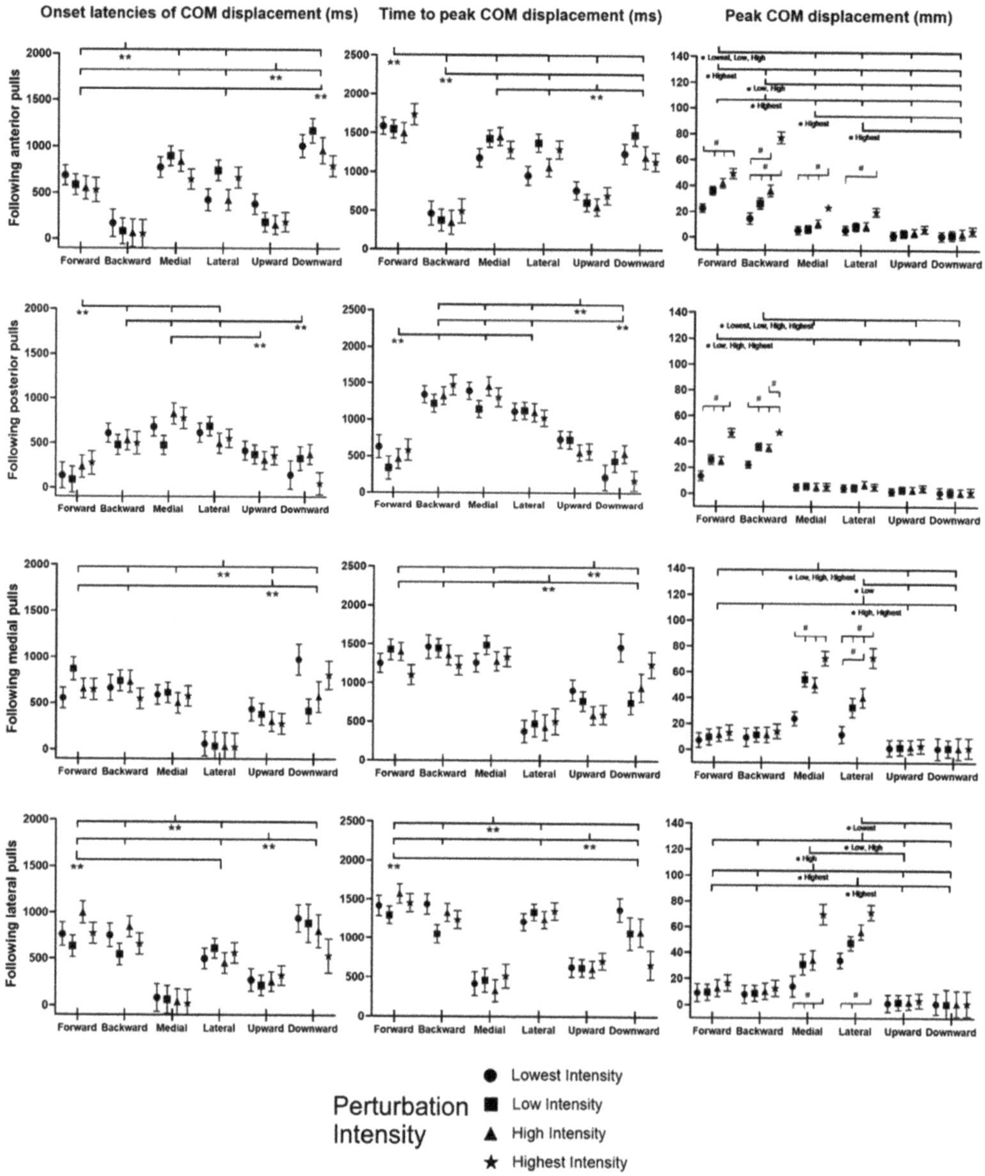

Figure 5. The onset latency of COM displacement, time to peak COM displacement, and peak COM displacement following unexpected horizontal perturbations (mean ± SE, n = 12). (Note: ⌐ or └ indicates post hoc pairwise comparison; **SE**, standard error; # indicates significant simple main effects of intensity factor; ** indicates significant main effects of postural sway factor; * indicates significant simple main effects of postural sway factor.)

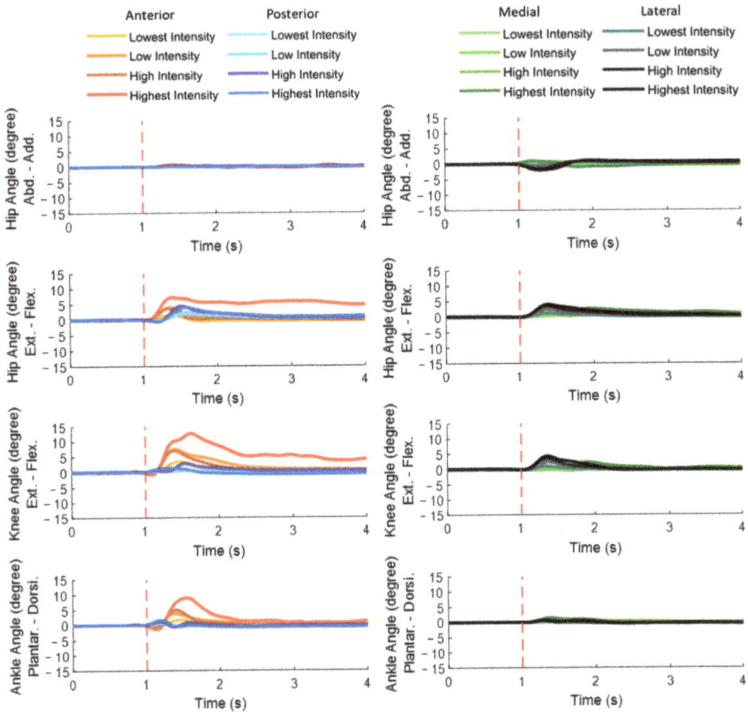

Figure 6. The mean dominant-leg joint angle changes of twelve subjects following the unexpected perturbations with four directions and four intensities ($n = 12$). (Note: **The red dotted line** specifies the start of the balance perturbation; **Add.**, adduction; **Abd**, abduction; **Flex.**, flexion; **Ext.**, extension; **Dorsi.**, dorsiflexion; **Plantar.**, plantarflexion.)

When anterior perturbation was induced, significant differences within joints existed in the angle-onset latencies (hip flexion < hip extension; hip adduction < hip abduction; $p < 0.05$) and in the time to peak angles (hip flexion < hip extension; hip adduction < hip abduction; knee flexion < knee extension; $p < 0.05$). Generally, the peak angles of hip flexion, knee flexion, and ankle dorsiflexion significantly increased with the perturbation intensity ($p < 0.05$).

When posterior perturbation was induced, ankle dorsiflexion had significantly earlier angle onset and significantly shorter time to peak angle than ankle plantarflexion ($p < 0.05$). Among the eight joint motions, the significantly largest joint motion occurred in hip flexion ($p < 0.05$). Generally, larger perturbation intensity induced larger dominant-leg joint motions ($p < 0.05$).

When medial perturbation was induced, hip adduction showed the significantly earliest angle onset among the eight joint motions ($p < 0.05$). Hip adduction also showed significantly shorter time to reach peak angle than hip abduction under the low, high, and highest perturbation intensities ($p < 0.05$), while ankle dorsiflexion showed significantly shorter time to reach peak angle than ankle plantarflexion under the highest perturbation intensity ($p < 0.05$). Generally, the peak angles of hip flexion, knee flexion, and ankle dorsiflexion significantly increased with the perturbation intensity ($p < 0.05$).

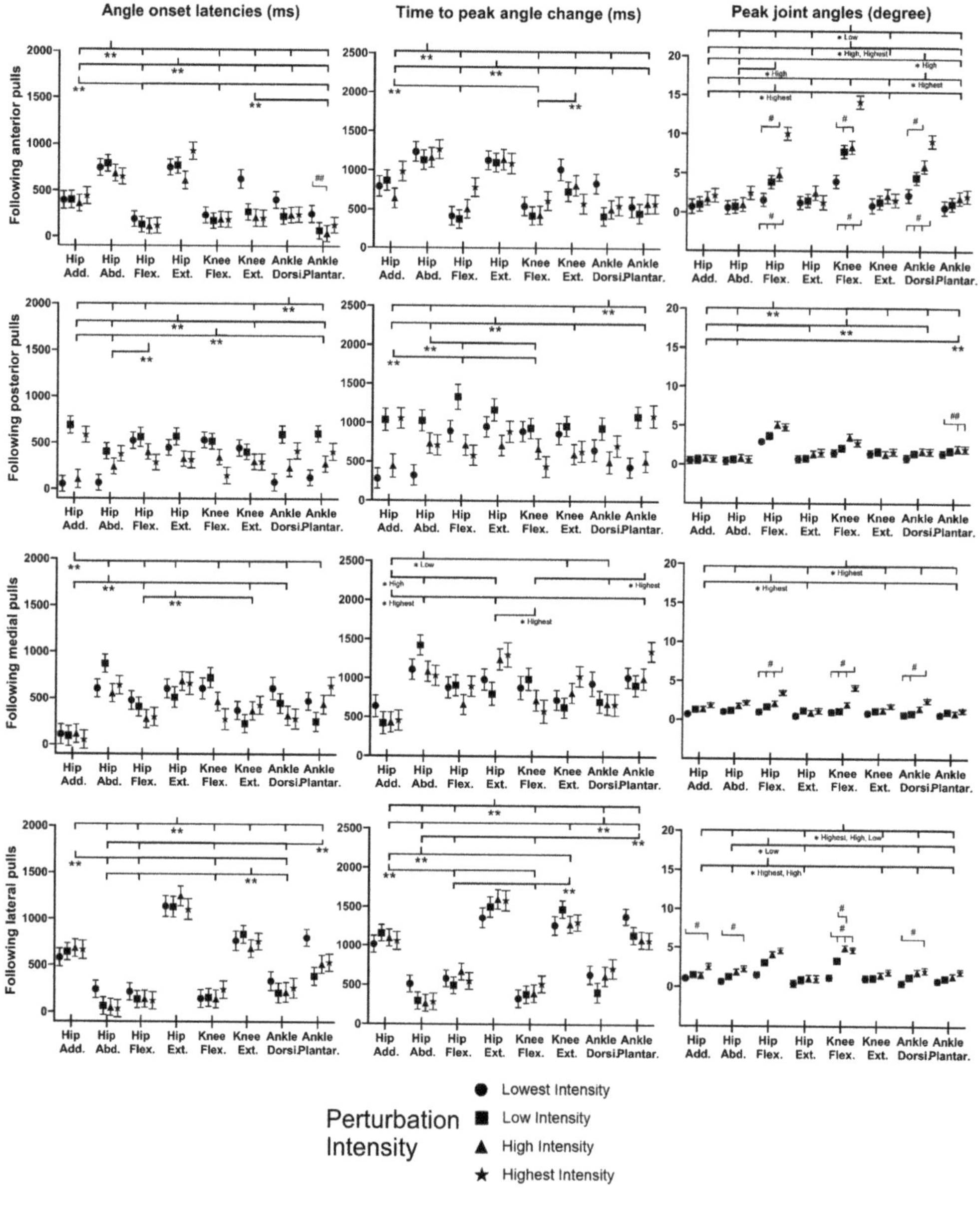

Figure 7. The angle-onset latencies, time to peak angle, and peak angles of eight lower-limb joint motions following unexpected horizontal perturbations (mean ± SE, n = 12). (Note: ⌐┘ or └┐ indicates post hoc pairwise comparison; **SE**, standard error. ## indicates significant main effects of intensity factor; # indicates significant simple main effects of intensity factor; ** indicates significant main effects of joint motion factor; * indicates significant simple main effects of joint motion factor.)

When lateral perturbation was induced, significant differences within joints existed in both the angle-onset latency and the time to peak angle (hip abduction < hip adduction; hip flexion < hip extension; knee flexion < knee extension; ankle dorsiflexion < ankle plantarflexion; $p < 0.05$). Under the low, high, and highest perturbation intensities, hip flexion and knee flexion had significantly larger peak angles than the rest of the joint motions ($p < 0.05$).

3.3. EMG Signals of Eight Dominant-Leg Muscles

Figure 8 shows the mean EMG signal of the twelve subjects for each of the eight dominant-leg muscles following the unexpected balance perturbations ($n = 12$). Figure 9 plots the mean and standard error (mean $\pm$ SE, $n = 12$) values of EMG-onset latencies, time to peak EMG amplitude, as well as rate of EMG rise against the eight dominant-leg muscles.

Following sudden anterior movement of the platform, significant differences within the agonist–antagonist muscle pairs were found in EMG-onset latency (ankle dorsiflexor < ankle plantarflexor for the lowest, low, and high perturbation intensities; hip flexor < hip extensor for the lowest perturbation intensity; $p < 0.05$) and in time to peak EMG amplitude (ankle dorsiflexor < ankle plantarflexor for all perturbation intensities; knee extensor < knee flexor for the lowest perturbation intensity; $p < 0.05$). The rate of EMG rise was remarkably highest for the ankle dorsiflexor compared to the other muscles ($p < 0.05$).

Following sudden posterior movement of the platform, the ankle plantarflexor had a significantly shorter EMG-onset latency compared to the knee extensor, hip extensor, and hip adductor ($p < 0.05$). Among the eight dominant-leg muscles, the ankle plantarflexor had the significantly largest rate of EMG rise ($p < 0.05$). Generally, larger perturbation intensities induced significantly shorter EMG-onset latencies ($p < 0.05$) and a significantly larger rate of EMG rise ($p < 0.05$).

Following sudden medial movement of the platform, significant differences within the agonist–antagonist muscle pairs were found in EMG-onset latency (hip abductor < hip adductor; $p < 0.05$) and time to EMG peak amplitude (hip abductor < hip adductor; knee extensor < knee flexor; $p < 0.05$). The ankle dorsiflexor had generally the largest rate of EMG rise among the eight dominant-leg muscles under the low, high, and highest perturbation intensities ($p < 0.05$). Generally, larger perturbation intensities induced significantly shorter EMG-onset latencies ($p < 0.05$) and significantly shorter time to EMG amplitude ($p < 0.05$); for the ankle dorsiflexor, ankle plantarflexor, and hip abductor, the rate of EMG rise also significantly increased with the perturbation intensity ($p < 0.05$).

Following sudden lateral movement of the platform, significant agonist–antagonist differences were found in EMG-onset latency (ankle dorsiflexor < ankle plantarflexor; knee extensor < knee flexor; hip flexor < hip extensor; $p < 0.05$) and in time to peak EMG amplitude (ankle dorsiflexor < ankle plantarflexor; hip adductor < hip abductor; hip flexor < hip extensor; $p < 0.05$). Among the eight dominant-leg muscles, the ankle dorsiflexor had the significantly largest rate of EMG rise ($p < 0.05$). Generally, larger perturbation intensities induced significantly shorter EMG-onset latencies ($p < 0.05$), a shorter time to peak EMG amplitude ($p < 0.05$), and a larger rate of EMG rise ($p < 0.05$).

3.4. MMG Signals of Eight Dominant-Leg Muscles

Figure 10 shows the mean MMG signal of the twelve subjects for each of the eight dominant-leg muscles following the unexpected balance perturbations ($n = 12$). Figure 11 plots the mean and standard error (mean $\pm$ SE, $n = 12$) values of MMG-onset latencies, time to peak MMG amplitude, as well as rate of MMG rise against the eight dominant-leg muscles.

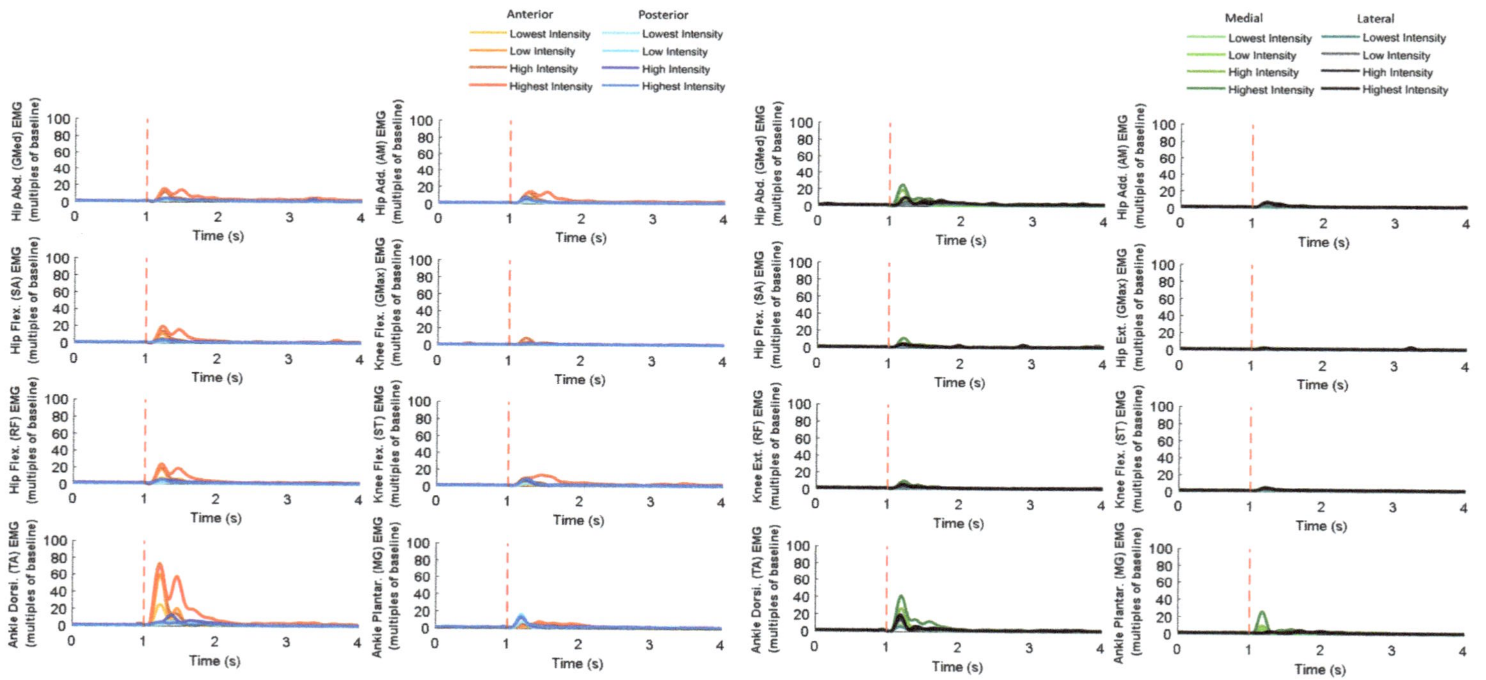

Figure 8. The mean EMG signal changes of twelve subjects for eight dominant-leg muscles following the unexpected perturbations with four directions and four intensities (n = 12). (Note: **The red dotted line** specifies the start of the balance perturbation; **EMG,** electromyography; **GMed**, gluteus medius; **AM**, adductor magus; **SA**, sartorius; **GMax**, gluteus maximus; **RF**, rectus femoris; **ST**, semitendinosus; **TA**, tibialis anterior; **MG**, gastrocnemius medialis.)

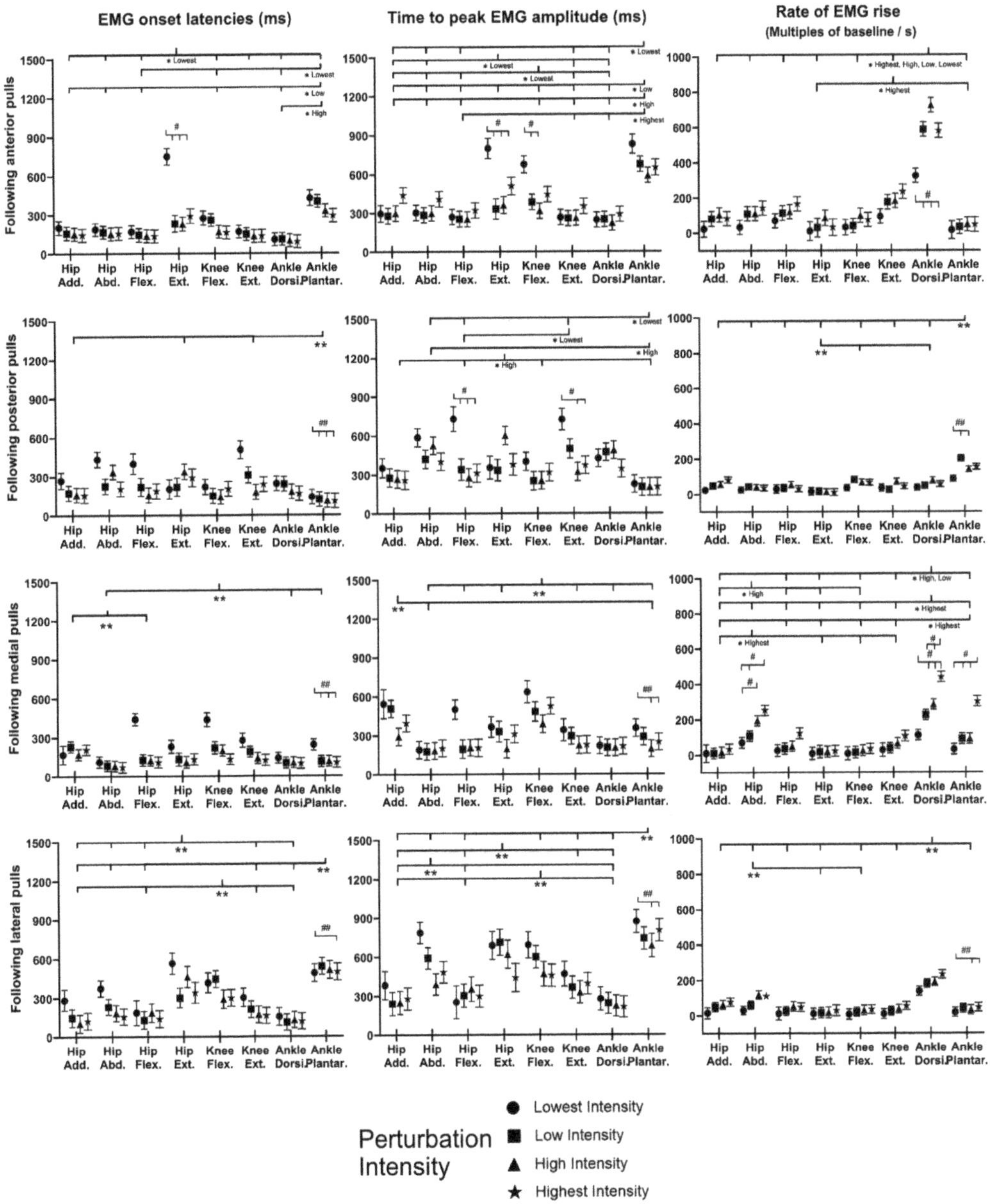

Figure 9. The EMG-onset latencies, time to peak EMG amplitude, and rate of EMG rise for eight dominant-leg muscles following unexpected horizontal perturbations (mean ± SE, n = 12). (Note: ⌐ or ⌙ represents post hoc pairwise comparison; **SE**, standard error; ## indicates significant main effects of intensity factor; # indicates significant simple main effects of intensity factor; ** indicates significant main effects of muscle factor; * indicates significant simple main effects of muscle factor.)

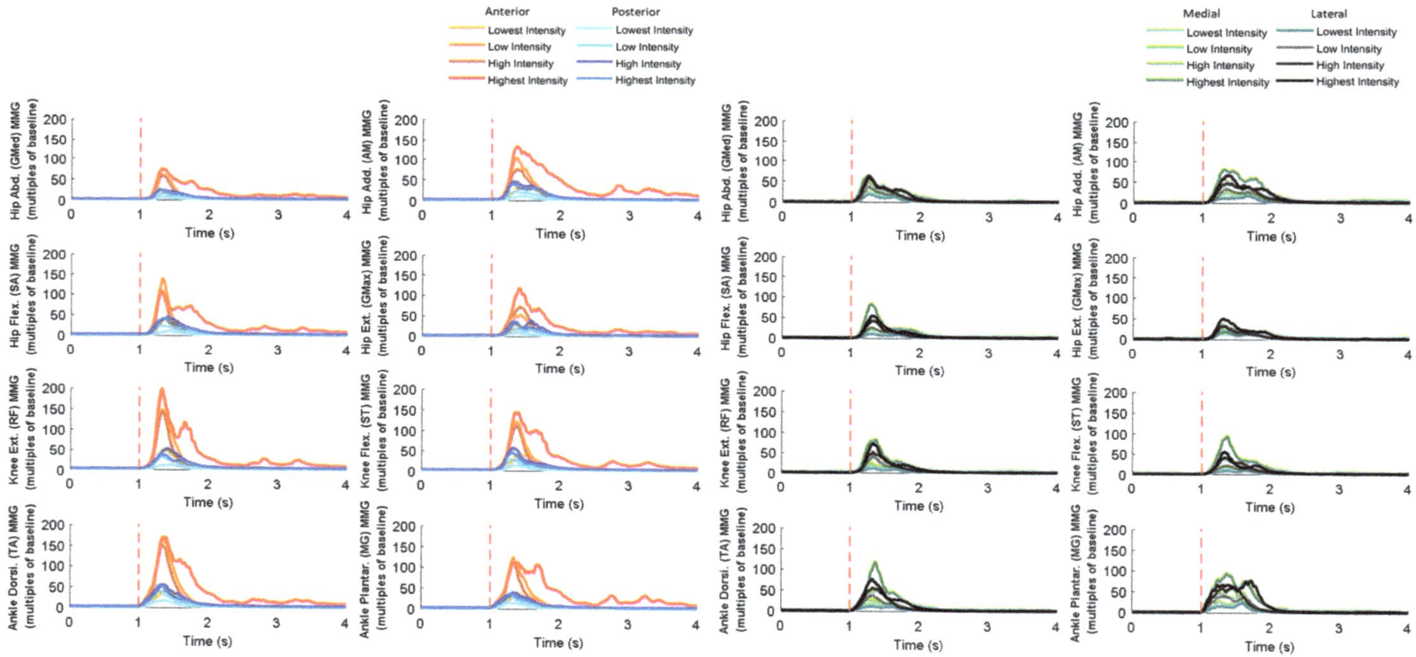

Figure 10. The mean MMG signal changes of twelve subjects for eight dominant-leg muscles following the unexpected perturbations with four directions and four intensities (n = 12). (Note: **The red dotted line** specifies the start of the balance perturbation; **MMG,** mechanomyography; **GMed,** gluteus medius; **AM,** adductor magus; **SA,** sartorius; **GMax,** gluteus maximus; **RF,** rectus femoris; **ST,** semitendinosus; **TA,** tibialis anterior; **MG,** gastrocnemius medialis.)

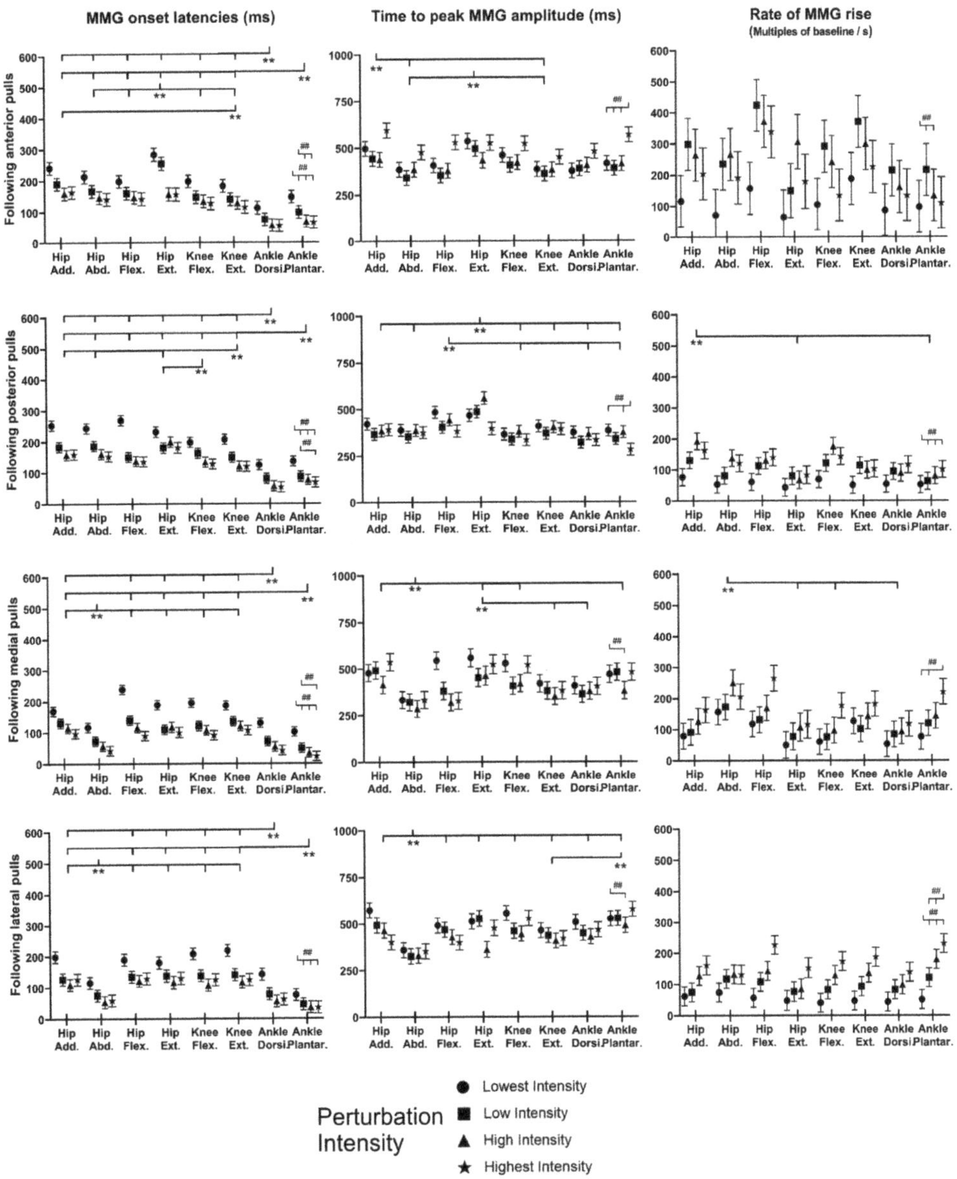

Figure 11. The MMG-onset latencies, time to peak MMG amplitude, and rate of MMG rise for eight dominant leg muscles following unexpected horizontal perturbations (mean ± SE, n = 12). (Note: ⌐┘ or └¬ represents post hoc pairwise comparison; **SE**, standard error; ## indicates significant main effects of intensity factor; ** indicates significant main effects of muscle factor.)

In general, the onset of MMG signals was significantly earlier in ankle muscles than in knee or hip muscles ($p < 0.05$). Such an MMG-onset pattern (activation started from distal to proximal lower limb) was observed following all the four directions of balance perturbations. Moreover, following the balance perturbations in the frontal plane, the hip abductor was in the queue with early onset of the MMG signal. Larger perturbation intensities induced significantly shorter MMG-onset latencies ($p < 0.05$), a shorter time to peak MMG amplitude ($p < 0.05$), and a larger rate of MMG rise ($p < 0.05$).

Following sudden anterior perturbation, the ankle dorsiflexor and ankle plantarflexor had the significantly shorter MMG-onset latencies compared to the remaining muscles ($p < 0.05$). Significant differences within the agonist–antagonist muscle pairs were found in MMG-onset latency (hip flexor < hip extensor; $p < 0.05$) and in time to peak MMG amplitude (hip abductor < hip adductor; $p < 0.05$). No specific trend was observed when comparing the rate of MMG rise among muscles.

Following sudden posterior perturbation, the ankle dorsiflexor and ankle plantarflexor had the significantly shorter MMG-onset latencies compared to the other muscles ($p < 0.05$).

Following sudden medial perturbation, the ankle dorsiflexor, ankle plantarflexor, and hip abductor had significantly shorter onset latencies than the remaining dominant-leg muscles ($p < 0.05$). Significant differences within the agonist–antagonist muscle pairs were found in both the MMG-onset latency and the time to peak MMG amplitude (hip abductor < hip adductor; $p < 0.05$).

Following sudden lateral perturbation, the ankle dorsiflexor, ankle plantarflexor, and hip abductor had significantly shorter onset latencies than the remaining dominant-leg muscles ($p < 0.05$). Additionally, among the eight dominant-leg muscles, the hip abductor had the shortest time to peak MMG amplitude ($p < 0.05$).

4. Discussion

Via the synchronized capture of eight dominant-leg muscles' electrical and mechanical activities (EMG and MMG signals), eight dominant-leg joint motions (angles), and whole-body postural sways (COM displacements), this study is novel in its comprehensive investigation of the timing and the speed of combined reactions in hip, knee, and ankle muscles and joints following unexpected horizontal/translational perturbations with different intensities and directions. In agreement with our hypothesis 1, this study has observed that (1) agonist muscles resisting the perturbation-induced postural sway activated more rapidly than antagonist muscles, and among the eight dominant-leg muscles, ankle muscles' large rate of activation contributed the most to resisting the perturbations in both sagittal and frontal planes. However, our hypotheses 2 and 3 were not entirely supported, as results showed that (2) fast responses existed not only in those lower-limb joint motions and COM displacements that were passively/involuntarily induced by the perturbation but could also occur in those actively/voluntarily generated ones to counteract the perturbation; and (3) a larger perturbation intensity evoked the more rapid muscle activities but did not induce faster joint motion or postural sway.

These findings build on our knowledge of how fast the hip/knee/ankle muscles can activate and how the lower-limb joints can coordinate to maintain reactive standing balance in healthy young adults. This potentially facilitates the understanding of strategies regarding how humans cope with the varying challenges of losing balance in daily life, which could provide further evidence and guidance for the development of fall-prevention approaches in the future; the details are discussed below.

4.1. Faster Activation Existed in Agonist Lower-Limb Muscles, Espaecially Ankle Muscles, to Resist the Induced Postural Sway (Hypothesis 1)

The primary finding of this study was that earlier EMG onset and shorter time to peak EMG amplitude occurred in muscles that could resist the involuntary COM shift induced by the unexpected moving-platform perturbations. On top of this, this study may highlight the great contribution of ankle muscles' large rate of activation in balance maintenance under unexpected perturbation in both the sagittal and frontal planes.

Following the unexpected anterior movement of the platform, while the COM had a firstly posterior shift relative to the BOS, the ventral muscles that could rotate the body forward (ankle dorsiflexor, knee extensor, and hip flexor) had a generally earlier onset of activation and shorter latency to reach peak activation compared to the dorsal muscles. These observations are consistent with the previously reported EMG-onset patterns (i.e., EMG-onset latency of ankle dorsiflexor < ankle plantarflexor; knee extensor < knee flexor) [12,14,45] and time to peak patterns (i.e., time to peak EMG amplitude in ankle dorsiflexor < ankle plantarflexor; knee extensor < knee flexor) [45,46]. On top of this, this study also observed that the ankle dorsiflexor had a remarkably large rate of activation after onset of perturbation (within 50 ms after onset) under all the perturbation intensities, while the knee extensor showed a large rate of activation under high perturbation intensity. This indicated the major contribution of the ventral muscles, especially the ankle dorsiflexor, in rapidly shifting the body forward to resist the unexpected anterior movement of the supporting platform. In addition, under the highest perturbation intensity, a second peak was commonly observed for the dominant-leg muscles' EMG signals, which might be related to the subjects' stepping action to recover postural balance. This observation is also in accordance with previous findings that a stepping strategy would be needed to increase the area of BOS and maintain balance when the ankle and/or hip strategies were insufficient [9].

Following the unexpected posterior movement of the platform, the dorsal muscle (ankle plantarflexor) showed an early onset of activation and quick reaching of peak activation to resist the induced forward COM displacement relative to BOS. This agreed with the previous findings that gastrocnemius and hamstrings had faster [10] and greater [15,46] muscle activities than the ventral muscles to prevent excessive forward postural sways. In addition, among the eight dominant-leg muscles, this study observed that the ankle plantarflexor had a notably large rising rate at the early phase of muscle activation. This corroborated the previous finding that the rate of the ankle plantarflexor's activation played a key role in resisting the forward waist-pull balance perturbations [22] and preventing the forward tripping [20].

Following the unexpected medial movement of the platform, the hip abductor was evoked earlier and reached the peak activation earlier than the hip adductor to resist the induced lateral moving of the COM relative to the BOS. The result is consistent with previous studies that reported the significant relationship between the hip abductor and balance recovery under lateral waist-pull perturbations [22,47,48]. In addition, this study observed that the ankle dorsiflexor had a generally larger rate of activation than the other dominant-leg muscles; under the high and the highest perturbation intensities, a large rate of activation was further evoked in the hip abductor and ankle plantarflexor, as the body weight was more quickly transferred to the dominant leg. The dominant-leg distal ankle muscles have been reported in previous studies to provide the immediate joint torque to regain balance under the medial perturbation of platform, followed by the proximal hip muscles with the increasing of perturbation intensity [49–51]. Such kinetic responses could partially be corroborated by the further neuromuscular evidence in this study.

Following the unexpected lateral movement of the platform, the hip adductor reached peak activation earlier than the hip abductor to counteract the sudden medial moving of the COM relative to the BOS. Moreover, among the eight dominant-leg muscles, the ankle dorsiflexor had the greatest rate of activation. These findings were consistent with previous studies that indicated the essential contributions of ankle and hip muscles in controlling mediolateral postural balance [21,22,49,52]. On top of this, in the sagittal plane, this study further observed that the ventral muscles (ankle dorsiflexor, knee extensor, and hip flexor) had earlier onset and shorter time to peak activation than the dorsal muscles. These rapid activation patterns might be related to the attempt at trying to counteract the body weight unloading from the dominant leg and prevent the excessive medial postural sway induced by the unexpected lateral moving of platform [53].

To the authors' knowledge, no previous study has investigated the activation pattern of all the major hip, knee, and ankle muscles to maintain balance over the unexpected platform movement. By examining the hip adductor/abductor, hip flexor/extensor, knee flexor/extensor, and ankle dorsiflexor/plantarflexor simultaneously, this study identified the essential importance of ankle muscles' rapid activation in resisting horizontal perturbations for young adults. It is also expected that this study's more comprehensive and in-depth investigation in the eight leg muscles' activities could facilitate the future development of programs and assistive devices to improve balance and prevent falls in older adults [53–64].

4.2. Rapid Kinematic Responses Varied with the Perturbation Direction (Hypothesis 2)

The secondary finding of this study was that the rapid responses of lower-limb joint motions and postural sways varied in different directions of balance perturbations. Following the unexpected platform movement, lower-limb joint motions caused by the inertia of body segments were generally the first to appear and are considered as passive/involuntary, while sometimes, other active/voluntary joint motions could also appear as early as the passive/involuntary ones. Among the six directions of COM displacement, COM moving toward the opposite direction of the balance perturbation was generally the earliest because of inertia, which is consistent with the previous studies' findings [10,58,65], while sometimes, the COM displacement in the vertical direction could also occur as early as in the horizontal direction either because of inertia or active/voluntary reactions.

Early onset of joint angles and short time to peak angles were generally observed in the passive/involuntary joint motions induced by the moving platform. Specifically, because of inertia, faster responses of ankle dorsiflexion (compared to ankle plantarflexion) [10], hip adduction (compared to hip abduction) [22,65], and hip abduction (compared to hip adduction) [22,65] were induced under the unexpected posterior, medial, and lateral perturbations, respectively. However, only under the medial perturbation was the onset of passively induced hip adduction found to be significantly earlier than the remaining seven lower-limb joint motions. For the anterior, posterior, and lateral directions, the passive/involuntary joint motion was usually accompanied by the fast responses of other active/voluntary joint motions to resist the balance perturbation.

The timing patterns of active/voluntary lower-limb joint motions were different following the four directions of unexpected balance perturbations. Specifically, under the unexpected <u>anterior</u> perturbation, the passively/involuntarily induced ankle plantarflexion was accompanied by the consistently early onset of hip flexion (compared to hip extension). A previous study also reported that early ankle plantarflexion was followed by the knee flexion, and hip flexion under the sudden forward movement of platform [14]. On top of it, this study observed that knee flexion (compared to knee extension) and hip flexion (compared to hip extension) reached peak angles more quickly, which further corroborates the finding in the onset of joint motions. Under the unexpected <u>posterior</u> perturbation, no consistently fast response within the knee or hip joint accompanied the passively/involuntarily induced ankle dorsiflexion. However, a previous study reported that young adults also had an earlier hip extension than hip flexion apart from the ankle joint motions following the posterior moving-platform perturbation [10]. This may be because the perturbation intensity induced by the posterior movement of the platform was not as large as that in the previous study [10,22]. Therefore, this study observed only the consistently later onset and peak in ankle joint motion (ankle dorsiflexion < ankle plantarflexion). The corrective reaction, i.e., ankle plantarflexion, was sufficient to recover from the induced forward loss of balance. Under the unexpected <u>medial</u> perturbation, all the active/voluntary joint motions appeared after the passively/involuntarily induced hip adduction. The hip abduction was corrective, as the muscle activity of the hip abductor was detected, which could work to oppose the passive hip adduction. This reaction was also supported by a previous study that found the corrective response of hip abduction momentarily following perturbations in frontal plane [22,65]. Under the unexpected <u>lateral</u> perturbation, the passively/involuntarily induced hip abduction was accompanied by the consistently early onset and short time to peak of hip flexion, knee extension, and ankle dorsiflexion. Similar to the medial perturbation, the hip adductor muscle worked to oppose the passive hip abduction and produce the later corrective hip abduction [22,65]. In addition, the observations of this study may suggest that when the body weight was unloaded from the dominant leg following lateral perturbations, fast joint motions in the sagittal plane were also required to maintain balance, while they were not required when the body weight was loaded on the dominant leg following medial perturbations.

The unexpected horizontal perturbation also induced the consistently faster response of COM in the vertical direction. As far as the authors know, previous studies have rarely compared the timing of postural sways in horizonal and vertical directions following a balance perturbation. Specifically, in this study, the faster upward COM displacements (compared to the downward direction) were observed following the anterior, medial, and lateral balance perturbations, while the posterior perturbation induced a faster downward COM displacement. Following the anterior perturbation, the earlier upward COM displacement (compared to downward direction) seemed to be related to the great proportion of subjects' stepping strategies and toe-rise strategies in the study. Following the medial or the lateral perturbation, the faster responses of hip flexion, knee flexion, and ankle dorsiflexion in the unloaded leg were observed. The fast upward COM displacement could be caused by the lifting of the unloaded leg. By contrast, following the posterior perturbation, the COM reached peak displacement more quicky in the downward direction than in the upward direction. This response was considered to be passive, as the downward and the passively induced forward postural sways had similar onset latencies and time to peak. The posterior displacement quickly induced the subject's forward inclined posture, so the COM had a firstly downward displacement and was followed by a later upward displacement to recover the upward posture. Difference in perturbation intensities may explain why the initial COM displacement in the vertical direction following posterior perturbations differed from that following anterior/medial/lateral perturbations. Posterior perturbations were set with smaller intensities than the anterior/medial/lateral perturbations in this study. The latter ones were challenging enough and induced the faster active/voluntary reactions that elevated the COM, while the former ones did not.

4.3. Larger Perturbation Intensity Evoked Faster Rosponse in Muscle Activation (Hypothesis 3)

The tertiary finding of this study was that larger perturbation intensity induced an earlier EMG onset, shorter time to peak EMG amplitude, and larger rate of EMG rise in the dominant-leg muscles but did not lead to faster responses in postural sways or lower-limb joint motions. This may suggest that under a larger unexpected challenge to loss of balance, the lower-limb muscles could activate earlier and more rapidly to restrict excessive joint motions and prevent excessive COM shifts out of the BOS.

The results in this study indicate that the response rate of lower-limb muscles could be related to perturbation intensity in general. EMG-onset latencies and time to peak EMG amplitude were significantly longer under the smaller perturbation intensities than under the higher ones. Previous studies have reported such a phenomenon mainly in the sagittal plane (anterior and posterior directions) [10,14,46,66]. Furthermore, this study suggests that this trend was also applicable to perturbation in the frontal plane (medial and lateral directions). In addition, this study observed a higher EMG rising rate under a larger perturbation intensity. Such effects of perturbation intensity seemed to be more prominent in the agonist muscles that could resist postural sways induced by the unexpected moving-platform perturbations (e.g., ankle dorsiflexor under the anterior perturbations; ankle muscles and hip abductor under the medial perturbations). However, the specific type of correlation between the muscle responses and perturbation intensities has remained unclear. It would be interesting to establish some models between the two factors in future studies.

A larger perturbation intensity could evoke larger responses in lower-limb joint motions and postural sways; however, it may not be able to evoke faster kinematic responses. For the postural sways, this study found that larger perturbation intensity generally induced larger COM displacement along the line of perturbation direction. An example was that both the forward and the backward peak COM displacements increased with the anterior perturbation intensity. This was understandable since the different perturbation intensities in the study were position-controlled. However, a larger intensity of perturbation did not evoke an earlier onset or shorter time to peak COM displacement. A similar amount of time was required to reach a larger postural sway under the greater perturbation intensity. This result partly agreed with a previous study that showed increasing peak COM velocity and peak COM acceleration with perturbation intensity [61]. For the lower-limb joint motions, it was found that ankle dorsiflexion, knee flexion, and hip flexion angles increased with the perturbation intensity for all the four perturbation directions. Such strategies seemed to be able to reduce the additional horizontal excursions when the challenge to loss of standing balance became larger [45]. However, the onset or the time to peak for neither the whole-body postural sways nor lower-limb joint motions were affected by the perturbation intensity. These may suggest that earlier and faster lower-limb muscle activation would be adequate for the successful maintenance of balance following a larger balance challenge. In addition, as these findings indicate that the neuromuscular reaction time (EMG-onset latency and time to EMG peak amplitude) could be modulated by the different intensities of perturbations, EMG temporal parameters could potentially be used as the training outcome or biofeedback in perturbation-based balance training [67].

4.4. MMG Signals Following Balance Perturbations Merit Further Study

Attempts have also been made to process and analyze the MMG signals, aiming to examine the possible delays between the electrical and mechanical muscle activities in response to unexpected balance perturbations. A new processing method was used upon optimizing the one reported in our previous study [22]. However, the MMG signals obtained in the current study may still not fully reflect the exact mechanical activities of muscles since the onset of MMG signal was not consistently later than that of EMG signal. The observed time delay between the EMG and MMG onset was not comparable with the previous studies either. The delay in the MMG signal after the EMG signal observed in previous studies ranged from 7 ms to 30 ms instead [68–72]. Thus, it should be noted that the following discussion of the MMG data might be affected by the current processing method of MMG signals used in this study. Further attempts are still needed to improve the MMG data processing method in future studies.

When comparing among the eight muscles, the onset of the MMG signal under all directions of perturbation was significantly earlier at distal than proximal muscles. Such onset might be caused by the perturbation induced from a moving platform supporting standing, i.e., at the distal side of subject's body. This is further supported by the result that the value of each parameter in MMG recorded greatly depended on pulling intensity but not for muscles or pulling directions. Although MMG showed considerable reliability to detect muscle activities in static conditions [72,73], it might not be effective in dynamic conditions, as the current processing method of MMG signals can still not effectively eliminate the noise caused by the moving platform and the movement of body segment. Further studies and optimization of the set-up are required for MMG technologies to be applied to muscle-activity measurement in dynamic situations.

4.5. Strengths and Limitations

This study has the below strengths. Firstly, the moving-platform perturbation system was synchronized with the Vicon system and the Trigno Wireless Biofeedback System, enabling our accurate analyses of the temporal parameters of multiple signals during balance control. Secondly, the perturbation intensity (i.e., pulling displacement) was set as a percentage of the subject's body height so that the perturbation was a consistent challenge to postural balance across different individuals. Thirdly, this study comprehensively analyzed how fast the eight major leg muscles' activation and eight lower-limb joint motions could occur during balance control. These findings in healthy young adults can serve as the foundation and reference for not only further studies of balance-controlling mechanisms in older adults with high fall risks, but also the further development of assistive/robotic devices for targeted balance training and fall prevention.

There are some potential limitations of this study. Firstly, only a small number of subjects were recruited for this pilot study. Future studies in older adults or a specific population should justify the sample size to make the findings more representative. Secondly, during the processing of EMG signals, this study used baseline EMG value in normal standing for normalization. Therefore, it should be noted that the rate of EMG rise in this study was based on the muscle-activation level in normal standing rather than the capacity of muscle activation. Maximal voluntary contraction (MVC) tests could be carried out in the future to examine if the amplitude-normalization methods affect the finding. Lastly, the current MMG processing method might still be not mature enough to extract the exact vibrations of lower-limb muscles. Further observation and development are needed. More tests could be performed on MMG to evaluate the reliability and validity of reflecting the mechanical muscle activities following the unexpected perturbation.

5. Conclusions

To conclude, among the eight dominant-leg muscles, the ankle muscles' rapid activation contributed the most to resisting the unexpectedly induced postural sways in both the sagittal and frontal planes. Fast responses of the lower-limb joint motions and the vertical postural sways were related to the perturbation direction. Under a larger perturbation intensity, muscles reacted more rapidly, while joint motions or postural sways were not necessarily faster. These findings provide new insights on the sequence or the fast responses of multiple lower-limb muscles/joints in coping with the different levels of balance challenges. The mechanisms underlying reactive standing balance are thus better understood, which may facilitate future research on developing targeted balance-training protocol and/or technology or devices for fall prevention in older adults.

Supplementary Materials: The following supporting information can be downloaded at: https://www.mdpi.com/article/10.3390/bioengineering10070831/s1, Figure S1: The mean platform displacements, velocities, and accelerations of twelve subjects following the unexpected anterior, posterior, medial, and lateral perturbations with four intensities (n = 12); Table S1: Mean and ICC values of pulling parameters examining the reliability of the moving-platform balance perturbation system (n = 12).

Author Contributions: Conceptualization, C.Y.T., R.T.-L.Z. and C.Z.-H.M.; methodology, R.T.-L.Z. and C.Z.-H.M.; software, C.Y.T., R.T.-L.Z. and Y.T.L.; validation, C.Y.T., R.T.-L.Z., H.F. and Y.T.L.; formal analysis, C.Y.T.; investigation, C.Y.T., R.T.-L.Z. and Y.T.L.; resources, C.Z.-H.M.; data curation, C.Y.T.; writing—original draft preparation, C.Y.T. and R.T.-L.Z.; writing—review and editing, C.Y.T., R.T.-L.Z., Y.T.L., F.M.H.L., E.M.S., H.F. and C.Z.-H.M.; visualization, C.Y.T., R.T.-L.Z. and E.M.S.; supervision, C.Z.-H.M.; project administration, C.Z.-H.M.; funding acquisition, C.Y.T. and C.Z.-H.M. All authors have read and agreed to the published version of the manuscript.

Funding: This research was funded by Hong Kong Research Grants Council (RGC) Direct Allocation Grant—Funding Support to Small Projects, grant number P0036830; Research Institute for Smart Ageing, The Hong Kong Polytechnic University, grant number P0038945; The Hong Kong Polytechnic University, grant number P0034491; Associated Money, The Hong Kong Polytechnic University, grant number G4Y56R006; and Service-Learning and Leadership Office, The Hong Kong Polytechnic University.

Institutional Review Board Statement: The study was conducted according to the guidelines of the Declaration of Helsinki and approved by the Institutional Review Board (IRB) of The Hong Kong Polytechnic University (Reference No.: HSEARS20201230002; Date of approval: 1 December 2020.

Informed Consent Statement: Written informed consent was obtained from each subject to publish this paper.

Data Availability Statement: Data are contained within the article and Supplementary Material.

Acknowledgments: We sincerely appreciate the support from Stephen Tsui, Pei-Zhao Lyu, and Shuai Li in the setting up of the moving-platform perturbation system, and Samy Leung's technical support in the use of the 3D Motion Capture and Analysis System.

Conflicts of Interest: The authors declare no conflict of interest.

References

1. World Health Organization. Falls. Available online: https://www.who.int/news-room/fact-sheets/detail/falls# (accessed on 30 April 2023).
2. Bergen, G.; Stevens, M.R.; Burns, E.R. Falls and fall injuries among adults aged ≥65 years—United States, 2014. *Morb. Mortal. Wkly. Rep.* **2016**, *65*, 993–998. [CrossRef] [PubMed]
3. Solis-Escalante, T.; Stokkermans, M.; Cohen, M.X.; Weerdesteyn, V. Cortical responses to whole-body balance perturbations index perturbation magnitude and predict reactive stepping behavior. *Eur. J. Neurosci.* **2021**, *54*, 8120–8138. [CrossRef] [PubMed]
4. Moreland, B.; Kakara, R.; Henry, A. Trends in nonfatal falls and fall-related injuries among adults aged ≥65 years—United States, 2012–2018. *Morb. Mortal. Wkly. Rep.* **2020**, *69*, 875. [CrossRef] [PubMed]
5. Rubenstein, L.Z. Falls in older people: Epidemiology, risk factors and strategies for prevention. *Age Ageing* **2006**, *35*, ii37–ii41. [CrossRef] [PubMed]
6. Rubega, M.; Di Marco, R.; Zampini, M.; Formaggio, E.; Menegatti, E.; Bonato, P.; Masiero, S.; Del Felice, A. Muscular and cortical activation during dynamic and static balance in the elderly: A scoping review. *Aging Brain* **2021**, *1*, 100013. [CrossRef]
7. Blenkinsop, G.M.; Pain, M.T.; Hiley, M.J. Balance control strategies during perturbed and unperturbed balance in standing and handstand. *R. Soc. Open Sci.* **2017**, *4*, 161018. [CrossRef]
8. Ono, H.; Sato, T.; Ohnishi, K. Balance Recovery of Ankle Strategy: Using Knee Joint for Biped Robot. In Proceedings of the 2011 1st International Symposium on Access Spaces (ISAS), Yokohama, Japan, 17–19 June 2011; pp. 236–241.
9. Kochoa, P. Balance Strategy Basics. Available online: https://www.professionalptandtraining.com/balance-strategy-basics/ (accessed on 1 June 2023).
10. Runge, C.; Shupert, C.; Horak, F.; Zajac, F. Ankle and hip postural strategies defined by joint torques. *Gait Posture* **1999**, *10*, 161–170. [CrossRef]
11. Bair, W.-N.; Prettyman, M.G.; Beamer, B.A.; Rogers, M.W. Kinematic and behavioral analyses of protective stepping strategies and risk for falls among community living older adults. *Clin. Biomech.* **2016**, *36*, 74–82. [CrossRef]
12. Tsai, Y.-C.; Hsieh, L.-F.; Yang, S. Age-related changes in posture response under a continuous and unexpected perturbation. *J. Biomech.* **2014**, *47*, 482–490. [CrossRef]
13. Chen, C.-L.; Lou, S.-Z.; Wu, H.-W.; Wu, S.-K.; Yeung, K.-T.; Su, F.-C. Effects of the type and direction of support surface perturbation on postural responses. *J. Neuroeng. Rehabil.* **2014**, *11*, 50. [CrossRef]
14. Hwang, S.; Tae, K.; Sohn, R.; Kim, J.; Son, J.; Kim, Y. The Balance Recovery Mechanisms Against Unexpected Forward Perturbation. *Ann. Biomed. Eng.* **2009**, *37*, 1629–1637. [CrossRef] [PubMed]
15. Baudry, S.; Lecoeuvre, G.; Duchateau, J. Age-related changes in the behavior of the muscle-tendon unit of the gastrocnemius medialis during upright stance. *J. Appl. Physiol.* **2012**, *112*, 296–304. [CrossRef] [PubMed]
16. Błaszczyszyn, M.; Szczęsna, A.; Piechota, K. sEMG activation of the flexor muscles in the foot during balance tasks by young and older women: A pilot study. *Int. J. Environ. Res. Public Health* **2019**, *16*, 4307. [CrossRef] [PubMed]
17. Cattagni, T.; Scaglioni, G.; Laroche, D.; Grémeaux, V.; Martin, A. The involvement of ankle muscles in maintaining balance in the upright posture is higher in elderly fallers. *Exp. Gerontol.* **2016**, *77*, 38–45. [CrossRef] [PubMed]
18. Sawers, A.; Pai, Y.-C.; Bhatt, T.; Ting, L.H. Neuromuscular responses differ between slip-induced falls and recoveries in older adults. *J. Neurophysiol.* **2017**, *117*, 509–522. [CrossRef] [PubMed]
19. Faulkner, K.A.; Redfern, M.S.; Cauley, J.A.; Landsittel, D.P.; Studenski, S.A.; Rosano, C.; Simonsick, E.M.; Harris, T.B.; Shorr, R.I.; Ayonayon, H.N. Multitasking: Association between poorer performance and a history of recurrent falls. *J. Am. Geriatr. Soc.* **2007**, *55*, 570–576. [CrossRef] [PubMed]
20. Pijnappels, M.; Bobbert, M.F.; van Dieën, J.H. Control of support limb muscles in recovery after tripping in young and older subjects. *Exp. Brain Res.* **2005**, *160*, 326–333. [CrossRef]
21. Inacio, M.; Creath, R.; Rogers, M.W. Effects of aging on hip abductor-adductor neuromuscular and mechanical performance during the weight transfer phase of lateral protective stepping. *J. Biomech.* **2019**, *82*, 244–250. [CrossRef]
22. Zhu, R.T.-L.; Lyu, P.-Z.; Li, S.; Tong, C.Y.; Ling, Y.T.; Ma, C.Z.-H. How Does Lower Limb Respond to Unexpected Balance Perturbations? New Insights from Synchronized Human Kinetics, Kinematics, Muscle Electromyography (EMG) and Mechanomyography (MMG) Data. *Biosensors* **2022**, *12*, 430. [CrossRef]
23. Cè, E.; Longo, S.; Limonta, E.; Coratella, G.; Rampichini, S.; Esposito, F. Peripheral fatigue: New mechanistic insights from recent technologies. *Eur. J. Appl. Physiol.* **2020**, *120*, 17–39. [CrossRef]
24. Woodward, R.B.; Stokes, M.J.; Shefelbine, S.J.; Vaidyanathan, R. Segmenting mechanomyography measures of muscle activity phases using inertial data. *Sci. Rep.* **2019**, *9*, 5569. [CrossRef] [PubMed]
25. Ma, C.Z.-H.; Ling, Y.T.; Shea, Q.T.K.; Wang, L.-K.; Wang, X.-Y.; Zheng, Y.-P. Towards Wearable Comprehensive Capture and Analysis of Skeletal Muscle Activity during Human Locomotion. *Sensors* **2019**, *19*, 195. [CrossRef] [PubMed]
26. Lyu, P.-Z.; Zhu, R.T.; Ling, Y.T.; Wang, L.-K.; Zheng, Y.-P.; Ma, C.Z. How Paretic and Non-Paretic Ankle Muscles Contract during Walking in Stroke Survivors: New Insight Using Novel Wearable Ultrasound Imaging and Sensing Technology. *Biosensors* **2022**, *12*, 349. [CrossRef] [PubMed]

27. Gerards, M.H.; Meijer, K.; Karamanidis, K.; Grevendonk, L.; Hoeks, J.; Lenssen, A.F.; McCrum, C. Adaptability to balance perturbations during walking as a potential marker of falls history in older adults. *Front. Sports Act. Living* **2021**, *3*, 132. [CrossRef]
28. VICON. Full Body Modeling with Plug-In Gait. Available online: https://docs.vicon.com/display/Nexus212/Full+body+modeling+with+Plug-in+Gait (accessed on 20 April 2022).
29. Quam, S. *Johnson Health Tech: EMG Sensor Holder for Heels and Center of Mass Approximation*; University of Wisconsin: Madison, WI, USA, 2020.
30. SENIAM. The SENIAM Project. Available online: http://seniam.org/sensor_location.htm (accessed on 20 April 2022).
31. Jiroumaru, T.; Kurihara, T.; Isaka, T. Measurement of muscle length-related electromyography activity of the hip flexor muscles to determine individual muscle contributions to the hip flexion torque. *SpringerPlus* **2014**, *3*, 624. [CrossRef]
32. Hides, J.A.; Beall, P.; Smith, M.M.F.; Stanton, W.; Miokovic, T.; Richardson, C. Activation of the hip adductor muscles varies during a simulated weight-bearing task. *Phys. Ther. Sport* **2016**, *17*, 19–23. [CrossRef]
33. Lee, P.H.; Macfarlane, D.J.; Lam, T.H.; Stewart, S.M. Validity of the International Physical Activity Questionnaire Short Form (IPAQ-SF): A systematic review. *Int. J. Behav. Nutr. Phys. Act.* **2011**, *8*, 115. [CrossRef]
34. Kempen, G.I.J.M.; Yardley, L.; Van Haastregt, J.C.M.; Zijlstra, G.A.R.; Beyer, N.; Hauer, K.; Todd, C. The Short FES-I: A shortened version of the falls efficacy scale-international to assess fear of falling. *Age Ageing* **2008**, *37*, 45–50. [CrossRef]
35. Swanenburg, J.; Nevzati, A.; Hager, A.G.M.; de Bruin, E.D.; Klipstein, A. The maximal width of the base of support (BSW): Clinical applicability and reliability of a preferred-standing test for measuring the risk of falling. *Arch. Gerontol. Geriatr.* **2013**, *57*, 204–210. [CrossRef]
36. Shao, X.R.; Wang, Z.; Luan, L.J.; Sheng, Y.L.; Yu, R.N.; Pranata, A.; Adams, R.; Zhang, A.R.; Han, J. Impaired ankle inversion proprioception during walking is associated with fear of falling in older adults. *Front. Aging Neurosci.* **2022**, *14*, 946509. [CrossRef]
37. Franchignoni, F.; Horak, F.; Godi, M.; Nardone, A.; Giordano, A. Using psychometric techniques to improve the Balance Evaluation Systems Test: The mini-BESTest. *J. Rehabil. Med.* **2010**, *42*, 323–331. [CrossRef] [PubMed]
38. Hoffman, M.; Schrader, J.; Applegate, T.; Koceja, D. Unilateral postural control of the functionally dominant and nondominant extremities of healthy subjects. *J. Athl. Train.* **1998**, *33*, 319–322. [PubMed]
39. Pai, Y.-C.; Rogers, M.W.; Patton, J.; Cain, T.D.; Hanke, T.A. Static versus dynamic predictions of protective stepping following waist–pull perturbations in young and older adults. *J. Biomech.* **1998**, *31*, 1111–1118. [CrossRef] [PubMed]
40. Luchies, C.W.; Alexander, N.B.; Schultz, A.B.; Ashton-Miller, J. Stepping responses of young and old adults to postural disturbances: Kinematics. *J. Am. Geriatr. Soc.* **1994**, *42*, 506–512. [CrossRef]
41. Singh, H.; Sanders, O.; McCombe Waller, S.; Bair, W.-N.; Beamer, B.; Creath, R.A.; Rogers, M.W. Relationship Between Head-Turn Gait Speed and Lateral Balance Function in Community-Dwelling Older Adults. *Arch. Phys. Med. Rehabil.* **2017**, *98*, 1955–1961. [CrossRef]
42. Caulcrick, C.; Huo, W.; Hoult, W.; Vaidyanathan, R. Human Joint Torque Modelling With MMG and EMG During Lower Limb Human-Exoskeleton Interaction. *IEEE Robot. Autom. Lett.* **2021**, *6*, 7185–7192. [CrossRef]
43. Borrelli, J.R.; Zabukovec, J.; Jones, S.; Junod, C.A.; Maki, B.E. Age-related changes in the capacity to select early-onset upper-limb reactions to either recover balance or protect against impact. *Exp. Gerontol.* **2019**, *125*, 110676. [CrossRef]
44. Cronin, N.J.; Barrett, R.S.; Lichtwark, G.; Mills, P.M.; Carty, C.P. Decreased lower limb muscle recruitment contributes to the inability of older adults to recover with a single step following a forward loss of balance. *J. Electromyogr. Kinesiol.* **2013**, *23*, 1139–1144. [CrossRef]
45. de Freitas, P.B.; Knight, C.A.; Barela, J.A. Postural reactions following forward platform perturbation in young, middle-age, and old adults. *J. Electromyogr. Kinesiol.* **2010**, *20*, 693–700. [CrossRef]
46. Krašna, S.; Keller, A.; Linder, A.; Silvano, A.P.; Xu, J.-C.; Thomson, R.; Klug, C. Human response to longitudinal perturbations of standing passengers on public transport during regular operation. *Front. Bioeng. Biotechnol.* **2021**, *9*, 680883. [CrossRef]
47. Afschrift, M.; Pitto, L.; Aerts, W.; van Deursen, R.; Jonkers, I.; De Groote, F. Modulation of gluteus medius activity reflects the potential of the muscle to meet the mechanical demands during perturbed walking. *Sci. Rep.* **2018**, *8*, 11675. [CrossRef]
48. Gilles, M.; Wing, A.M.; Kirker, S.G. Lateral balance organisation in human stance in response to a random or predictable perturbation. *Exp. Brain Res.* **1999**, *124*, 137–144. [CrossRef] [PubMed]
49. Jeon, W.; Griffin, L.; Hsiao, H.-Y. Effects of initial foot position on postural responses to lateral standing surface perturbations in younger and older adults. *Gait Posture* **2021**, *90*, 449–456. [CrossRef]
50. Freyler, K.; Gollhofer, A.; Colin, R.; Brüderlin, U.; Ritzmann, R. Reactive balance control in response to perturbation in unilateral stance: Interaction effects of direction, displacement and velocity on compensatory neuromuscular and kinematic responses. *PLoS ONE* **2015**, *10*, e0144529. [CrossRef]
51. Winter, D.A.; Patla, A.E.; Frank, J.S.; Walt, S.E. Biomechanical walking pattern changes in the fit and healthy elderly. *Phys. Ther.* **1990**, *70*, 340–347. [CrossRef]
52. Kovacikova, Z.; Zemkova, E.; Neumannova, K.; Jelen, M.; Jelen, K.; Janura, M. The role of lateral preference of lower limbs in a postural stabilization task. *Neuroendocrinol. Lett.* **2015**, *36*, 91–95. [PubMed]
53. Ma, C.Z.-H.; Chung, A.K.-L.; Ling, Y.T.; Huang, Z.-H.; Cheng, C.L.-K.; Zheng, Y.-P. A Newly-Developed Smart Insole System with Instant Reminder: Paves the Way towards Integrating Artificial Intelligence (AI) Technology to Improve Balance and Prevent Falls. *Age Ageing* **2019**, *48*, iv28–iv33. [CrossRef]

54. Ma, C.Z.-H.; Bao, T.; DiCesare, C.A.; Harris, I.; Chambers, A.; Shull, P.B.; Zheng, Y.-P.; Cham, R.; Sienko, K.H. Reducing Slip Risk: A Feasibility Study of Gait Training with Semi-Real-Time Feedback of Foot–Floor Contact Angle. *Sensors* **2022**, *22*, 3641. [CrossRef]
55. Ma, C.Z.-H.; Lam, W.-K.; Chang, B.-C.; Lee, W.C.-C. Can Insoles Be Used to Improve Static and Dynamic Balance of Community-Dwelling Older Adults? A Systematic Review on Recent Advances and Future Perspectives. *J. Aging Phys. Act.* **2020**, *28*, 971–986. [CrossRef]
56. Ma, C.Z.-H.; Zheng, Y.-P.; Lee, W.C.-C. Changes in gait and plantar foot loading upon using vibrotactile wearable biofeedback system in patients with stroke. *Top. Stroke Rehabil.* **2018**, *25*, 20–27. [CrossRef]
57. Ma, C.Z.-H.; Wong, D.W.-C.; Wan, A.H.-P.; Lee, W.C.-C. Effects of orthopedic insoles on static balance of older adults wearing thick socks. *Prosthet. Orthot. Int.* **2018**, *42*, 357–362. [CrossRef] [PubMed]
58. Ma, C.Z.-H.; Lee, W.C.-C. A wearable vibrotactile biofeedback system improves balance control of healthy young adults following perturbations from quiet stance. *Hum. Mov. Sci.* **2017**, *55*, 54–60. [CrossRef] [PubMed]
59. Ma, C.Z.-H.; Wong, D.W.-C.; Lam, W.K.; Wan, A.H.-P.; Lee, W.C.-C. Balance improvement effects of biofeedback systems with state-of-the-art wearable sensors: A systematic review. *Sensors* **2016**, *16*, 434. [CrossRef] [PubMed]
60. Wan, A.H.; Wong, D.W.; Ma, C.Z.; Zhang, M.; Lee, W.C. Wearable vibrotactile biofeedback device allowing identification of different floor conditions for lower-limb amputees. *Arch. Phys. Med. Rehabil.* **2016**, *97*, 1210–1213. [CrossRef] [PubMed]
61. Ma, C.Z.-H.; Wan, A.H.-P.; Wong, D.W.-C.; Zheng, Y.-P.; Lee, W.C.-C. A vibrotactile and plantar force measurement-based biofeedback system: Paving the way towards wearable balance-improving devices. *Sensors* **2015**, *15*, 31709–31722. [CrossRef]
62. Wang, H.; Gao, C.; Fu, H.; Ma, C.Z.-H.; Wang, Q.; He, Z.; Li, M. Automated Student Classroom Behaviors' Perception and Identification Using Motion Sensors. *Bioengineering* **2023**, *10*, 127. [CrossRef]
63. Huang, Z.-H.; Ma, C.Z.-H.; Wang, L.-K.; Wang, X.-Y.; Fu, S.-N.; Zheng, Y.-P. Real-time visual biofeedback via wearable ultrasound imaging can enhance the muscle contraction training outcome of young adults. *J. Strength Cond. Res.* **2022**, *36*, 941. [CrossRef]
64. Elhadi, M.M.O.; Ma, C.Z.-H.; Lam, W.K.; Lee, W.C.-C. Biomechanical approach in facilitating long-distance walking of elderly people using footwear modifications. *Gait Posture* **2018**, *64*, 101–107. [CrossRef]
65. Rietdyk, S.; Patla, A.; Winter, D.; Ishac, M.; Little, C. Balance recovery from medio-lateral perturbations of the upper body during standing. *J. Biomech.* **1999**, *32*, 1149–1158. [CrossRef]
66. Lin, S.-I.; Woollacott, M.H. Postural muscle responses following changing balance threats in young, stable older, and unstable older adults. *J. Mot. Behav.* **2002**, *34*, 37–44. [CrossRef]
67. Gerards, M.; Marcellis, R.; Senden, R.; Poeze, M.; de Bie, R.; Meijer, K.; Lenssen, A. The effect of perturbation-based balance training on balance control and fear of falling in older adults: A single-blind randomised controlled trial. *BMC Geriatr.* **2023**, *23*, 305. [CrossRef]
68. Cè, E.; Coratella, G.; Bisconti, A.V.; Venturelli, M.; Limonta, E.; Doria, C.; Rampichini, S.; Longo, S.; Esposito, F. Neuromuscular versus mechanical stretch-induced changes in contralateral versus ipsilateral muscle. *Med. Sci. Sports Exerc.* **2020**, *52*, 1294–1306. [CrossRef] [PubMed]
69. Cè, E.; Rampichini, S.; Agnello, L.; Limonta, E.; Veicsteinas, A.; Esposito, F. Effects of temperature and fatigue on the electromechanical delay components. *Muscle Nerve* **2013**, *47*, 566–576. [CrossRef]
70. Uchiyama, T.; Hori, Y.; Suzuki, K. Estimation of Tibialis Anterior Muscle Stiffness during the Swing Phase of Walking with Various Footwear. In Proceedings of the 2017 39th Annual International Conference of the IEEE Engineering in Medicine and Biology Society (EMBC), Jeju Island, South Korea, 11–15 July 2017; pp. 4131–4134.
71. Fukawa, T.; Uchiyama, T. System Identification of Evoked Mechanomyogram to Clarify Lower Limb Muscle Stiffness in Treadmill Walking. *Adv. Biomed. Eng.* **2016**, *5*, 1–6. [CrossRef]
72. Smith, C.M.; Housh, T.J.; Hill, E.C.; Johnson, G.O.; Schmidt, R.J. Dynamic versus isometric electromechanical delay in non-fatigued and fatigued muscle: A combined electromyographic, mechanomyographic, and force approach. *J. Electromyogr. Kinesiol.* **2017**, *33*, 34–38. [CrossRef] [PubMed]
73. Ling, Y.T.; Ma, C.Z.-H.; Shea, Q.T.K.; Zheng, Y.-P. Sonomechanomyography (SMMG): Mapping of Skeletal Muscle Motion Onset during Contraction Using Ultrafast Ultrasound Imaging and Multiple Motion Sensors. *Sensors* **2020**, *20*, 5513. [CrossRef] [PubMed]

bioengineering

MDPI

Article

Gender Differences in Lower Extremity Stiffness during a Single-Leg Landing Motion in Badminton

Yanan Zhang [1,†], Zhe Hu [1,†], Bairan Li [2], Xuan Qiu [3], Ming Li [1], Xiangwei Meng [1], Sukwon Kim [1,*] and Youngsuk Kim [1,*]

1 Department of Physical Education, Jeonbuk National University, Jeonju 54896, Republic of Korea; 202055397@jbnu.ac.kr (Y.Z.); huzhe0710@jbnu.ac.kr (Z.H.); lming@jbnu.ac.kr (M.L.); mengx@jbnu.ac.kr (X.M.)
2 Department of Physical Education, Putian University, Putian 351100, China; libairan0526@ptu.edu.cn
3 Department of Physical Education, Yichun University, Yichun 336000, China; 208144@jxycu.edu.cn
* Correspondence: rockwall@jbnu.ac.kr (S.K.); ys43530@jbnu.ac.kr (Y.K.); Tel.: +82-63-270-2860 (S.K.); +82-63-270-2849 (Y.K.); Fax: +82-63-270-2850 (S.K. & Y.K.)
† These authors contributed equally to this work.

Abstract: In general, at the same level of exercise, female athletes are three to six times more likely to injure an anterior cruciate ligament (ACL) than male athletes. Female athletes also had higher rates of ACL injury than males in a single-leg landing task after a backcourt backhand side overhead stroke in badminton. In many previous studies, stiffness of the musculoskeletal system in the lower limbs has been reported as a potential factor contributing to differences in ACL injury rates between genders. The purpose of this study was to describe the differences between genders in leg and knee stiffness in male and female athletes during a single-leg landing action after the backhand side overhead shot in the backcourt. Eight male athletes and eight female athletes participated in this test. Leg stiffness and knee stiffness were calculated separately for male and female athletes during the landing phase. The results showed that both absolute and normalized leg stiffness were lower in female athletes than in male athletes ($p < 0.05$). And both absolute and normalized knee stiffness were also lower than male athletes ($p < 0.05$). The low leg stiffness and knee stiffness demonstrated by females in this single-leg drop task compared to male athletes may indicate that females have lower dynamic leg stability than males during the drop, which may lead to hypermobility of the knee joint and may put females at a higher risk of injury in this high-risk maneuver for non-contact cruciate ligament injuries.

Keywords: badminton; single-leg landing; ACL injury; lower extremity stiffness

1. Introduction

Previous investigations have shown that anterior cruciate ligament (ACL) injuries may be the most severe lower limb injuries in badminton [1,2]. The most common type of injury among lower extremity ACL injuries is the non-contact ACL injury, accounting for seventy percent of all cases. This type of injury typically occurs more frequently in rapid sports that involve lateral cutting, twisting, and landing [3]. Competitive badminton is a complex sport involving high-frequency, high-intensity sudden stops, changes of direction, and landing. Furthermore, studies have indicated that female athletes typically experience ACL injury rates three to six times higher than their male counterparts at the same level of exercise [4]. Previous studies have shown that ACL injuries often occur when most or all of the body weight is transferred to one foot [5]. Through analysis of videos of badminton competitions, some academics have found that non-contact ACL injuries are most commonly suffered when a player lands on a single leg after performing a backhand side overhead stroke in the backcourt [6]. Additionally, epidemiological studies have indicated that in the sport of badminton, female athletes are at a higher risk of sustaining injuries during single-leg landing actions after executing backhand side overhead shots, compared to males. These injuries appear to occur most frequently during the landing phase [6,7].

Previous studies have identified both intrinsic and extrinsic risk factors for the occurrence of cruciate ligament injuries in different genders. Most authors have proposed various factors, including the influence of hormones and menstrual cycles, as well as anatomical, genetic, and neuromuscular differences between male and female athletes [8–10]. However, as the cause of ACL injury may be attributed to a complex interplay of risk factors, several studies have suggested that biomechanical factors may partially explain the gender difference in the incidence of ACL injury [11], and it is believed that stiffness of the musculoskeletal system is one of the biomechanical factors that may contribute to the sex differences in ACL injury rates [12].

The stiffness of the human body reflects its capacity to withstand the deformations caused by the ground reaction force (GRF) [13,14]. The spring-mass model reflects the characteristics of human jumping motion and is employed to approximate the musculoskeletal system of the lower extremity [15]. The term 'leg stiffness' is used to describe the resistance to change in the overall length of the leg following the application of an internal or external force. Leg stiffness can be controlled by adjusting the stiffness of individual joints. Joint stiffness is controlled by a variety of biomechanical factors, including muscle activation and strength [16–18], reflexes [19], antagonist co-activation, and lower limb kinematics during ground contact [20–23]. Joint stiffness can be controlled by altering the range of motion of the lower limb joints and the associated muscle activity [24]. Leg stiffness has been shown to be an important indicator of the risk of sports injury. Through numerous studies, an increasing amount of evidence indicates that both excessively high and excessively low stiffness can significantly contribute to a higher incidence of musculoskeletal injuries [7,12,25]. Previous studies have shown that excessive leg stiffness may increase peak forces and reduce the lower limb range of motion, the combination of which usually increases loading rates [26]. The combination of increased peak forces, loading rates, and impact forces can make people more susceptible to skeletal injuries [27]. Moreover, insufficient leg stiffness may lead to increased pressure on the passive supporting structures of the knee during the landing process, compromising joint stability and resulting in excessive joint motion. This can elevate the risk of non-contact soft tissue injuries, particularly knee ligament injuries [13].Women exhibit lower muscle stiffness than men when controlled open-chain measurements are performed on the isolated knee [25,28]. In addition, a prospective study found that bilateral differences in preseason leg stiffness increased the likelihood of non-contact lower limb injuries [29]. Some scholars have found that lower limb stiffness was generally lower in female than in male athletes when comparing male and female athletes performing jump landings and volleyball block jump landings. They suggest that the reduced stiffness in female athletes may result in reduced knee stability, causing excessive joint motion at the moment of landing, which may put female athletes at higher risk of ACL injury [30,31]. Therefore, by measuring the variables of lower limb leg stiffness and joint stiffness, we can gain more insight into the potential risk factors for multiple cruciate ligament injuries in female athletes than in male athletes during sports. Previous studies have investigated gender differences in lower extremity stiffness in some two-legged jumping events [32], however, no gender differences in lower limb stiffness were investigated during the movement of landing on one leg after a backhand overhead stroke in the backcourt of badminton, where female athletes are at higher risk of ACL injury (6 male and 15 female badminton players) [6]. To gain more insight into the possible factors that place female athletes at a higher risk of ACL injury than male athletes in single-leg landings after backcourt lateral backhand overhead strokes, a high-risk movement for ACL injury in badminton, and to provide injury prevention strategies for athletes, coaches, and rehabilitation practitioners, it is necessary to examine the gender bias in leg stiffness and knee stiffness during single-leg landings in both male and female athletes.

Therefore, we hypothesized that when badminton players landed on a single leg after a backhand overhead shot in the backcourt, female athletes may exhibit relatively less lower extremity stiffness compared with male athletes.

2. Materials and Methods

2.1. Subjects

In our study, we recruited 16 experienced badminton players, comprising 8 male and 8 female players (Table 1). All participants were members of the university's badminton team and trained at least 6 times per week, with each training session lasting for 3 h. None of the participants had a history of surgery or injury to the trunk, spine, or extremities, limited range of motion in any joint, or muscle weakness, as confirmed by a review of their medical records. All subjects held the racket with their right hand. Prior to participating in the study, all subjects read and signed the informed consent form. This study received approval from the ethics committee of Jeonbuk University (JBNU2022-04-008-001).

Table 1. Basic information of male and female athletes participating in the experiment.

	Males (n = 8)	Females (n = 8)
Age (years)	21.5 ± 2.57	20.38 ± 2.19
Height (cm)	178.5 ± 2.21	167.6 ± 5.76
Body weight (Kg)	70.63 ± 6.17	61.38 ± 6.98
Experiences (years)	9.62 ± 1.95	10.75 ± 2.87

2.2. Preparation for Testing

The three-dimensional motion data use a motion capture analysis system (OptiTrack, NaturalPoint, Inc., Corvallis, OR, USA) including 13 high-speed infrared cameras, and collects experimental data from each participating subject at a sampling frequency of 120 HZ. Each subject's anatomical landmarks were equipped with 57 reflective markers. Ground reaction forces were collected by a force plate embedded in the floor (OR6-6-2000 force platform, AMTI Inc., Plano, TX, USA) at a sampling frequency of 1200 Hz. The motion analysis system and force plate were set up simultaneously before testing. After each test, the 3D motion data were transferred to Visual3D software (Professional 6.0, C-Motion Inc., Germantown, MD, USA) for data analysis of joint angles and other features.

2.3. Test Procedure

We provided clear explanations of the test procedure and purpose to each subject prior to the commencement of the official test. Additionally, we recorded the subjects' basic information, including gender, age, weight, height, and years of experience playing badminton (Table 1). Based on previous research, the actions described by Kimura in badminton with a higher risk of ACL injury were simulated (Figure 1) [5]. Each subject performed a task associated with a high-risk posture for ACL injury, which involved taking one step back to the backhand side of the badminton court to perform an overhead stroke followed by a single-leg landing. Considering that ACL injuries seem to frequently occur during the landing phase, we defined the landing phase in this study as the period from the initial contact point on the force plate to the point of maximum knee flexion during the testing [33].

To minimize individual differences and ensure the accuracy of our experimental results, we enlisted the help of an experienced trainer to demonstrate the proper test movements to all participants. To ensure consistency in every movement, we marked lines at a 45-degree angle on the badminton court and instructed each participant to land on the force measuring plate with one leg after hitting the backhand over the ball in the badminton backcourt. They were then required to quickly return to the starting point (see Figure 2). To reduce the risk of injury during the test, each participant was asked to perform a 15 min warm-up session consisting of jogging, jumping, and several high-clear swings prior to the formal test. Participants were then asked to perform three to five successful trials, with a 30 s rest period in between each test to avoid fatigue. To further minimize potential errors in the experiment, we provided each participant with the same badminton racket and shuttlecock, as well as the same experimental equipment.

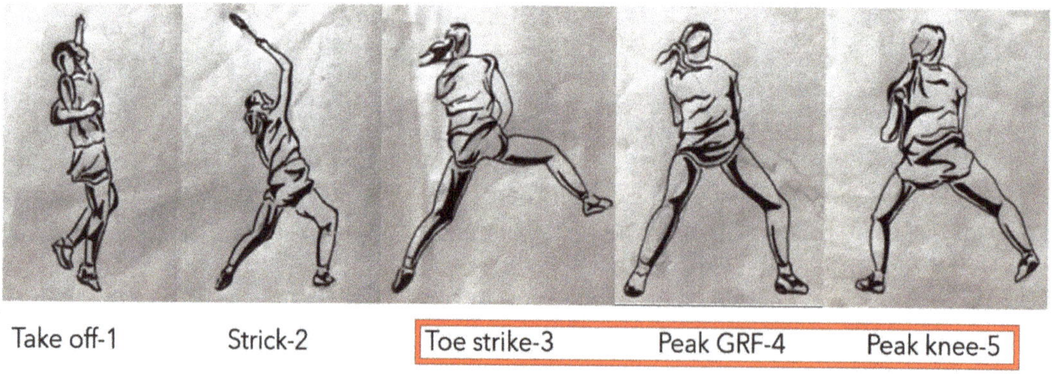

Figure 1. The single-leg landing motion after the backhand side overhead shot in the backcourt of badminton is divided into five stages: take off, strick, toe strike, peak GRF, and peak knee [5]. Red boxes indicate the landing stages analysed in this study.

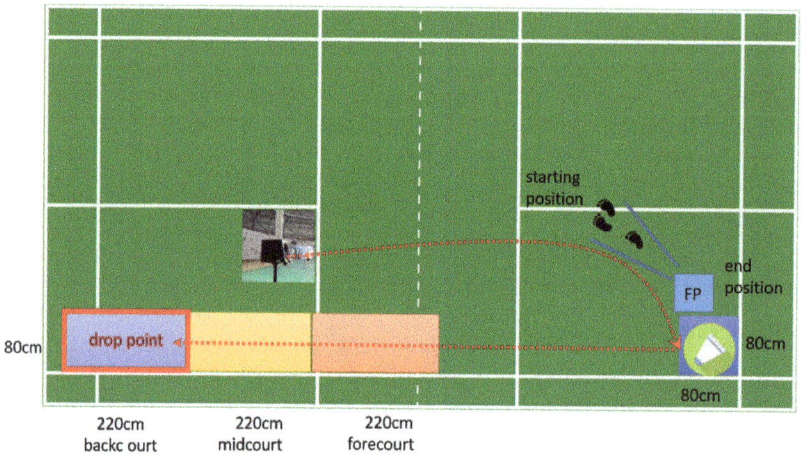

Figure 2. The shuttlecock service machine delivers the shuttlecock to the same location at the same speed and frequency. The subjects stepped back from the starting point to the backhand side of the badminton backcourt to perform the landing task. On landing, they dropped their left foot into the force plate and hit the badminton to the designated area. And quickly return to the starting position within 3 s of the end of the action. The red dotted lines show the sending line of the shuttlecock, and the flight path of the shuttlecock after it has been hit, respectively. The different boxes indicate where the shuttlecock will land and we require that the shuttlecock must land in the blue box after being struck to be recorded as a successful experiment.

2.4. Leg and Knee Stiffness Calculations

The spring-mass model consists of a body and linear leg springs supporting the body. Calculations of lower extremity leg stiffness and knee stiffness were performed using a spring-mass model as presented in previous studies [34]. Leg stiffness is defined as the ratio of the maximum ground reaction force (GRF) to the maximum leg pressure during the landing phase. The calculation formula is as follows:

$$\text{Kleg (N/m)} = \text{peak GRF vertical}/\Delta L_{COM}$$

where peak GRF is the maximum vertical ground reaction force. ΔLCOM is the vertical displacement of the center of mass (COM) from initial contact to maximum knee flexion. We will calculate the center of mass in Visual3D using a full-body biomechanical model based on the position and inertial properties of each body part. GRF data were normalized to body weight (BW), COM shifts were additionally normalized to height, and Kleg was normalized to weight and height. Both will be reported as absolute values and normalized values, respectively.

Joint stiffness was defined as the ratio of the joint moment changes to joint flexion during the landing phase. Knee joint stiffness is calculated using the formula:

$$\text{Kjoint (Nm/rad)} = \Delta\text{Mjoint}/\Delta\theta\text{joint}$$

In this formula, ΔMjoint represents the change in joint moment between the moment of initial touchdown and the peak knee moment, and Δθjoint is the angular displacement of the knee joint between the moment of initial touchdown and the peak knee moment.

2.5. Data Processing and Analysis

All marker trajectory data were recorded and digitized using 3D motion capture system MotiveBody 2.2.0 software (OptiTrack, LEYARD, Buffalo Grove, IL, USA). Sagittal, frontal, and horizontal kinematic and kinetic data of the left hip, left knee, and left ankle were processed using Visual 3D Professional 6.0 software (C-Motion, Inc., Germantown, MD, USA) and presented as mean and standard deviation (SD) of the test. The impact phase of landing was analyzed first, as it is the critical period for non-contact ACL injuries, which commonly occur during the early stages of landing [35]. In this study, the landing phase was defined as the period from initial contact with the force plate to the point of maximum knee flexion in the test, considering that ACL injuries usually occur during this phase [33]. The angular position of the knee is defined as the calf relative to the thigh and using X (flexion/extension), Y (adduction/abduction), and Z (internal rotation/external rotation), using the right-hand convention. Directions are fixed by sign, being positive for flexion, negative for extension, positive for adduction, negative for abduction, positive for internal rotation, and negative for external rotation. Joint torque is calculated using the inverse dynamics method by combining force plate data with kinematic data. We analyzed the data collected in the experiment using SPSS19 software. After calculating the data collected from badminton players, the calculated kinematic and kinetic data were compared statistically using independent *t*-tests. $p < 0.05$ was considered statistically significant.

Absolute leg stiffness and leg stiffness normalized to height and weight, as well as absolute knee stiffness and knee stiffness normalized to height and weight, were separately calculated for each subject, including eight male athletes and eight female athletes. Before conducting an independent sample *t*-test, normality analysis and chi-square tests were performed on the data of the male and female athletes. The two sets of data are from normally distributed populations with flush variance and satisfy independence. Subsequently, independent sample *t*-tests were performed on the data from the male and female athletes to examine gender differences between initial ground contact and maximum knee flexion. The tests included changes in vertical GRF, vertical COM displacement, leg stiffness, knee moment change, knee flexion angle displacement, and knee stiffness.

3. Results

3.1. Leg Stiffness

In Table 2, we observe that the absolute change GRF is significantly higher in male athletes compared to female athletes ($p < 0.05$). There is no significant difference in the vertical displacement of the center of gravity between male and female athletes. However, the calculated absolute leg stiffness in men is significantly higher than that in women, and this difference is statistically significant ($p < 0.05$).

Table 2. Absolute change in vertical GRF, absolute vertical COM displacement, absolute leg stiffness (mean ± SD).

	Males	Females	*p* Value
Change in vertical GRF (N)	2339.16 ± 549.50	1235.44 ± 316.87	0.0002 *
Vertical COM displacement (m)	0.141 ± 0.025	0.131 ± 0.024	0.3852
Leg stiffness (KN/m)	16.95 ± 4.17	9.45 ± 1.98	0.0004 *

"*" indicates a significant difference $p < 0.05$.

From Table 3, we can see that the normalized variation in GRF was also significantly greater in males than in female athletes ($p < 0.05$). There was no significant difference between male and female athletes in terms of normalized vertical displacement of the COM. However, there was also a significant difference in normalized leg stiffness between male and female athletes ($p < 0.05$).

Table 3. Normalized change in vertical GRF, normalized vertical COM displacement, normalized leg stiffness (mean ± SD).

	Males	Females	*p* Value
Change in vertical GRF (BW)	3.29 ± 0.73	2.03 ± 0.38	0.0006 *
Vertical COM displacement (ht)	0.079 ± 0.014	0.078 ± 0.013	0.9954
Leg stiffness (KN/m)	16.95 ± 4.17	9.45 ± 1.98	0.0004 *

"*" indicates a significant difference $p < 0.05$.

3.2. Knee Joint Stiffness

In Table 4, we can see that there is a significant difference in the absolute change in knee torque between male and female athletes ($p < 0.05$). In addition, the absolute change in knee flexion angle was significantly smaller in male athletes compared to female athletes, a significant difference ($p < 0.05$). Additionally, the absolute knee stiffness calculated from these measurements was significantly greater in male athletes than in female athletes, a significant difference ($p < 0.05$).

Table 4. Absolute change in knee joint moment, absolute knee flexion displacement, absolute knee stiffness (mean ± SD).

	Males	Females	*p* Value
Change in knee joint moment (N.m)	158.46 ± 32.31	106.67 ± 51.57	0.0304 *
Knee flexion displacement (°)	30.511 ± 3.442	40.989 ± 6.770	0.0015 *
Knee stiffness (N.m/°)	5.179 ± 0.789	2.57 ± 1.099	0.0002 *

"*" indicates a significant difference $p < 0.05$.

In Table 5, we can see that there is no difference between male and female athletes in the amount of change in knee moment after normalization, but there is a significant difference between male and female athletes in the calculated normalized knee stiffness ($p < 0.05$). Female athletes had significantly lower knee stiffness than male athletes and there was a significant difference ($p < 0.05$).

Table 5. Normalized change in knee joint moment, normalized knee flexion displacement, normalized knee stiffness (mean ± SD).

	Males	Females	*p* Value
Change in knee joint moment (BW.ht)	0.125 ± 0.022	0.104 ± 0.045	0.2713
Knee flexion displacement (°)	30.511 ± 3.442	40.988 ± 6.769	0.0015 *
Knee stiffness (BW.ht/°)	0.0041 ± 0.0008	0.0026 ± 0.001	0.0034 *

"*" indicates a significant difference $p < 0.05$.

4. Discussion

This study aimed to investigate the differences between genders in regard to leg and knee stiffness among male and female athletes during single-leg landing after a backhand overhead shot in the backcourt of badminton. The results of this study support our hypothesis, as we found that female athletes exhibited lower leg and knee stiffness in this landing task compared to males. This could be a potential factor contributing to the higher risk of non-contact ACL injuries among female athletes in this type of landing task compared to males.

In our study, we observed that during a single-leg landing after a backhand overhead shot in the backcourt of badminton, male athletes exhibited significantly higher absolute leg stiffness (16.95 KN/m $\pm$ 4.17) and normalized leg stiffness (42.56 BW/ht $\pm$ 10.66) compared to female athletes, who had lower absolute leg stiffness (9.45 KN/m $\pm$ 1.98) and normalized leg stiffness (26.07 BW/ht $\pm$ 4.72). Similar results have been seen in previous studies on two-legged landing tasks. Ward, Rachel E et al. compared the stiffness of male and female dancers and male and female athletes during jumping and landing tasks and they also found that female athletes had less leg stiffness than male athletes [33]. A previous study by Padua et al. also found that, compared to males, female athletes had significantly less stiffness in the lower limbs during jumping compared to males [12]. However, the mean leg stiffness values for the male and female athletes in this study were higher than in previous studies, which may be due to differences in our single-leg landing task.

In the single-leg landing task, we investigated and we observed that males had a larger absolute vertical GRF variation compared to females. This difference may be attributed to the fact that males generally have significantly higher body weight. However, even after normalizing the data based on weight, males still exhibited a higher vertical GRF compared to females. Additionally, there were no significant differences in both absolute and normalized vertical COM displacement between males and females. However, when examining both absolute and normalized leg stiffness, calculated based on these variables, we found that female athletes had significantly lower values than male athletes. When performing high-intensity functional tasks, the stiffness of muscles and joints plays a critical role in the stability of the functional joint [36]. Stiffer muscles can more quickly and effectively resist sudden joint displacement, possibly as a protective mechanism to prevent acute knee joint injuries [13]. In addition, the passive and dynamic resistance to joint displacement of larger muscles is associated with a greater muscle cross-sectional area [37,38].In the same task, female athletes exhibit lower leg stiffness compared to male athletes, which may indicate a weaker ability for females to resist external compressive and resistance forces during functional single-leg landing tasks, leading to lower dynamic stability of the legs than males. As dynamic leg stability can be reflected in leg stiffness, stiffness is interpreted as the ability of the leg to resist compressive forces from external forces, such as flexion of the hip, knee, or ankle during landing [31]. And this may be related to anatomical differences between males and females, as males typically have greater muscle mass than females. And exhibiting low leg stiffness may increase the stress on the passive support structures of the knee during landings in women, leading to hypermobility of the joint and thus increasing the likelihood of non-contact cruciate ligament injuries in female athletes [31]. However, Granata, Padua, and Wils in their study [12] it is not clear whether the cause of the gender difference in leg stiffness is due to the physical characteristics of male and female athletes. However, in our results, the male athletes still had significantly higher leg stiffness than female athletes even after normalizing for weight and height.

In the single-leg landing motion following a backhand overhead shot in the backcourt of badminton, female athletes showed a significant difference in absolute knee joint stiffness (2.57 N.m/° $\pm$ 1.099) compared to male athletes (5.17 N.m/° $\pm$ 0.789). Additionally, the normalized knee joint stiffness of female athletes (0.0026 BW.ht/° $\pm$ 0.0001) was significantly lower than that of male athletes (0.0041 BW.ht/° $\pm$ 0.0008). This finding supports our hypothesis that in this single-leg landing task, female athletes exhibit lower leg stiffness and knee joint stiffness compared to male athletes. These findings in our study align with similar results observed in another investigation on volleyball blocking jumps [31]. These results suggest that lower knee joint stiffness may be a potential risk factor for ACL injury in female athletes during single-leg landings. In this study, the decrease in normalized knee joint stiffness among female athletes compared to males may be attributed to their less leg stiffness (absolute and normalized values). Joint stiffness (Kjoint) is a fundamental measure for all lower extremity tasks, as the stiffness of joint components within the system ultimately affects the overall system stiffness (i.e., Kvert or Kleg) [39–41]. Joint stiffness is influenced by various factors, including the stiffness of each tendon unit that crosses the joint. The stiffness of muscle-tendon units, in turn, depends on both muscle stiffness and tendon stiffness [20]. It is important to note that muscle stiffness is determined by the level of muscle activation; in other words, muscle stiffness can be indicated by the degree of muscle activation [18,42]. During high-intensity lower extremity exercise, the combined contraction of the hamstrings and quadriceps increases joint contact force, limits intra-articular motion (thus keeping the joint stable), and provides protection to the knee joint against movements that carry a high risk of injury, such as knee abduction and twisting movements [43]. During high-load functional tasks, the greater the resistance of the muscles to knee joint rotation, the higher the likelihood of maintaining dynamic stability and increased stiffness in the knee joint. Consequently, there is a reduced likelihood of stressing passive structures, such as the cruciate ligaments. Therefore, knee joint stiffness may be a significant factor in preventing cruciate ligament injuries. In our study, the lower knee joint stiffness observed in female athletes may be associated with insufficient activation of the knee joint antagonist muscles. Co-activation of the lower limb antagonist muscles is part of a strategy that can increase muscle stiffness and stability [44,45]. Previous studies have shown that during jump landing tasks, females attempt to partially alter lower limb stiffness by recruiting more quadriceps, and while large quadriceps activation may be an effective mechanism for modulating lower limb stiffness during jumping, it may have a detrimental effect on knee joint stability [32]. In addition, a previous study had found that an unbalanced recruitment strategy of the quadriceps and hamstrings was used more significantly in females compared to males during the landing task [32], previous studies have shown that when the hamstrings are stiffer it may be able to limit tibial anterior translation and shear forces and can relatively reduce the external forces exerted on the cruciate ligament [37].

In this single-leg landing task, we observed a significant difference in the knee flexion angle displacement between female athletes (36.97° $\pm$ 7.38) and males (28.88° $\pm$ 4.92). This disparity may be attributed to weaker hamstring strength and lower muscle activation, which limits the ability of muscle contraction to protect the ligaments, leading to reduced joint stiffness and lack of stability upon landing. Consequently, female athletes face a higher risk of cruciate ligament injury compared to their male counterparts during landing. Notably, our study also found significantly lower normalized knee stiffness in females compared to males, contradicting some conflicting results in the published literature [32]. This may also be caused by the fact that our present study was a single-leg landing task, unlike the previous two-leg landing task. Previous research showed that when knee stiffness was normalized for body weight, the differences between male and female athletes were not evident, indicating that the increased net external knee flexion moment after normalization could maintain similar normalized knee stiffness in female athletes compared to males [46,47]. Moreover, other studies have demonstrated that humans can autonomously control joint stiffness through muscle recruitment, thereby enhancing dynamic joint stability by adjusting the joint stiffness [48]. As previously mentioned, female athletes who used these strategies while jumping showed a more dominant recruitment pattern for the quadriceps compared to male athletes [32]. A lower knee flexion moment in female athletes may contribute to lower extremity stiffness and higher injury rates due to the limited ability of the quadriceps to balance [49].

When interpreting the results of this study, it is important to acknowledge and consider certain limitations. Firstly, the average age of the athletes we recruited was 20 years, which is probably younger than the age used in previous studies. As leg stiffness is influenced by the combined effects of hip, knee, and ankle stiffness [12], we focused solely on knee stiffness in this study. Furthermore, torsional joint stiffness is regulated by various biomechanical factors, including muscle activation and strength [16–18], reflexes [19], antagonist co-activation, and lower limb kinematics during ground contact [20–23]. In this study, we solely examined lower limb kinematic and kinetic data from male and female athletes during ground contact. However, it is important to supplement these findings with lower limb muscle surface electromyography to assess muscle strength and function during exercise tasks [50,51]. Additionally, future investigations could explore different muscle activation and exercise strategies to modulate lower limb stiffness under functional loading conditions.

5. Conclusions

In the single-leg landing motion, after a backhand overhead shot in the backcourt of badminton, compared with male athletes, female athletes showed significantly less absolute and normalized leg stiffness and less absolute and normalized knee stiffness during landing. This suggests that female athletes may be more susceptible to factors than males to non-contact ACL injuries during landing motion, as female athletes exhibit lower leg low dynamic stability and high knee hypermobility during landing than male athletes. In future training, female athletes should appropriately increase the stiffness of their lower limbs. However, further research is needed to determine the "optimal" stiffness level required to achieve functional tasks.

Author Contributions: Conceptualization, Y.Z. and Z.H.; methodology, Y.Z. and S.K.; software, B.L., M.L., X.Q. and X.M.; validation, Y.K. and S.K.; formal analysis, Y.Z., Z.H., B.L., M.L. and X.M.; investigation, Y.Z. and Z.H.; data curation, Y.Z., Z.H., S.K. and Y.K.; writing—original draft preparation, Y.Z. and Z.H.; writing—review and editing, S.K. and Y.K.; visualization, S.K.; supervision, S.K.; project administration, Y.K. All authors have read and agreed to the published version of the manuscript.

Funding: This research received no external funding.

Institutional Review Board Statement: The study was conducted in accordance with the Declaration of Helsinki, and approved by the Institutional Review Board of Jeonbuk National University (JBNU2022-04-008-001).

Informed Consent Statement: Informed consent was obtained from all subjects involved in the study.

Data Availability Statement: The data presented in this study are available on request from the corresponding author.

Conflicts of Interest: The authors declare no conflict of interest.

References

1. Nagano, Y.; Sasaki, S.; Higashihara, A.; Ichikawa, H. Movements with greater trunk accelerations and their properties during badminton games. *Sports Biomech.* **2020**, *19*, 342–352. [CrossRef] [PubMed]
2. Shao, E.; Lu, Z.; Cen, X.; Zheng, Z.; Sun, D.; Gu, Y. The Effect of Fatigue on Lower Limb Joint Stiffness at Different Walking Speeds. *Diagnostics* **2022**, *12*, 1470. [CrossRef] [PubMed]
3. Griffin, L.Y. Anterior cruciate ligament injuries in female athletes: Prevention strategies. *Instr. Course Lect.* **2002**, *51*, 311–314. [PubMed]
4. Arendt, E.; Dick, R. Knee injury patterns among men and women in collegiate basketball and soccer: NCAA data and review of literature. *Am. J. Sports Med.* **1995**, *23*, 694–701. [CrossRef] [PubMed]
5. Olsen, O.-E.; Myklebust, G.; Engebretsen, L.; Bahr, R. Injury mechanisms for anterior cruciate ligament injuries in team handball: A systematic video analysis. *Am. J. Sports Med.* **2004**, *32*, 1002–1012. [CrossRef]
6. Kimura, Y.; Ishibashi, Y.; Tsuda, E.; Yamamoto, Y.; Tsukada, H.; Toh, S. Mechanisms for anterior cruciate ligament injuries in badminton. *Br. J. Sports Med.* **2010**, *44*, 1124–1127. [CrossRef]

7. Griffin, L.Y.; Albohm, M.J.; Arendt, E.A.; Bahr, R.; Beynnon, B.D.; DeMaio, M.; Dick, R.W.; Engebretsen, L.; Garrett, W.E.; Hannafin, J.A.; et al. Understanding and preventing noncontact anterior cruciate ligament injuries: A review of the Hunt Valley II meeting, January 2005. *Am. J. Sports Med.* **2006**, *34*, 1512–1532. [CrossRef]
8. Biedert, R.; Bachmann, M. Women's soccer. Injuries, risks, and prevention. *Orthopade* **2005**, *34*, 448–453. [CrossRef]
9. Hewett, T.E.; Myer, G.D.; Ford, K.R. Reducing knee and anterior cruciate ligament injuries among female athletes: A systematic review of neuromuscular training interventions. *J. Knee Surg.* **2005**, *18*, 82–88. [CrossRef]
10. Posthumus, M.; September, A.V.; O'Cuinneagain, D.; van der Merwe, W.; Schwellnus, M.P.; Collins, M. The COL5A1 gene is associated with increased risk of anterior cruciate ligament ruptures in female participants. *Am. J. Sports Med.* **2009**, *37*, 2234–2240. [CrossRef]
11. Griffin, L.Y.; Agel, J.; Albohm, M.J.; Arendt, E.A.; Dick, R.W.; Garrett, W.E.; Garrick, J.G.; Hewett, T.E.; Huston, L.; Ireland, M.L. Noncontact anterior cruciate ligament injuries: Risk factors and prevention strategies. *J. Am. Acad. Orthop. Surg.* **2000**, *8*, 141–150. [CrossRef] [PubMed]
12. Granata, K.; Padua, D.; Wilson, S.; Kinesiology. Gender differences in active musculoskeletal stiffness. Part II. Quantification of leg stiffness during functional hopping tasks. *J. Electromyogr. Kinesiol.* **2002**, *12*, 127–135. [CrossRef]
13. Butler, R.J.; Crowell III, H.P.; Davis, I.M. Lower extremity stiffness: Implications for performance and injury. *Clin. Biomech.* **2003**, *18*, 511–517. [CrossRef] [PubMed]
14. Latash, M.L.; Zatsiorsky, V.M. Joint stiffness: Myth or reality? *Hum. Mov. Sci.* **1993**, *12*, 653–692. [CrossRef]
15. Blickhan, R. The spring-mass model for running and hopping. *J. Biomech.* **1989**, *22*, 1217–1227. [CrossRef]
16. Hunter, I.; Kearney, R. Dynamics of human ankle stiffness: Variation with mean ankle torque. *J. Biomech.* **1982**, *15*, 747–752. [CrossRef]
17. Julian, F.J.; Sollins, M.R. Variation of muscle stiffness with force at increasing speeds of shortening. *J. Gen. Physiol.* **1975**, *66*, 287–302. [CrossRef]
18. Weiss, P.; Hunter, I.; Kearney, R. Human ankle joint stiffness over the full range of muscle activation levels. *J. Biomech.* **1988**, *21*, 539–544. [CrossRef]
19. Kearney, R.; Stein, R.; Parameswaran, L. Identification of intrinsic and reflex contributions to human ankle stiffness dynamics. *IEEE Trans. Biomed. Eng.* **1997**, *44*, 493–504. [CrossRef]
20. Farley, C.T.; Morgenroth, D.C. Leg stiffness primarily depends on ankle stiffness during human hopping. *J. Biomec.* **1999**, *32*, 267–273. [CrossRef]
21. Greene, P.R.; McMahon, T.A. Reflex stiffness of man's anti-gravity muscles during kneebends while carrying extra weights. *J. Biomech.* **1979**, *12*, 881–891. [CrossRef] [PubMed]
22. McMahon, T.A.; Valiant, G.; Frederick, E.C. Groucho running. *J. Appl. Physiol.* **1987**, *62*, 2326–2337. [CrossRef] [PubMed]
23. Zhang, L.-Q.; Nuber, G.; Butler, J.; Bowen, M.; Rymer, W.Z. In vivo human knee joint dynamic properties as functions of muscle contraction and joint position. *J. Biomech.* **1997**, *31*, 71–76. [CrossRef] [PubMed]
24. Serpell, B.G.; Ball, N.; Scarvell, J.; Smith, P.N. A review of models of vertical, leg, and knee stiffness in adults for running, jumping or hopping tasks. *J. Sports Sci.* **2012**, *30*, 1347–1363. [CrossRef] [PubMed]
25. Granata, K.P.; Wilson, S.E.; Padua, D.A. Gender differences in active musculoskeletal stiffness. Part I.: Quantification in controlled measurements of knee joint dynamics. *J. Electromyogr. Kinesiol.* **2002**, *12*, 119–126. [CrossRef] [PubMed]
26. Hennig, E.M.; Lafortune, M.A. Relationships between ground reaction force and tibial bone acceleration parameters. *J. Biomech.* **1991**, *7*, 303–309. [CrossRef]
27. Grimston, S.K.; Engsberg, J.R.; Kloiber, R.; Hanley, D.A. Bone Mass, External Loads, and Stress Fracture in Female Runners. *Int. J. Sport. Biomech.* **1991**, *7*, 293–302. [CrossRef]
28. Blackburn, J.; Riemann, B.L.; Padua, D.A.; Guskiewicz, K.M. Sex comparison of extensibility, passive, and active stiffness of the knee flexors. *Clin. Biomech.* **2004**, *19*, 36–43. [CrossRef]
29. Watsford, M.L.; Murphy, A.J.; McLachlan, K.A.; Bryant, A.L.; Cameron, M.L.; Crossley, K.M.; Makdissi, M. A Prospective Study of the Relationship between Lower Body Stiffness and Hamstring Injury in Professional Australian Rules Footballers. *Am. J. Sports Med.* **2010**, *38*, 2058–2064. [CrossRef]
30. Wang, I.-L.; Wang, S.-Y.; Wang, L.-I. Sex differences in lower extremity stiffness and kinematics alterations during double-legged drop landings with changes in drop height. *Sports Biomech.* **2015**, *14*, 404–412. [CrossRef]
31. Hughes, G.; Watkins, J. Lower limb coordination and stiffness during landing from volleyball block jumps. *Res. Sports Med.* **2008**, *16*, 138–154. [CrossRef] [PubMed]
32. Padua, D.A.; Carcia, C.R.; Arnold, B.L.; Granata, K.P. Gender Differences in Leg Stiffness and Stiffness Recruitment Strategy During Two-Legged Hopping. *J. Mot. Behav.* **2005**, *37*, 111–126. [CrossRef] [PubMed]
33. Ward, R.E.; Yan, A.F.; Orishimo, K.F.; Kremenic, I.J.; Hagins, M.; Liederbach, M.; Hiller, C.E.; Pappas, E. Comparison of lower limb stiffness between male and female dancers and athletes during drop jump landings. *Scand. J. Med. Sci. Sports* **2019**, *29*, 71–81. [CrossRef] [PubMed]
34. Hobara, H.; Kimura, K.; Omuro, K.; Gomi, K.; Muraoka, T.; Sakamoto, M.; Kanosue, K. Differences in lower extremity stiffness between endurance-trained athletes and untrained subjects. *J. Sci. Med. Sport.* **2010**, *13*, 106–111. [CrossRef]

35. Kimura, Y.; Ishibashi, Y.; Tsuda, E.; Yamamoto, Y.; Hayashi, Y.; Sato, S. Increased knee valgus alignment and moment during single-leg landing after overhead stroke as a potential risk factor of anterior cruciate ligament injury in badminton. *Br. J. Sports Med.* **2012**, *46*, 207–213. [CrossRef]
36. Riemann, B.L.; Lephart, S.M.J.J.o.a.t. The sensorimotor system, part II: The role of proprioception in motor control and functional joint stability. *J. Athl. Train.* **2002**, *37*, 80.
37. Blackburn, J.T.; Bell, D.R.; Norcross, M.F.; Hudson, J.D.; Engstrom, L.A.; Kinesiology. Comparison of hamstring neuromechanical properties between healthy males and females and the influence of musculotendinous stiffness. *J. Electromyogr. Kinesiol.* **2009**, *19*, e362–e369. [CrossRef]
38. Herda, T.J.; Costa, P.B.; Walter, A.A.; Ryan, E.D.; Hoge, K.M.; Kerksick, C.; Stout, J.R.; Cramer, J. Effects of Two Modes of Static Stretching on Muscle Strength and Stiffness. *Med. Sci. Sports Exerc.* **2011**, *43*, 1777–1784. [CrossRef]
39. Ferris, D.P.; Louie, M.; Farley, C.T. Running in the real world: Adjusting leg stiffness for different surfaces. *Proc. R. Soc. B: Boil. Sci.* **1998**, *265*, 989–994. [CrossRef]
40. Kuitunen, S.; Komi, P.V.; Kyröläinen, H. Knee and ankle joint stiffness in sprint running. *Med. Sci. Sports Exerc.* **2002**, *34*, 166–173. [CrossRef]
41. Hobara, H.; Muraoka, T.; Omuro, K.; Gomi, K.; Sakamoto, M.; Inoue, K.; Kanosue, K. Knee stiffness is a major determinant of leg stiffness during maximal hopping. *J. Biomech.* **2009**, *42*, 1768–1771. [CrossRef] [PubMed]
42. Nielsen, J.B.; Toft, E.; Kagamihara, Y. Segmental reflexes and ankle joint stiffness during co-contraction of antagonistic ankle muscles in man. *Exp. Brain Res.* **1994**, *102*, 350–358. [CrossRef] [PubMed]
43. Solomonow, M.; Baratta, R.; Zhou, B.; Shoji, H.; Bose, W.; Beck, C.; D'Ambrosia, R. The synergistic action of the anterior cruciate ligament and thigh muscles in maintaining joint stability. *Am. J. Sports Med.* **1987**, *15*, 207–213. [CrossRef] [PubMed]
44. Lavender, S.A.; Tsuang, Y.-H.; Hafezi, A.; Anderson, G.B.J.; Chaffin, D.B.; Hughes, R.E. Coactivation of the Trunk Muscles during Asymmetric Loading of the Torso. *Hum. Factors: J. Hum. Factors Ergon. Soc.* **1992**, *34*, 239–247. [CrossRef]
45. Granata, K.P.; Marras, W.S. The Influence of Trunk Muscle Coactivity on Dynamic Spinal Loads. *Spine* **1995**, *20*, 913–919. [CrossRef]
46. Fagenbaum, R.; Darling, W.G. Jump landing strategies in male and female college athletes and the implications of such strategies for anterior cruciate ligament injury. *Am. J. Sports Med.* **2003**, *31*, 233–240. [CrossRef]
47. Huston, L.; Vibert, B.; Ashton-Miller, J.A.; Wojtys, E.M. Gender differences in knee angle when landing from a drop-jump. *Am. J. knee Surg.* **2001**, *14*, 215–219; discussion 219–220.
48. Zhang, L.-Q.; Xu, D.; Wang, G.; Hendrix, R.W. Muscle strength in knee varus and valgus. *Med. Sci. Sports Exerc.* **2001**, *33*, 1194–1199. [CrossRef]
49. Zazulak, B.T.; Paterno, M.; Myer, G.D.; Romani, W.A.; Hewett, T.E. The Effects of the Menstrual Cycle on Anterior Knee Laxity. *Sports Med.* **2006**, *36*, 847–862. [CrossRef]
50. Lloyd, D.G.; Buchanan, T.S. Strategies of muscular support of varus and valgus isometric loads at the human knee. *J. Biomec.* **2001**, *34*, 1257–1267. [CrossRef]
51. Besier, T.F.; Lloyd, D.G.; Ackland, T.R. Muscle Activation Strategies at the Knee during Running and Cutting Maneuvers. *Med. Sci. Sports Exerc.* **2003**, *35*, 119–127. [CrossRef] [PubMed]

bioengineering

MDPI

Article

Pallidal Recordings in Chronically Implanted Dystonic Patients: Mitigation of Tremor-Related Artifacts

Jasmin Del Vecchio Del Vecchio [1,*], Ibrahem Hanafi [1], Nicoló Gabriele Pozzi [1], Philipp Capetian [1], Ioannis U. Isaias [1,2], Stefan Haufe [3,4,5,†] and Chiara Palmisano [1,†]

1 Department of Neurology, University Hospital of Würzburg and Julius-Maximilian-University Würzburg, 97080 Würzburg, Germany; hanafi_i@ukw.de (I.H.); pozzi_n2@ukw.de (N.G.P.); capetian_p@ukw.de (P.C.); isaias_i@ukw.de (I.U.I.); palmisano_c@ukw.de (C.P.)
2 Centro Parkinson e Parkinsonismi, ASST G. Pini-CTO, 20122 Milano, Italy
3 Uncertainty, Inverse Modeling and Machine Learning Group, Technische Universität Berlin, 10623 Berlin, Germany; stefan.haufe@charite.de
4 Physikalisch-Technische Bundesanstalt Braunschweig und Berlin, 10587 Berlin, Germany
5 Berlin Center for Advanced Neuroimaging, Charité—Universitätsmedizin Berlin, 10117 Berlin, Germany
* Correspondence: delvecchio_j@ukw.de
† These authors contributed equally to this work.

Abstract: Low-frequency oscillatory patterns of pallidal local field potentials (LFPs) have been proposed as a physiomarker for dystonia and hold the promise for personalized adaptive deep brain stimulation. Head tremor, a low-frequency involuntary rhythmic movement typical of cervical dystonia, may cause movement artifacts in LFP signals, compromising the reliability of low-frequency oscillations as biomarkers for adaptive neurostimulation. We investigated chronic pallidal LFPs with the Percept™ PC (Medtronic PLC) device in eight subjects with dystonia (five with head tremors). We applied a multiple regression approach to pallidal LFPs in patients with head tremors using kinematic information measured with an inertial measurement unit (IMU) and an electromyographic signal (EMG). With IMU regression, we found tremor contamination in all subjects, whereas EMG regression identified it in only three out of five. IMU regression was also superior to EMG regression in removing tremor-related artifacts and resulted in a significant power reduction, especially in the theta-alpha band. Pallido-muscular coherence was affected by a head tremor and disappeared after IMU regression. Our results show that the Percept PC can record low-frequency oscillations but also reveal spectral contamination due to movement artifacts. IMU regression can identify such artifact contamination and be a suitable tool for its removal.

Keywords: dystonia; tremor; local field potentials; globus pallidus; deep brain stimulation

1. Introduction

Dystonia is a movement disorder characterized by patterned, directional, and often sustained involuntary muscle contractions that produce abnormal postures or repetitive movements [1]. Tremor can be a basic feature of a dystonic contraction and is reported in up to 87% of patients [2]. One of the most common dystonic tremors is head tremor in patients with cervical dystonia (CD) [3], in which it causes a severe reduction in quality of life.

The pathophysiology of CD and dystonic tremor (DT) is not entirely known. It is still unclear whether tremor in dystonia has its own pathophysiology unrelated to dystonia or shares some mechanisms. It is also still debated whether DT, which is the presence of tremor in a body part affected by dystonia, and tremor associated with dystonia (TAWD), defined as tremor in a body part not affected by dystonia [4], are distinct entities or similar syndromes [5,6]. Previous studies revealed increased intermuscular coherence in DT because of a loss of reciprocal inhibition [7–9], indicating that DT shares some dystonia pathophysiology [10–12]. Functional imaging studies further showed the involvement of the basal ganglia, thalamus, midbrain, and sensory-motor cortex in DT, similar to dystonia without tremor [13,14]. Recently, there has been increasing evidence of cerebellar involvement and interactions between the cerebellum and basal ganglia in DT and dystonia, and most of the literature converges in supporting the involvement of both basal ganglia-thalamo-cortical and cerebello-thalamo-cortical pathways in dystonia [15–27]. In particular, the cerebellum has a critical role in the generation and expression of tremor and CD [28]. Neuroimaging studies showed greater activation of the anterior cerebellar regions ipsilateral to the direction of head rotation and decreased activation in the posterior cerebellar regions [29,30]. Patients with CD and head tremor showed higher clinical scores of cerebellar dysfunctions, e.g., ataxia, than those without tremor [28], and dystonic tremor improved after deep brain stimulation (DBS) of the cerebellar thalamus (ventralis intermediate nucleus [VIM]) [31]. On the other hand, a recent study comparing patients with CD without tremor, CD with jerky head oscillations, and sinusoidal head oscillations showed a distinct pallidal dysfunction in the group with sinusoidal oscillations [32]. This would favor the hypothesis of a specific contribution of the basal ganglia to the pathophysiology of DT [15].

Chronic DBS of the globus pallidus pars interna (GPi) is a safe and effective treatment for advanced, disabling dystonia [33–36]. Despite successful results, pallidal stimulation for dystonia remains a poorly standardized therapy with variable clinical outcomes [37]. A significant challenge remains the variability of treatment benefits at an individual level. An added complexity is that improvement after DBS is typically delayed or progressive over months or years [35,38,39].

New implantable devices capable of chronically recording local field potentials (LFPs) during stimulation will enable a better understanding of disease-related brain activity patterns, their evolution over time, and their modulation in response to therapies [40]. This could dramatically improve tailoring treatment to each patient by adapting stimulation parameters (adaptive DBS, aDBS) in response to an input signal that can represent symptoms, motor activity, or other behavioral features [41]. In this regard, two aspects are particularly relevant: (i) the ability to identify robust biomarkers reflecting symptoms and their fluctuations in the context of activities of daily living and (ii) the reliability of the device for real-time monitoring of artifact-free recordings and online adjustment of one or more stimulation parameters [40].

One of the most promising biomarkers for dystonia is an increase in the magnitude of oscillatory activity in the theta-alpha range (3–12 Hz) embedded in GPi-LFPs [42–44]. Neumann et al. showed a correlation between these oscillations and the severity of dystonia [42], but their acute suppression might not be followed by a direct change in symptom severity [45]. Additionally, the reliability of this biomarker in chronically stimulated patients has yet to be fully explored. Piña-Fuentes et al. observed a significantly lower theta-alpha frequency power in (still symptomatic) dystonic patients chronically treated with DBS in comparison to newly implanted patients, even when stimulation was suspended [45].

The aim of the present study was to investigate pallidal low-frequency oscillatory activity in our first series of dystonic patients chronically stimulated with the Percept^{TM} PC device (Medtronic PLC). This is one of the first commercially available devices for chronic DBS able to continuously record LFP in real time and transmit them wirelessly to a storage device (a tablet-user interface) [46].

In this study, we particularly focused on dystonic tremor as a possible source of artifactual contamination of GPi-LFP recordings. Indeed, consistent and rhythmic movements are particularly likely to contaminate the power spectrum [47]. This would be critical in subjects with CD as they may present head tremor at a frequency of 1–6 Hz, which falls in the same range as the GPi-LFP's clinically relevant spectral power [48,49].

2. Materials and Methods

2.1. Subjects, Surgery, and Clinical Evaluation

We reviewed data collected from eight patients with idiopathic dystonia implanted in the GPi with the Percept PC device (Medtronic, PLC), who were routinely evaluated at our center. Demographic and clinical data are listed in Table 1. Four patients had CD, three had myoclonus dystonia (DM), and one had segmental dystonia primarily affecting the head and the (left and right) arm (MFD). Five of these patients showed dystonic tremors of the head. This was defined as a spontaneous oscillatory, rhythmical head movement [1].

Table 1. Demographic and clinical data. Abbreviations: T+—patients with head tremor; T−—patients without head tremor; CD—cervical dystonia; MFD—multifocal dystonia; DM—dystonia with myoclonus; TWSTRS—Toronto Western Spasmodic Torticollis Rating Scale; DBS—Deep Brain Stimulation; NA—not available. * Identifies patients studied at battery replacement. ** Age at battery replacement.

Patients		DW01 (T+)	DW02 (T+)	DW06 (T+)	DW07 * (T+)	DW08 (T+)	DW03 * (T−)	DW04 * (T−)	DW05 (T−)
Sex		F	F	F	F	F	M	M	F
Age		52	44	57	50	33	74	62	65
Age at onset, years		38	36	42	Childhood	Childhood	42	Childhood	Childhood
Age at surgery		50	43	56	48 **	31	72 **	62 **	63
Disease		CD	CD	CD	MFD	DM	CD	DM	DM
TWSTRS pre-DBS, score		18	19	13	NA	22	22	NA	18
TWSTRS post-DBS, score	Stim-off	16	18	8	17	19	16	21	18
TWSTRS post-DBS, score	Stim-on	15	14	6	8	NA	5	13	6

All patients were implanted with standard non-directional DBS leads (3389, Medtronic, PLC). The surgical procedure for DBS implantation has been described previously. Briefly, patients underwent simultaneous bilateral stereotactic implantation of DBS electrodes into the posteroventrolateral internal globus pallidus. The DBS electrode used was model 3389 (Medtronic, PLC), with four platinum-iridium cylindrical contacts of 1.5 mm each and a contact-to-contact separation of 0.5 mm. The DBS electrodes were connected to an implantable pulse generator (IPG) during the same or a subsequent surgery [39,50]. Three out of eight patients received the Percept PC as a battery replacement. Along with GPi-DBS, one patient with DM received DBS of the motor thalamus (i.e., VIM).

We assessed the severity of symptoms with the Toronto Western Spasmodic Torticollis Rating Scale (TWSTRS, severity subscale [51,52]). The evaluations were performed before and after DBS implantation (i.e., on the day of GPi-LFP recordings). After DBS, evaluations were performed in both stimulation-off (stim-off) and stimulation-on (stim-on) conditions with the clinically optimized stimulation parameters.

The local Institutional Review Board approved the study and waived review for the data collection. Informed consent was obtained from all subjects involved in the study according to the Declaration of Helsinki.

2.2. Experimental Setup and Recordings

We recorded GPi-LFPs from the chronically implanted electrodes in stim-off condition at least six months after DBS implant. The stimulation was paused for at least 30 min before the experiment. During the recordings, patients were at rest, comfortably sitting in a chair. They were asked to keep their eyes open without speaking or performing any voluntary movement. The average (±standard deviation) recording length was 233.62 s (±141.68 s), ranging from 66.8 s (patient DW02) to 451.48 s (patient DW03). According to the clinical evaluation of a neurologist expert in movement disorders (N.P.), the subject was considered a tremor (T+) or non-tremor (T−) patient. The presence of tremor was further confirmed by inspecting the video recordings of the experiment (VIXTA, BTS).

For one T+ patient (DW02), we performed three additional recordings aimed at investigating the effect of head tremor on LFPs. First, during the execution of an alleviating maneuver (sensory trick or geste antagoniste) [53], namely, a light touch of the face performed with the left hand. This is a peculiar feature of dystonia that enables a temporary relief of dystonic muscle contractions upon sensory stimulation [53,54]. Second, during voluntary alternating (left to right and back) rhythmic movements of the head with small and, third, large amplitude. We limited this second set of recordings to only patient DW02 as she was the only one among the T+ patients with a clinically effective sensory trick.

GPi LFPs were recorded bilaterally from all non-adjacent contact pairs (i.e., 0–3, 0–2, 1–3, where 0 is the lowermost and 3 the uppermost contact, respectively) at a sampling frequency of 250 Hz (*indefinite streaming* mode) [46].

Head tremor was recorded bilaterally with surface electromyography (FREEEMG, BTS) of the sternocleidomastoid and trapezius muscles at a sampling frequency of 1000 Hz. We chose these two muscles because they were affected by tremor in all patients and could be easily recorded. Additionally, we placed one EMG probe on the left chest to record heart activity and remove cardiac artifacts from the LFPs [55] and one on the neck close to the cable connecting the implantable pulse generator (IPG) with the DBS electrodes for synchronization purposes [46,55]. The method for synchronizing LFP and EMG recordings has previously been described in [46,56,57]. Briefly, a transcutaneous electrical nerve stimulation (TENS) burst was delivered at the level of the neck (f = 80 Hz) at the beginning and at the end of each recording session. We used the abrupt drop-off of the TENS artifact simultaneously recorded by the DBS electrodes and EMG probe to align the two signals.

In the T+ group, head tremor was recorded with a triaxial inertial measurement unit (IMU) (Opal, APDM) placed on the forehead at a sampling frequency of 128 Hz. IMU and EMG signals were synchronized by aligning the data with respect to the rising edge of a transistor-transistor logic (TTL) signal going from 0 to 5 V.

2.3. Data Analysis

2.3.1. Data Preprocessing

All data were imported to MATLAB (R2022b, The Mathworks, Natick, MA, USA) and analyzed offline using custom codes.

EMG recordings were down-sampled to the LFP sampling frequency, i.e., 250 Hz. Although the IPG was located in the right subclavicular region in five out of eight patients [58], all LFP signals were contaminated by cardiac activity. The cardiac artifacts were removed from the LFP signals by means of singular value decomposition (SVD). We first detected the cardiac QRS peaks as recorded by the EMG probe placed on the chest. We then divided the LFP signals into epochs centered on each QRS peak. For each epoch, we computed the SVD of the LFP signals and visually identified all the eigenvectors corresponding to the ECG artifact. We then reconstructed the cardiac artifact from these components and subtracted it from the raw LFP [55].

To characterize tremor, EMGs were band-pass filtered in the band 1–120 Hz (second order IIR filter). We used the absolute value of the Hilbert transform of the EMG signals for the subsequent analysis. The IMU signals were high-pass filtered at 1 Hz (second-order Butterworth filter).

Figure 1 shows an example of the synchronized recordings of EMG, IMU, and LFP in one patient (DW08).

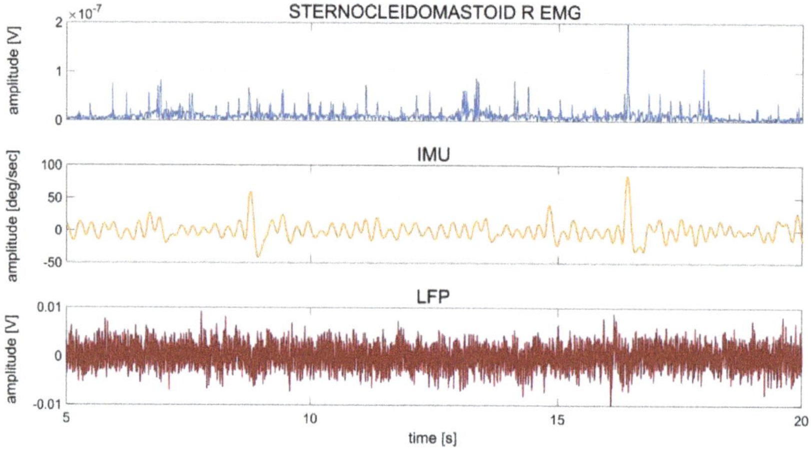

Figure 1. Patient DW08: time series of 20 s of recording of the right sternocleidomastoid muscle (first row), IMU (second row), and LFP (third row) during rest. The IMU time series were averaged over the three axes (x, y, z), and the LFP time series were averaged over the six contact pairs (0–3, 0–2, 1–3, left and right). The patient showed a dystonic tremor during the acquisition, as also confirmed by clinical notes and a video evaluation of the recording. The waveform of the tremor peaks captured by the IMU can also be observed in the LFPs.

2.3.2. Spectral Analyses

The power spectral density (PSD) of all signals was computed using Welch's method with 1-s windows and a 50% overlap.

The LFP power spectra were characterized by the presence of an aperiodic part following a 1/f power law. Following Donoghue et al. [55,59], we modeled the observed PSD as the sum of putative, periodic oscillatory components parameterized by their center frequency, power, and bandwidth, as measured from Gaussian model fits, plus an aperiodic component parameterized by the offset and slope of an exponentially decaying (1/f shaped) function. Following the parameterization procedure, we removed the 1/f aperiodic component from the PSD to analyze only the true oscillatory components. The resulting LFP power spectra were then normalized to the standard deviation of the spectrum in the range 5–95 Hz to de-emphasize spectral features prone to movement artifacts [42,60]. LFP PSDs were averaged over all contact pairs and over trials.

IMU and EMG power spectra were normalized to the standard deviation of the spectra in the range 1–64 Hz and 1–125 Hz, respectively. EMG power spectra were averaged over the four recorded muscles and over trials. IMU power spectra were averaged over the three recorded axes and over trials.

2.3.3. Assessment of Tremor-Artifacts in LFP Recording and Comparison of IMU vs. EMG Regression Analysis

We investigated eventual dystonic tremor contamination in the LFP by (i) comparing PSDs across modalities and (ii) regressing multiple time-lagged copies of the EMG and the IMU out of the LFP and evaluating the effect on LFP–PSDs.

With regards to PSD comparison, individual averaged power spectra were visually inspected for peaks in the theta-alpha band (3–12 Hz), which corresponds to the range of tremor [61]. We focused on the theta-alpha frequency peaks as computed on LFP, EMG, and IMU PSDs. LFP spectra were considered contaminated by dystonic tremor when the peak in theta-alpha power aligned across LFPs, EMGs, and IMUs.

To perform the regression, all recordings were down-sampled to the lowest available sampling frequency: 128 Hz when IMUs were used, 250 Hz when EMG signals were used.

To regress the temporal dynamics of the EMG and IMU channels capturing head-tremor out of the LFPs, a temporal embedding of the EMG and IMU time series was performed. To this end, each time series $x_m(t)$ was complemented by temporally shifted versions $\tilde{x}_m(t) = [x_m(t + \tau_1), \ldots, x_m(t + \tau_K)]^T$, $m = 1, \ldots, M$, where, $x_m(t + \tau)$ was the activity of the m-th EMG or IMU sensor at time $t + \tau$. In this work, we used K = 51 equally spaced shifts for the EMGs, ranging from $\tau_1 = -250$ samples to $\tau_K = 250$ samples in steps of 10 samples, and K = 52 equally spaced shifts ranging from $\tau_1 = -128$ samples to $\tau_K = 128$ samples in steps of 5 samples for the IMU. Thus, the tremor dynamics of both EMG and IMU were extracted within a window of two seconds and regressed out of LFP. The relation between the embedded signal of all M EMG and/or IMU sensors, $\tilde{x}(t) = [\tilde{x}_1(t), \ldots, \tilde{x}_M(t), 1]^T$ (including an offset term) and the LFP signal $y(t)$ was modeled to be linear according to the equation $y(t) = \beta^T \tilde{x}(t) + y^{clean}(t)$, where $y^{clean}(t)$ denotes residual (genuine) LFP activity not explained by EMG or IMU. The $(K \cdot M + 1)$-dimensional vector of regression coefficients $\beta^{OLS} = (\tilde{X}\tilde{X}^T)^{-1}\tilde{X}y^T$ was estimated using ordinary least-squares (OLS) regression, where $\tilde{X} = [\tilde{x}(1), \ldots, \tilde{x}(T)]$, $y = [y(1), \ldots, y(T)]$, and T denoted the number of available paired measurements of EMG/IMU and LFP activity. Using the fitted model, the part of the LFP signal that could be predicted from EMG/IMU was obtained as $\hat{y}(t) = \beta^{OLS^T}\tilde{x}(t)$ [62]. The cleaned LFP signal was then obtained as the residual $y^{clean}(t) = y(t) - \hat{y}(t)$.

Cleaned LFPs were used to compute PSDs, which were compared with those obtained before performing the regression. The reduction in theta-alpha peak power after performing the regression was used as the criterion to assess the degree of contamination of LFPs by head tremor.

Because we were most interested in the theta-alpha band, we also computed the theta-alpha peak power by integrating the LFP–PSDs over a 4 Hz wide band surrounding the patient-specific theta-alpha peak (peak frequency $\pm$ 2 Hz; 4 bins) (i) without regression, (ii) with EMG regression, and (iii) with IMU regression.

2.3.4. Evaluation of Pallido-Muscular Coherence with IMU-Regression

Coherence (COH) is a frequency-domain measure of the linear phase and amplitude relationships between signals. It can reveal spectrally specific functional connectivity, and it is an established method in neuroscience [63].

To investigate whether EMG and IMU carry different information about tremor, we computed COH between LFP and EMG before and after IMU regression. We postulated that the reduction in coherence after IMU regression indicates that EMG and IMU signals would carry to some extent overlapping information. As such, the LFP–EMG coherence would be due to tremor contamination, thus artifactual.

Additionally, we computed (i) LFP–IMU COH without and with IMU regression and (ii) LFP–EMG COH without and with EMG regression.

We computed coherence at frequency f as $COH(X, Y, f) = |S_{XY}(f)|^2./S_{XX}(f)S_{YY}(f)$, where S_{XX}, S_{YY} represent the auto-spectrum of signals X and Y, respectively, and S_{XY} represents the cross-spectrum [57]. Note that, being already normalized, coherence spectra do not require additional normalization for across-patient analysis and do not have a prominent 1/f aperiodic component [42].

2.3.5. Statistical Analysis

Statistically significant differences between (i) LFPs theta-alpha peak power with and without IMU regression, (ii) theta-alpha LFP–IMU COH with and without IMU regression, and (iii) theta-alpha pallido-muscular COH with and without IMU or EMG regression were assessed by means of a matched-pairs Wilcoxon signed rank test with a significance level of 0.05.

Significant values of pallido-muscular COH were determined by statistical comparison with a population of 1000 surrogate COH values in which any COH was destroyed. Surrogate data were obtained by randomly shifting the EMG signal 1000 times by a random offset of at least 2 s before computing the LFP–EMG COH. The significance level was set to 0.05.

3. Results

3.1. Clinical and Demographic Data

All but one patient (DW08) significantly benefited from GPi-DBS. The improvement for this patient was limited by the development of typical GPi-DBS side effects (i.e., bradykinesia). The overall average benefit from GPi-DBS was about 40% (TWSTRS score stim-off: 16.62 ± 3.85 and stim-on: 9.57 ± 4.27, mean ± standard deviation) (Table 1).

3.2. Tremor Contamination of LFP Recordings and Comparison of IMU vs. EMG Regression Analysis

Two patients (DW01 and DW08) showed tremor contamination of the LFP, as suggested by the alignment of the frequency peaks in the PSDs around the head tremor frequency (DW01: f = 4 Hz, DW08: f = 4 Hz) (Figure 2).

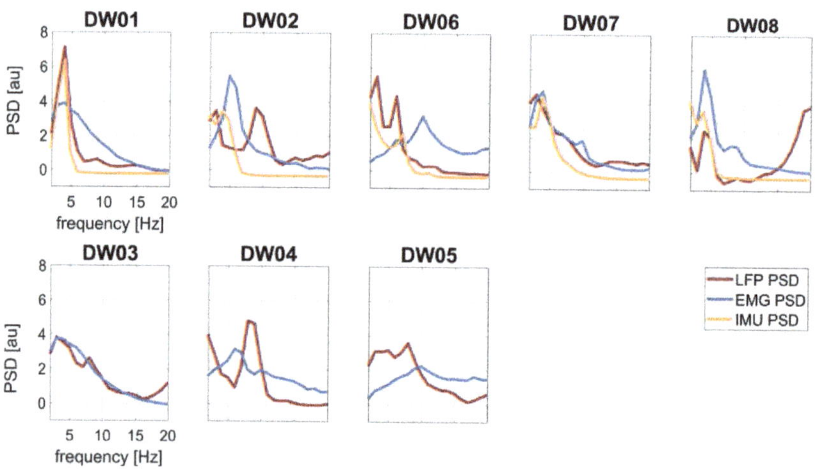

Figure 2. Spectral profiles of the LFP (red line), EMG (blue line), and IMU (yellow line) recordings of all patients. First row: patients with tremor (T+); second row: patients without tremor (T−).

Regression-based removal of IMU signals from LFPs led to power reduction, especially in the theta-alpha band, in all T+ patients (Figure 3). Regression of the EMG signal was instead not affecting LFP theta-alpha peak power except for three patients (DW02, DW06, and DW08) (Figure 3 and Table 2).

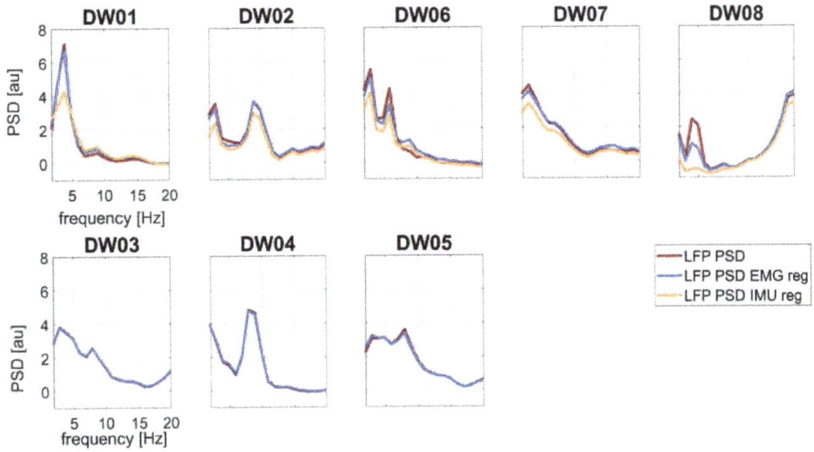

Figure 3. LFP spectral profiles before regression (red line), after EMG regression (blue line), and after IMU regression (yellow line). First row: patients with tremor (T+); second row: patients without tremor (T−). Abbreviation: reg (regression).

Table 2. Columns 2–4: theta-alpha peak power [au] without and with EMG or IMU regression. Differences (Δ) between LFP theta-alpha peak power without and with EMG or IMU regression are shown in brackets. Columns 5–6: averaged theta-alpha pallido-muscular COH without and with IMU regression. The differences (Δ) between LFP and EMG COH without and with IMU regression are shown in brackets. Abbreviations: COH—coherence; EMG—electromyographic recording; IMU—inertial measurement unit recording; LFP—local field potential; reg—regression; NA—not available.

Patient	LFP θ-α Power	LFP θ-α Power EMG Reg (Δ)	LFP θ-α Power IMU Reg (Δ)	LFP-EMG θ-α COH	LFP-EMG θ-α COH—IMU Reg (Δ)
DW01	17.84	17.93 (−0.09)	15.01 (2.83)	0.015	0.008 (0.007)
DW02	8.16	7.03 (1.13)	4.50 (3.66)	0.020	0.007 (0.013)
DW06	14.34	12.85 (1.49)	9.78 (4.56)	0.002	0.002 (0)
DW07	14.56	13.70 (0.86)	10.59 (3.97)	0.007	0.007 (0)
DW08	6.07	2.66 (3.41)	−2.21 (8.28)	0.010	0.002 (0.008)
DW03	16.32	16.22 (0.10)	NA	NA	NA
DW04	11.06	10.88 (0.18)	NA	NA	NA
DW05	7.33	8.00 (0.67)	NA	NA	NA

The LFP theta-alpha peak power of each patient before and after EMG and IMU regression are shown in Table 2. IMU regression reduced the theta-alpha peak power more in comparison to EMG regression. Differences between LFPs theta-alpha peak power with and without IMU regression were statistically significant (4.66 ± 2.12 au (mean ± standard deviation)).

3.3. Pallido-Muscular Coherence after Cleaning

LFP–IMU and LFP–EMG COH profiles are shown in Figure 4. The COH drop after regression analysis was significant for both LFP–IMU COH and LFP–EMG COH.

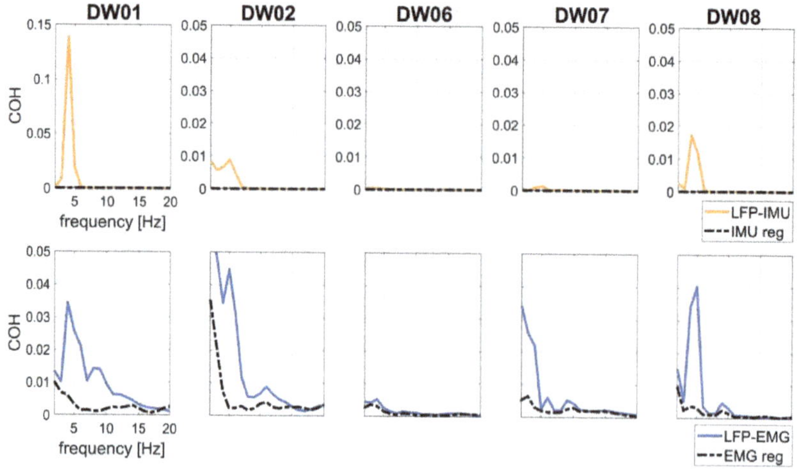

Figure 4. LFP–IMU COH (first row) without (continuous, yellow line) and with (dotted, black line) IMU regression in patients T+. LFP–EMG COH (second row) without (continuous, blue line) and with (dotted, black line) EMG regression in patients T+.

To investigate the effects of tremor-related artifacts on pallido-muscular COH, we computed LFP–EMG COH with and without regressing the IMU out of the LFP signals. LFP–EMG COH before IMU regression was small but significant with respect to shuffled data (Figure 5). IMU regression significantly reduced pallido-muscular COH in all but two subjects (DW06 and DW07) (Table 2 and Figure 5).

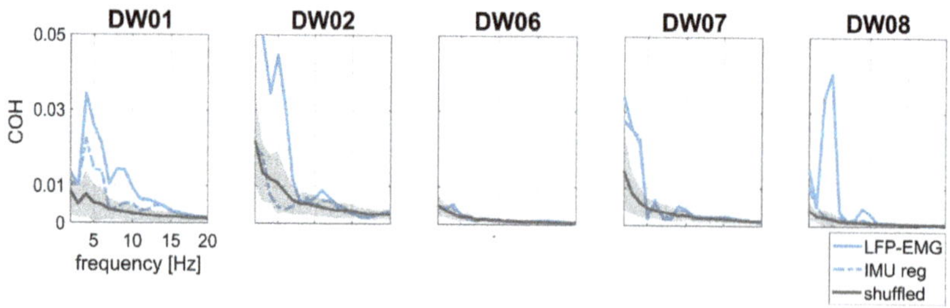

Figure 5. Pallido-muscular COH without (continuous, light blue line) and with (dotted, light blue line) IMU regression. Surrogate data are shown in gray as the mean (continuous line) ±2 standard deviations (shaded area).

3.4. Sensory Trick and Voluntary Rhythmic Movement

In one patient (DW02) with a clinically effective sensory trick (i.e., maneuver alleviating dystonic tremor), we computed the PSD during the sensory trick and voluntary alternating head movements with small and large amplitude. For each condition, we performed the regression of IMU and EMG.

The sensory trick reduced the theta-alpha peak power in the LFP–PSDs as compared to baseline (i.e., dystonic tremor condition) (Figure 6). However, both EMG and IMU detected residual tremor activity (Figure 6), which was effectively removed from LFP–PSDs with IMU regression. Of note, the PSDs of the IMU and LFP do not show an aligned peak (Figure 6), thus suggesting that LFPs manifest harmonics of the artifactual frequency.

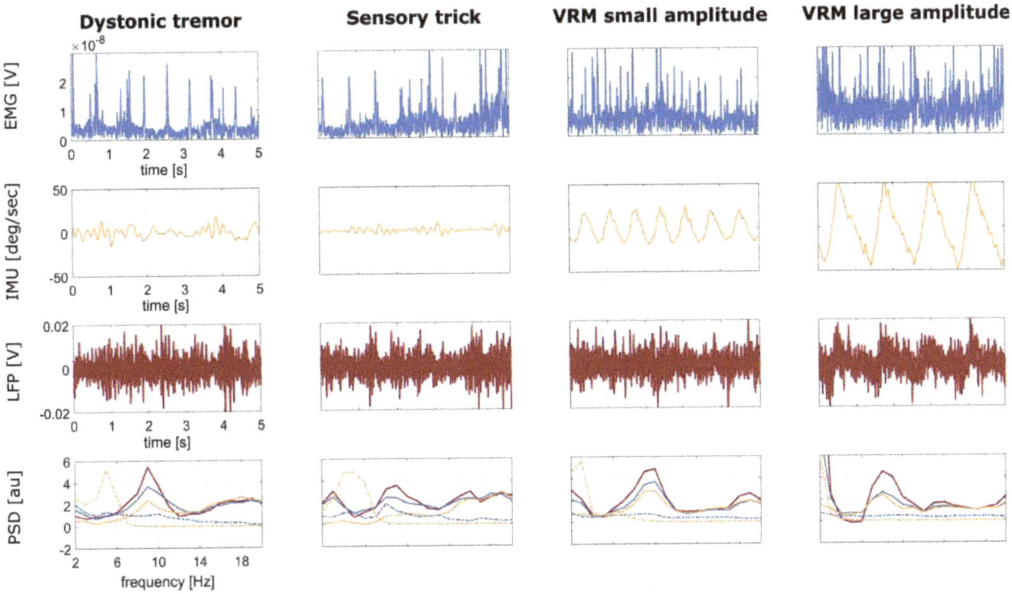

Figure 6. Patient DW02: time series of 5 s recordings at rest (first column), while performing the sensory trick (second column), during voluntary alternating rhythmic movement of the head with small amplitude (third column), and with large amplitude (fourth column), of the right sternocleidomastoid EMG (first row), IMU (second row), and LFP (third row) without regression. IMU and LFP time series were averaged over channels, i.e., over the three axes (x, y, z) and over the six contact pairs (0–3, 0–2, 1–3 left and right), respectively. The corresponding PSDs are shown in the fourth row: LFP without regression (continuous red line), LFP with EMG regression (continuous blue line), LFP with IMU regression (continuous yellow line), EMG (dotted blue line), and IMU (dotted yellow line). Abbreviations: VRM—voluntary rhythmic movement.

When looking at voluntary movements, LFP–PSDs showed movement-related artifacts at the head oscillation frequency (Figure 6).

4. Discussion

New DBS devices with sensing capabilities open new opportunities to improve the clinical effectiveness of DBS by optimizing stimulation parameters in response to an input signal representing symptoms, motor activity, or other behavioral characteristics [40]. Pallidal theta-alpha oscillatory activity is a promising biomarker for dystonia [45] and for future therapeutic development [46], such as improving efficacy and the timing of the therapeutic response while reducing side effects and battery consumption.

Our results show that the Percept PC is capable of recording low-frequency oscillations in chronically stimulated patients with CD but also confirm a spectral contamination due to movement artifacts (voluntary and pathological) [46].

Already, a visual inspection of the PSDs suggested artifact contamination in two subjects with dystonic tremor, with GPi-LFPs and both EMG and IMU PSDs exhibiting spectral peaks at the tremor frequency (Figure 2). When applying the IMU regression, all T+ subjects showed a reduction in power, indicating a tremor-related contamination of the raw GPi-LFP signals (Figure 3).

In our study, we showed that IMU regression was superior to EMG regression in removing the tremor-related artifact from the GPi-LFPs (Figure 3). This difference in effectiveness may be due to the greater capacity of IMUs to record a composite and irregular tremor such as dystonic tremor more distinctly [64]. Furthermore, EMG signals can be affected by skin conductance and probe placement, two aspects that increase intra- and inter-subject variability. However, we made sure that all EMG probes were adherent to the skin and placed near the bellies of selected muscles. Before electrode placement, the skin was cleaned with alcohol.

It should be noted that the EMG signal carries more information than just the kinematic (and artifactual) component of tremor, such as cross-talk from different muscles or a pathological dystonic activity [65]. To evaluate this issue, we computed pallido-muscular COH to estimate the information carried by IMU and EMG signals. After IMU regression, we observed a decrease in LFP–EMG COH at the tremor frequency in three out of five subjects (Figure 5), thus supporting the idea, in our case, of an artifactual origin of theta-alpha pallido-muscular COH.

Finally, we tested IMU and EMG-based multiple regression under different conditions, namely voluntary rhythmic head movement of small and large amplitude. This additional evaluation was performed only on the patient who showed a clinically effective sensory trick, a maneuver able to reduce tremor severity (Figure 6). We showed that both IMU and EMG regressions were effective in capturing voluntary head movements and led to a correction of GPi-LFPs proportional to the movement's amplitude. Averna et al. [66] also showed a drastic increase in the theta frequency range during neck tilting and upper limb movement. This might refer to the higher susceptibility of some implants to contamination. Moreover, IMU regression captured the residual tremor activity present during the sensory trick maneuver that was not clinically visible. The sensory trick did not affect the rhythmic spiking of the EMG, as expected [53,67], but EMG regression led to a marginal correction of GPi-LFPs (Figure 6).

This study has some limitations. First, the limited number of patients reduced the number of recordings that were available for our analysis. Considering the low prevalence of the disease (16.3 per 100,000 [68]), the limited number of dystonic patients implanted with DBS [69], and the recent release of the Percept PC device on the market (2020), the sample size is still considerable and comparable with previous studies on dystonia [45,70]. The same limiting factors prevented the recruitment of patients with similar clinical presentations. However, we do not expect clinical features other than tremor to be relevant for the technical aims of the current work. Second, we used relatively short recordings, with lengths ranging from one to four minutes. Nevertheless, this was considered sufficient to calculate power and coherence measurements, as Popov et al. have observed good to excellent test-retest reliability of resting-state power and coherence in a large sample based on recordings that were just 100 s long [71]. Potential biases of coherence on recording length [72] were not addressed here, as all statistical comparisons were performed within subjects on data of the same length. Third, we could not record and compare tremor-free GPi-LFP recordings for the same patients. Nevertheless, we documented the performance of IMU regression in one patient with a clinically effective sensory trick. Lastly, the observed theta-alpha power reduction is not sufficient proof of the cleaning efficacy. It represents the neural activity after removal of the component that is coherent with the head tremor, which appears to introduce artifactual spectral content in this low frequency range. Although a possible desynchronization of a genuine neural component associated with tremor cannot be ruled out, this interpretation is less likely because, to the best of our knowledge, dystonic tremor has not been associated with any oscillatory activity of the LFPs to date [47].

5. Conclusions

LFP-based biomarker detection will become standard in clinical practice, thus enabling better understanding and monitoring of distinctive neural signatures associated with specific symptoms or behaviors. Pallidal theta-alpha oscillations may be critical for understanding the pathophysiology of dystonia. They could act as a useful biomarker not only for programming stimulation parameters but also for adaptive DBS. However, critical use of newly available technologies is necessary to address possible drawbacks. Our work suggests caution when considering LFP recordings, as they may be susceptible to contamination by movement artifacts. This is particularly the case for head tremor in dystonia but also applies to patients with repetitive involuntary movements such as essential tremor, Tourette syndrome, or Parkinson's disease. Neglecting this contamination can lead to misinterpretation or hiding significant findings. We here provide methodological guidance on how to clean LFP recordings from head tremor artifacts. Regressing out head motions concurrently recorded with IMU might substantially alleviate LFP contamination and facilitate the neurophysiological interpretation of LFP analyses.

Author Contributions: Conceptualization, J.D.V.D.V., I.U.I., S.H. and C.P.; methodology, J.D.V.D.V., S.H. and C.P.; software, J.D.V.D.V. and S.H.; validation, J.D.V.D.V. and I.H.; formal analysis, J.D.V.D.V. and C.P.; investigation, J.D.V.D.V., I.H., N.G.P., P.C., I.U.I. and C.P.; resources, I.U.I.; data curation, N.G.P., I.H. and P.C.; writing—original draft preparation, J.D.V.D.V., I.H. and N.G.P. writing—review and editing, P.C., I.U.I., S.H. and C.P.; visualization, J.D.V.D.V. and C.P.; supervision, I.U.I., S.H. and C.P.; project administration, I.U.I. and C.P.; funding acquisition, I.U.I. All authors have read and agreed to the published version of the manuscript.

Funding: The study was sponsored by the Deutsche Forschungsgemeinschaft (DFG, German Research Foundation)—Project-ID 424778381-TRR 295 and the Fondazione Grigioni per il Morbo di Parkinson. IUI was supported by a grant from the New York University School of Medicine and The Marlene and Paolo Fresco Institute for Parkinson's and Movement Disorders, which was made possible with support from Marlene and Paolo Fresco. This publication was supported by the Open Access Publication Fund of the University of Würzburg. J.D.V.D.V. and I.H. received financial support from the Graduate School of Life Sciences, University of Würzburg. I.H. was supported by a scholarship from the German Academic Exchange Service (DAAD; Deutscher Akademischer Austauschdienst). S.H. received funding from the European Research Council (ERC) under the European Union's Horizon 2020 research and innovation program (Grant agreement No. 758985).

Institutional Review Board Statement: The study was conducted in accordance with the Declaration of Helsinki and approved by the Ethical Committee of the University Hospital Würzburg (n. 20230120 01).

Informed Consent Statement: Written informed consent was obtained from the patients to publish this paper.

Data Availability Statement: The data presented in this study are available upon request. The data are not publicly available due to privacy reasons. Inquiries can be filed to the corresponding author (Jasmin Del Vecchio Del Vecchio, University Hospital Würzburg, Department of Neurology; Josef-Schneider-Straße 11, 97080 Würzburg; phone: +49-(0)931/201-23605; fax: +49-(0)931/201-24901; E-Mail: delvecchio_j@ukw.de).

Acknowledgments: The authors would like to thank P. Fricke, C. Matthies and R. Nickl for the neurosurgical information and J. Volkmann for the valuable comments.

Conflicts of Interest: J.D.V.D.V., I.H., N.G.P., P.C., I.U.I., S.H. and C.P. declare no conflicts of interest related to this study. The Percept PC (Medtronic, PLC) and the related hardware and software for programming and readout are commercially available. The companies had no impact on study design, patient selection, data analysis, or reporting of the results.

References

1. Albanese, A.; Bhatia, K.; Bressman, S.B.; DeLong, M.R.; Fahn, S.; Fung, V.S.C.; Hallett, M.; Jankovic, J.; Jinnah, H.A.; Klein, C.; et al. Phenomenology and Classification of Dystonia: A Consensus Update: Dystonia: Phenomenology and Classification. *Mov. Disord.* **2013**, *28*, 863–873. [CrossRef] [PubMed]
2. Pandey, S.; Sarma, N. Tremor in dystonia. *Park. Relat. Disord.* **2016**, *29*, 3–9. [CrossRef] [PubMed]
3. Shaikh, A.G.; Beylergil, S.B.; Scorr, L.; Kilic-Berkmen, G.; Freeman, A.; Klein, C.; Junker, J.; Loens, S.; Brüggemann, N.; Münchau, A.; et al. Dystonia and Tremor. *Neurology* **2021**, *96*, e563–e574. [CrossRef] [PubMed]
4. Bhatia, K.P.; Bain, P.; Bajaj, N.; Elble, R.J.; Hallett, M.; Louis, E.D.; Raethjen, J.; Stamelou, M.; Testa, C.M.; Deuschl, G.; et al. Consensus Statement on the classification of tremors. from the task force on tremor of the International Parkinson and Movement Disorder Society: IPMDS Task Force on Tremor Consensus Statement. *Mov. Disord.* **2018**, *33*, 75–87. [CrossRef]
5. Defazio, G.; Conte, A.; Gigante, A.F.; Fabbrini, G.; Berardelli, A. Is tremor in dystonia a phenotypic feature of dystonia? *Neurology* **2015**, *84*, 1053. [CrossRef]
6. Panyakaew, P.; Cho, H.J.; Lee, S.W.; Wu, T.; Hallett, M. The Pathophysiology of Dystonic Tremors and Comparison With Essential Tremor. *J. Neurosci. Off. J. Soc. Neurosci.* **2020**, *40*, 9317–9326. [CrossRef]

7. Hallett, M. Neurophysiology of dystonia: The role of inhibition. *Neurobiol. Dis.* **2011**, *42*, 177–184. [CrossRef]
8. Atkinson-Clement, C.; Pinto, S.; Eusebio, A.; Coulon, O. Diffusion tensor imaging in Parkinson's disease: Review and meta-analysis. *Neuroimage Clin.* **2017**, *16*, 98–110. [CrossRef]
9. Quartarone, A.; Ruge, D. How Many Types of Dystonia? Pathophysiological Considerations. *Front. Neurol.* **2018**, *9*, 12. [CrossRef] [PubMed]
10. Münchau, A.; Schrag, A.; Chuang, C.; MacKinnon, C.D.; Bhatia, K.P.; Quinn, N.P.; Rothwell, J.C. Arm tremor in cervical dystonia differs from essential tremor and can be classified by onset age and spread of symptoms. *Brain J. Neurol.* **2001**, *124*, 1765–1776. [CrossRef]
11. Tinazzi, M.; Fasano, A.; Di Matteo, A.; Conte, A.; Bove, F.; Bovi, T.; Peretti, A.; Defazio, G.; Fiorio, M.; Berardelli, A. Temporal discrimination in patients with dystonia and tremor and patients with essential tremor. *Neurology* **2013**, *80*, 76. [CrossRef]
12. Conte, A.; Ferrazzano, G.; Belvisi, D.; Manzo, N.; Battista, E.; Voti, P.L.; Nardella, A.; Fabbrini, G.; Berardelli, A. Somatosensory temporal discrimination in Parkinson's disease, dystonia and essential tremor: Pathophysiological and clinical implications. *Clin. Neurophysiol.* **2018**, *129*, 1849–1853. [CrossRef] [PubMed]
13. Cerasa, A.; Nisticò, R.; Salsone, M.; Bono, F.; Salvino, D.; Morelli, M.; Arabia, G.; Quattrone, A. Neuroanatomical correlates of dystonic tremor: A cross-sectional study. *Park. Relat. Disord.* **2014**, *20*, 314–317. [CrossRef]
14. Kirke, D.N.; Battistella, G.; Kumar, V.; Rubien-Thomas, E.; Choy, M.; Rumbach, A.; Simonyan, K. Neural correlates of dystonic tremor: A multimodal study of voice tremor in spasmodic dysphonia. *Brain Imaging Behav.* **2017**, *11*, 166–175. [CrossRef]
15. Madelein van der Stouwe, A.M.; Nieuwhof, F.; Helmich, R.C. Tremor pathophysiology: Lessons from neuroimaging. *Curr. Opin. Neurol.* **2020**, *33*, 474–481. [CrossRef] [PubMed]
16. Tsuboi, T.; Wong, J.K.; Eisinger, R.S.; Okromelidze, L.; Burns, M.R.; Ramirez-Zamora, A.; Almeida, L.; Wagle Shukla, A.; Foote, K.D.; Okun, M.S.; et al. Comparative connectivity correlates of dystonic and essential tremor deep brain stimulation. *Brain* **2021**, *144*, 1774–1786. [CrossRef] [PubMed]
17. Nieuwhof, F.; Panyakaew, P.; van de Warrenburg, B.P.; Gallea, C.; Helmich, R.C. The patchy tremor landscape: Recent advances in pathophysiology. *Curr. Opin. Neurol.* **2018**, *31*, 455–461. [CrossRef] [PubMed]
18. Panyakaew, P.; Jinnah, H.A.; Shaikh, A.G. Clinical features, pathophysiology, treatment, and controversies of tremor in dystonia. *J. Neurol. Sci.* **2022**, *435*, 120199. [CrossRef]
19. DeSimone, J.C.; Archer, D.B.; Vaillancourt, D.E.; Wagle Shukla, A. Network-level connectivity is a critical feature distinguishing dystonic tremor and essential tremor. *Brain* **2019**, *142*, 1644–1659. [CrossRef]
20. van den Berg, K.R.E.; Helmich, R.C. The Role of the Cerebellum in Tremor–Evidence from Neuroimaging. *Tremor Hyperkinetic Mov.* **2021**, *11*, 49. [CrossRef]
21. Ma, H.; Chen, H.; Fang, J.; Gao, L.; Ma, L.; Wu, T.; Hou, Y.; Zhang, J.; Feng, T. Resting-state functional connectivity of dentate nucleus is associated with tremor in Parkinson's disease. *J. Neurol.* **2015**, *262*, 2247–2256. [CrossRef]
22. Battaglia, S.; Thayer, J.F. Functional interplay between central and autonomic nervous systems in human fear conditioning. *Trends Neurosci.* **2022**, *45*, 504–506. [CrossRef]
23. Ippolito, G.; Bertaccini, R.; Tarasi, L.; Di Gregorio, F.; Trajkovic, J.; Battaglia, S.; Romei, V. The Role of Alpha Oscillations among the Main Neuropsychiatric Disorders in the Adult and Developing Human Brain: Evidence from the Last 10 Years of Research. *Biomedicines* **2022**, *10*, 3189. [CrossRef] [PubMed]
24. Alongi, P.; Iaccarino, L.; Perani, D. PET Neuroimaging: Insights on Dystonia and Tourette Syndrome and Potential Applications. *Front. Neurol.* **2014**, *5*, 183. [CrossRef] [PubMed]
25. Poston, K.L.; Eidelberg, D. Functional brain networks and abnormal connectivity in the movement disorders. *NeuroImage* **2012**, *62*, 2261–2270. [CrossRef]
26. Lehéricy, S.; Tijssen, M.A.J.; Vidailhet, M.; Kaji, R.; Meunier, S. The anatomical basis of dystonia: Current view using neuroimaging. *Mov. Disord.* **2013**, *28*, 944–957. [CrossRef] [PubMed]
27. Carbon, M.; Argyelan, M.; Eidelberg, D. Functional imaging in hereditary dystonia. *Eur. J. Neurol.* **2010**, *17*, 58–64. [CrossRef]
28. Merola, A.; Dwivedi, A.K.; Shaikh, A.G.; Tareen, T.K.; Da Prat, G.A.; Kauffman, M.A.; Hampf, J.; Mahajan, A.; Marsili, L.; Jankovic, J.; et al. Head tremor at disease onset: An ataxic phenotype of cervical dystonia. *J. Neurol.* **2019**, *266*, 1844–1851. [CrossRef]
29. Prudente, C.N.; Stilla, R.; Singh, S.; Buetefisch, C.; Evatt, M.; Factor, S.A.; Freeman, A.; Hu, X.P.; Hess, E.J.; Sathian, K.; et al. A Functional Magnetic Resonance Imaging Study of Head Movements in Cervical Dystonia. *Front. Neurol.* **2016**, *7*, 201. [CrossRef]
30. Filip, P.; Gallea, C.; Lehéricy, S.; Bertasi, E.; Popa, T.; Mareček, R.; Lungu, O.V.; Kašpárek, T.; Vaníček, J.; Bareš, M. Disruption in cerebellar and basal ganglia networks during a visuospatial task in cervical dystonia. *Mov. Disord.* **2017**, *32*, 757–768. [CrossRef]
31. Tsuboi, T.; Jabarkheel, Z.; Foote, K.D.; Okun, M.S.; Wagle Shukla, A. Importance of the initial response to GPi deep brain stimulation in dystonia: A nine year quality of life study. *Park. Relat. Disord.* **2019**, *64*, 249–255. [CrossRef] [PubMed]
32. Sedov, A.; Usova, S.; Semenova, U.; Gamaleya, A.; Tomskiy, A.; Beylergil, S.B.; Jinnah, H.A.; Shaikh, A.G. Pallidal Activity in Cervical Dystonia with and Without Head Tremor. *Cerebellum Lond. Engl.* **2020**, *19*, 409–418. [CrossRef]
33. Kiss, Z.H.T.; Doig-Beyaert, K.; Eliasziw, M.; Tsui, J.; Haffenden, A.; Suchowersky, O. The Canadian multicentre study of deep brain stimulation for cervical dystonia. *Brain* **2007**, *130*, 2879–2886. [CrossRef]
34. Volkmann, J.; Wolters, A.; Kupsch, A.; Müller, J.; Kühn, A.A.; Schneider, G.-H.; Poewe, W.; Hering, S.; Eisner, W.; Müller, J.-U.; et al. Pallidal deep brain stimulation in patients with primary generalised or segmental dystonia: 5-year follow-up of a randomised trial. *Lancet Neurol.* **2012**, *11*, 1029–1038. [CrossRef]

35. Isaias, I.U.; Alterman, R.L.; Tagliati, M. Deep Brain Stimulation for Primary Generalized Dystonia: Long-term Outcomes. *Arch. Neurol.* **2009**, *66*, 465–470. [CrossRef] [PubMed]
36. Kaelin-Lang, A.; You, H.; Burgunder, J.-M.; Lönnfors-Weitze, T.; Loher, T.J.; Taub, E.; Isaias, I.U.; Krauss, J.K.; Michael Schüpbach, W.M. Bilateral pallidal stimulation improves cervical dystonia for more than a decade. *Park. Relat. Disord.* **2020**, *81*, 78–81. [CrossRef]
37. Tisch, S. Deep brain stimulation in dystonia: Factors contributing to variability in outcome in short and long term follow-up. *Curr. Opin. Neurol.* **2022**, *35*, 510–517. [CrossRef]
38. Isaias, I.U.; Volkmann, J.; Kupsch, A.; Burgunder, J.-M.; Ostrem, J.L.; Alterman, R.L.; Mehdorn, H.M.; Sch?necker, T.; Krauss, J.K.; Starr, P.; et al. Factors predicting protracted improvement after pallidal DBS for primary dystonia: The role of age and disease duration. *J. Neurol.* **2011**, *258*, 1469–1476. [CrossRef] [PubMed]
39. Reich, M.M.; Horn, A.; Lange, F.; Roothans, J.; Paschen, S.; Runge, J.; Wodarg, F.; Pozzi, N.G.; Witt, K.; Nickl, R.C.; et al. Probabilistic mapping of the antidystonic effect of pallidal neurostimulation: A multicentre imaging study. *Brain* **2019**, *142*, 1386–1398. [CrossRef]
40. Vissani, M.; Isaias, I.U.; Mazzoni, A. Deep brain stimulation: A review of the open neural engineering challenges. *J. Neural Eng.* **2020**, *17*, 051002. [CrossRef] [PubMed]
41. Pozzi, N.G.; Isaias, I.U. Adaptive deep brain stimulation: Retuning Parkinson's disease. *Handb. Clin. Neurol.* **2022**, *184*, 273–284.
42. Neumann, W.; Horn, A.; Ewert, S.; Huebl, J.; Brücke, C.; Slentz, C.; Schneider, G.; Kühn, A.A. A localized pallidal physiomarker in cervical dystonia. *Ann. Neurol.* **2017**, *82*, 912–924. [CrossRef] [PubMed]
43. Piña-Fuentes, D.; van Dijk, J.M.C.; Drost, G.; van Zijl, J.C.; van Laar, T.; Tijssen, M.A.J.; Beudel, M. Direct comparison of oscillatory activity in the motor system of Parkinson's disease and dystonia: A review of the literature and meta-analysis. *Clin. Neurophysiol.* **2019**, *130*, 917–924. [CrossRef] [PubMed]
44. Zhu, G.-Y.; Zhang, R.-L.; Chen, Y.-C.; Liu, Y.-Y.; Liu, D.-F.; Wang, S.-Y.; Jiang, Y.; Zhang, J.-G. Characteristics of globus pallidus internus local field potentials in generalized dystonia patients with TWNK mutation. *Clin. Neurophysiol.* **2020**, *131*, 1453–1461. [CrossRef]
45. Piña-Fuentes, D.; Beudel, M.; Van Zijl, J.C.; Van Egmond, M.E.; Oterdoom, D.L.M.; Van Dijk, J.M.C.; Tijssen, M.A.J. Low-frequency oscillation suppression in dystonia: Implications for adaptive deep brain stimulation. *Park. Relat. Disord.* **2020**, *79*, 105–109. [CrossRef]
46. Thenaisie, Y.; Palmisano, C.; Canessa, A.; Keulen, B.J.; Capetian, P.; Jiménez, M.C.; Bally, J.F.; Manferlotti, E.; Beccaria, L.; Zutt, R.; et al. Towards adaptive deep brain stimulation: Clinical and technical notes on a novel commercial device for chronic brain sensing. *J. Neural Eng.* **2021**, *18*, 042002. [CrossRef] [PubMed]
47. Sirica, D.; Hewitt, A.L.; Tarolli, C.G.; Weber, M.T.; Zimmerman, C.; Santiago, A.; Wensel, A.; Mink, J.W.; Lizárraga, K.J. Neurophysiological biomarkers to optimize deep brain stimulation in movement disorders. *Neurodegener. Dis. Manag.* **2021**, *11*, 315–328. [CrossRef] [PubMed]
48. Hess, C.W.; Pullman, S.L. Tremor: Clinical Phenomenology and Assessment Techniques. *Tremor Hyperkinetic Mov.* **2012**, *2*, 02. [CrossRef]
49. Lalli, S.; Albanese, A. Dystonic Tremor. In *Mechanisms and Emerging Therapies in Tremor Disorders*; Grimaldi, G., Manto, M., Eds.; Springer: New York, NY, USA, 2013; pp. 203–218. ISBN 978-1-4614-4026-0.
50. Volkmann, J.; Mueller, J.; Deuschl, G.; Kühn, A.A.; Krauss, J.K.; Poewe, W.; Timmermann, L.; Falk, D.; Kupsch, A.; Kivi, A.; et al. Pallidal neurostimulation in patients with medication-refractory cervical dystonia: A randomised, sham-controlled trial. *Lancet Neurol* **2014**, *13*, 875–884. [CrossRef] [PubMed]
51. Jost, W.H.; Hefter, H.; Stenner, A.; Reichel, G. Rating scales for cervical dystonia: A critical evaluation of tools for outcome assessment of botulinum toxin therapy. *J. Neural Transm. Vienna Austria 1996* **2013**, *120*, 487–496. [CrossRef]
52. Boyce, M.J.; Canning, C.G.; Mahant, N.; Morris, J.; Latimer, J.; Fung, V.S.C. The Toronto Western Spasmodic Torticollis Rating Scale: Reliability in neurologists and physiotherapists. *Park. Relat. Disord.* **2012**, *18*, 635–637. [CrossRef] [PubMed]
53. Masuhr, F.; Wissel, J.; Müller, J.; Scholz, U.; Poewe, W. Quantification of sensory trick impact on tremor amplitude and frequency in 60 patients with head tremor. *Mov. Disord.* **2001**, *15*, 960–964. [CrossRef]
54. Deuschl, G.; Heinen, F.; Kleedorfer, B.; Wagner, M.; Lücking, C.H.; Poewe, W. Clinical and polymyographic investigation of spasmodic torticollis. *J. Neurol.* **1992**, *239*, 9–15. [CrossRef] [PubMed]
55. Canessa, A.; Palmisano, C.; Isaias, I.U.; Mazzoni, A. Gait-related frequency modulation of beta oscillatory activity in the subthalamic nucleus of parkinsonian patients. *Brain Stimul.* **2020**, *13*, 1743–1752. [CrossRef] [PubMed]
56. Canessa, A.; Pozzi, N.G.; Arnulfo, G.; Brumberg, J.; Reich, M.M.; Pezzoli, G.; Ghilardi, M.F.; Matthies, C.; Steigerwald, F.; Volkmann, J.; et al. Striatal Dopaminergic Innervation Regulates Subthalamic Beta-Oscillations and Cortical-Subcortical Coupling during Movements: Preliminary Evidence in Subjects with Parkinson's Disease. *Front. Hum. Neurosci.* **2016**, *10*, 611. [CrossRef]
57. Arnulfo, G.; Pozzi, N.G.; Palmisano, C.; Leporini, A.; Canessa, A.; Brumberg, J.; Pezzoli, G.; Matthies, C.; Volkmann, J.; Isaias, I.U. Phase matters: A role for the subthalamic network during gait. *PLoS ONE* **2018**, *13*, e0198691. [CrossRef] [PubMed]
58. Neumann, W.-J.; Memarian Sorkhabi, M.; Benjaber, M.; Feldmann, L.K.; Saryyeva, A.; Krauss, J.K.; Contarino, M.F.; Sieger, T.; Jech, R.; Tinkhauser, G.; et al. The sensitivity of ECG contamination to surgical implantation site in brain computer interfaces. *Brain Stimul.* **2021**, *14*, 1301–1306. [CrossRef] [PubMed]

59. Donoghue, T.; Haller, M.; Peterson, E.J.; Varma, P.; Sebastian, P.; Gao, R.; Noto, T.; Lara, A.H.; Wallis, J.D.; Knight, R.T.; et al. Parameterizing Neural Power Spectra into Periodic and Aperiodic Components. *Nat. Neurosci.* **2020**, *23*, 1655–1665. [CrossRef]
60. Barow, E.; Neumann, W.J.; Brücke, C.; Huebl, J.; Horn, A.; Brown, P.; Krauss, J.K.; Schneider, G.H.; Kühn, A.A. Deep brain stimulation suppresses pallidal low frequency activity in patients with phasic dystonic movements. *Brain* **2014**, *137*, 3012–3024. [CrossRef]
61. Sharott, A.; Grosse, P.; Kühn, A.A.; Salih, F.; Engel, A.K.; Kupsch, A.; Schneider, G.H.; Krauss, J.K.; Brown, P. Is the synchronization between pallidal and muscle activity in primary dystonia due to peripheral afferance or a motor drive? *Brain* **2008**, *131*, 473–484. [CrossRef]
62. Haufe, S.; Isaias, I.; Pellegrini, F.; Palmisano, C. Gait event prediction from surface electromyography in parkinsonian patients. *medRxiv* **2023**. [CrossRef]
63. Schnitzler, A.; Gross, J. Normal and pathological oscillatory communication in the brain. *Nat. Rev. Neurosci.* **2005**, *6*, 285–296. [CrossRef] [PubMed]
64. Shaikh, A.G.; Jinnah, H.A.; Tripp, R.M.; Optican, L.M.; Ramat, S.; Lenz, F.A.; Zee, D.S. Irregularity distinguishes limb tremor in cervical dystonia from essential tremor. *J. Neurol. Neurosurg. Psychiatry* **2008**, *79*, 187–189. [CrossRef] [PubMed]
65. Chen, C.C.; Kühn, A.A.; Hoffmann, K.T.; Kupsch, A.; Schneider, G.H.; Trottenberg, T.; Krauss, J.K.; Wöhrle, J.C.; Bardinet, E.; Yelnik, J.; et al. Oscillatory pallidal local field potential activity correlates with involuntary EMG in dystonia. *Neurology* **2006**, *66*, 418–420. [CrossRef]
66. Averna, A.; Arlotti, M.; Rosa, M.; Chabardès, S.; Seigneuret, E.; Priori, A.; Moro, E.; Meoni, S. Pallidal and Cortical Oscillations in Freely Moving Patients With Dystonia. *Neuromodulation Technol. Neural Interface* **2022**, S1094715922000162. [CrossRef] [PubMed]
67. Schramm, A.; Reiners, K.; Naumann, M. Complex mechanisms of sensory tricks in cervical dystonia. *Mov. Disord.* **2004**, *19*, 452–458. [CrossRef] [PubMed]
68. Steeves, T.D.; Day, L.; Dykeman, J.; Jette, N.; Pringsheim, T. The prevalence of primary dystonia: A systematic review and meta-analysis. *Mov. Disord. Off. J. Mov. Disord. Soc.* **2012**, *27*, 1789–1796. [CrossRef]
69. Ortiz, R.M.; Scheperjans, F.; Pekkonen, E. Deep brain stimulation for dystonia in Finland during 2007–2016. *BMC Neurol.* **2019**, *19*, 137. [CrossRef]
70. Scheller, U.; Lofredi, R.; Wijk, B.C.M.; Saryyeva, A.; Krauss, J.K.; Schneider, G.; Kroneberg, D.; Krause, P.; Neumann, W.; Kühn, A.A. Pallidal low-frequency activity in dystonia after cessation of long-term deep brain stimulation. *Mov. Disord.* **2019**, *34*, 1734–1739. [CrossRef]
71. Popov, T.; Tröndle, M.; Baranczuk, Z.; Pfeiffer, C.; Haufe, S.; Langer, N. Test–retest reliability of resting-state EEG in young and older adults. *Psychophysiology* **2023**, e14268. [CrossRef]
72. Pellegrini, F.; Delorme, A.; Nikulin, V.; Haufe, S. Identifying best practices for detecting inter-regional functional connectivity from EEG. *bioRxiv* **2022**. [CrossRef]

bioengineering

MDPI

Article

A Comparison of Inertial Measurement Units and Overnight Videography to Assess Sleep Biomechanics

Nicholas Buckley [1,2,*], Paul Davey [1], Lynn Jensen [3], Kevin Baptist [4], Angela Jacques [5], Bas Jansen [4], Amity Campbell [1] and Jenny Downs [1,2]

1 Curtin School of Allied Health, Curtin University, Perth 6102, Australia
2 Telethon Kids Institute, Perth 6009, Australia
3 Physiotherapy Department, Perth Children's Hospital, Perth 6009, Australia
4 Ace Therapy Services, Perth 6021, Australia
5 Institute for Health Research, University of Notre Dame Australia, Fremantle 6160, Australia
* Correspondence: nicholas.buckley@telethonkids.org.au; Tel.: +61-0421183721

Abstract: Purpose: The assessment of sleep biomechanics (comprising movement and position during sleep) is of interest in a wide variety of clinical and research settings. However, there is no standard method by which sleep biomechanics are measured. This study aimed to (1) compare the intra- and inter-rater reliability of the current clinical standard, manually coded overnight videography, and (2) compare sleep position recorded using overnight videography to sleep position recorded using the XSENS DOT wearable sensor platform. Methods: Ten healthy adult volunteers slept for one night with XSENS DOT units in situ (on their chest, pelvis, and left and right thighs), with three infrared video cameras recording concurrently. Ten clips per participant were edited from the video. Sleeping position in each clip was coded by six experienced allied health professionals using the novel Body Orientation During Sleep (BODS) Framework, comprising 12 sections in a 360-degree circle. Intra-rater reliability was assessed by calculating the differences between the BODS ratings from repeated clips and the percentage who were rated with a maximum of one section of the XSENS DOT value; the same methodology was used to establish the level of agreement between the XSENS DOT and allied health professional ratings of overnight videography. Bennett's S-Score was used to assess inter-rater reliability. Results: High intra-rater reliability (90% of ratings with maximum difference of one section) and moderate inter-rater reliability (Bennett's S-Score 0.466 to 0.632) were demonstrated in the BODS ratings. The raters demonstrated high levels of agreement overall with the XSENS DOT platform, with 90% of ratings from allied health raters being within the range of at least 1 section of the BODS (as compared to the corresponding XSENS DOT produced rating). Conclusions: The current clinical standard for assessing sleep biomechanics, manually rated overnight videography (as rated using the BODS Framework) demonstrated acceptable intra- and inter-rater reliability. Further, the XSENS DOT platform demonstrated satisfactory levels of agreement as compared to the current clinical standard, providing confidence for its use in future studies of sleep biomechanics.

Keywords: overnight videography; XSENS DOTs; sleep biomechanics

1. Introduction

The assessment of movement and position during sleep (collectively, sleep biomechanics) is of clinical utility in a wide variety of conditions, including Obstructive Sleep Apnoea [1] and Parkinson's Disease [2]. Assessment of sleep biomechanics is of particular relevance to those with neurodisability, as insufficient overnight repositioning has long been suspected as contributing to the development of body shape distortion. First proposed by Fulford and Brown [3], the theory posits that those with severe physical disability (such as individuals with cerebral palsy, Gross Motor Function Classification System [4] levels IV and V) are less able to vary their position throughout the night through movement (typically by rolling over), and so spend more time in fewer positions compared to their typically developing peers [5]. This lack of positional variation results in uneven exposure to gravity, causing bone and connective tissues to be laid down asymmetrically [6]. Resulting body shape distortions (primarily presenting in cerebral palsy as scoliosis, pelvic obliquity, hip migration and chest wall deformity [7]) have negative health impacts, including pain, [8] impairment of respiratory function [9], sleep disturbance [10] and overall loss of function [11]. However, confirmatory evidence of this proposed difference in sleep biomechanics and the inability to reposition between people with severe physical disability and the general population is lacking. There are two main reasons: (1) an absence of an accepted data capture tool, and (2) no standard format to report sleep biomechanics.

There is no commonly accepted methodology for capturing sleep biomechanics data. Particular attention has been paid to sleep position; studies that have examined sleep position are methodologically diverse, with a variety of methods such as videography [12], pressure sensors [13] and wearable accelerometers [14] being used, rendering a synthesis of findings difficult. The current standard clinical assessment of sleep position is overnight infrared videography (typically, recorded video footage from a single camera angle), that is then visually inspected and coded by a clinician (typically, as supine/prone/left side lying/right side lying [15]). For example, Cary et al. investigated the relationship between sleep postures and lower back pain in adult participants, utilizing infrared cameras [16]. While this method provides valuable information [17] there are several limitations; data analysis is time consuming, relies on the availability of a skilled clinician, is constrained by the physical sleep environment (lighting, bedroom dimensions) and is inherently subjective, so is vulnerable to rater error. Further, there is no standard methodology of processing, analysing and presenting sleep biomechanical data once it is captured. Comparison of studies in this area is vexed by a lack of consistency in defining what constitutes a 'repositioning' event. For example, both 45 degree trunk rotation [5] and the movement of at least three limbs [18] have been proposed as definitions of 'repositioning'. Other studies have proposed more complex analysis methods; Wrzus et al., for example, utilized a decision tree paired with an angle-based segmentation algorithm [19]. While methodologically sound this is complex and so may render its implementation as a clinical tool (for use and interpretation by clinicians, patients and families) difficult. Additionally, many of these methods only include axial trunk rotation and do not capture limb movement, limiting understanding of how body segments may influence each other's position during sleep.

There is a need for an easily implemented, objective measure of sleep biomechanics that can be used as the standard assessment tool in research and clinical practice—a need currently unmet by the available methods. A set of wearable Inertial Measurement Units (IMUs) is putatively more efficient, has a lower skill requirement and is more objective and replicable than clinician-rated overnight videography. These devices have been used to good effect previously for the measurement of sleep position in children [14] and adults [19]. In addition, there is a need for a novel classification system for sleep biomechanics that (a) can be applied broadly across diverse research and clinical applications, (b) comprehensively describes the orientation of multiple body segments in relation to each other, and (c) has a streamlined, automated analysis process, providing results that are easily interpreted by clinicians, patients and their families—such an analysis process does not currently exist.

This study aimed to validate the use of a novel wearable sensor system (XSENS DOTs), paired with a new classification of position during sleep, the Body Orientation During Sleep (BODS) Framework. We aimed to answer the following questions:

What is the intra-rater reliability of sleep position measured using overnight infrared videography?

What is the inter-rater reliability of sleep position measured using overnight infrared videography?

What is the level of agreement between clinician-rated overnight infrared videography and a novel automated system (XSENS DOT orientation data, coded through the BODS Framework) in assessment of sleep position?

2. Methods

2.1. Working Definitions

The working definitions for the terms used in this paper are shown in the Box 1.

Box 1. A list of working definitions for terms used in this paper.

Sleep Biomechanics: Collective term for movements made and positions adopted during sleep.
(Body) Segment: Referring to a given anatomical region of the body—for this study, particularly referring to the attachment areas for the DOTs: sternum (anterior chest), pelvis (anterior abdomen) and left and right thighs (immediately superior to the patella).
DOTs: Small, multipurpose IMUs from XSENS (Enschede, Netherlands), programmed using a smartphone with the native DOT app installed.
BODS: The Body Orientation During Sleep Framework. A novel classification system for sleep biomechanics, splitting the 360° of orientation in the transverse plane into component sections to describe lying position (lying being the usual sleeping position).
(BODS) Section: One of the component sections making up the BODS. In the embodiment of the BODS used for this study, there are twelve sections in total. Each cardinal position (supine/prone/left side lying/right side lying) is 5° in size, and the other 8 sections are 42.5° in size.
(Sleep) Position: As defined by the BODS, the orientation of the given body segment in the transverse plane at a given point in time.
(Sleep) Movement: As defined by the BODS, a change in orientation of sufficient amplitude that it results in a change of one of more BODS sections.
Cardinal Positions: Collective term for sections 12 (supine), 3 (left side lying), 6 (prone) and 9 (right side lying).
Rater: An experienced clinician, reviewing captured video footage to assess and code the sleep position according to the BODS.
Difference Score: When comparing two data capture systems' outputs (in this case, the DOTs and human-rated overnight videography) and the sum of the BODS sections, the two data sets differ by when classifying the same sleeping position using the BODS Framework.

2.2. Ethics

This study received approval from Human Research Ethics Committee at Curtin University (HRE2020-0138).

Participants

Ten healthy volunteer adults (18–60 years old) were recruited via convenience sampling for monitoring of sleep positions. Adults were recruited to optimise compliance with specific instructions on the study procedures and provide consent for overnight video. Exclusion criteria included the presence of acute or chronic injuries or pain that would have limited mobility when lying, as well as allergy/irritation from adhesive dressings.

Raters were approached by the lead author to participate in the study. All those asked to participate provided oral consent with the understanding that this was voluntary, and they could change their mind at any time. Three occupational therapists and three physiotherapists were recruited to rate the captured video footage. All clinicians were experienced in the neurodisability field with >15 years of clinical experience and were all skilled in clinical postural assessments of people in the lying position, typically for the prescription of sleep support equipment.

2.3. Assessment Instruments

2.3.1. XSENS DOT Platform

The XSENS DOTs (XENS, Enschede, The Netherlands) (Version 2.0, 4 Hz sample, ±2000°/s gyroscope, ±16 g accelerometer, ±8 Gauss magnetometer) are a set of small

IMUs (36 × 30 × 11 mm, 10.8 g). XSENS DOTs (abbreviated to 'DOTs') were placed on the sternum, pelvis, left thigh and right thigh (one sensor per body segment, see Figure 1 for placement locations) and were used to collect the orientation of each of those body segments. The DOTs were programmed by and logged data via Bluetooth to a Samsung Galaxy S9 Smartphone (Samsung, Seoul, Republic of Korea) using the native XSENS DOT application (v.1.6, XENS, Enschede, The Netherlands). The DOTs were secured using 100 mm × 100 mm Tegaderm (3M, Saint Paul, MA, USA) transparent film dressing over the top of each DOT.

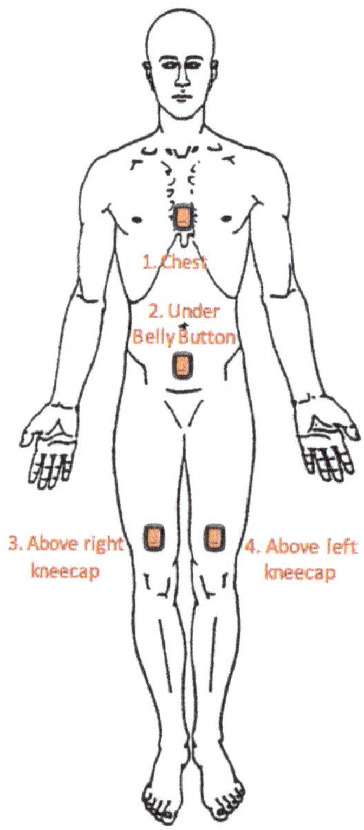

Figure 1. Locations of XSENS DOT Placement on Participants.

2.3.2. Body Orientation during Sleep Framework (BODS)

The Body Orientation During Sleep Framework (BODS) is a novel method of classifying body position developed specifically for the quantification of sleep biomechanics (Figure 2). The BODS divides the 360° of possible transverse rotation (in lying) into 12 sections; division into 12 sections was initially chosen for ease of visual reference (similar to a clock face). When a person is lying down the DOT orientation will always be in one of the sections. For example, the output of a DOT attached to the sternum of a participant lying in supine would be coded as being in Section 12. When the participant is lying in prone, the output of the DOT would be coded as being in Section 6 (Figure 2).

The cardinal positions of supine (Section 12), prone (Section 6), left side lying (Section 3) and right side lying (Section 9) were given smaller 5-degree sections to document symmetrical lying. The sections in between the cardinal positions were divided into two, comprising 42.5° each. The BODS is classified from the perspective of the rater being at the foot of the bed.

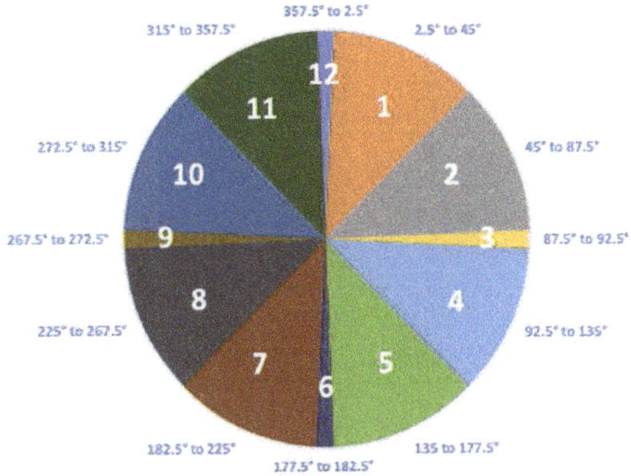

Figure 2. The Body Orientation During Sleep Framework (BODS).

2.3.3. Video Cameras

Overnight video footage was captured by three FDRAX33 digital video cameras (SONY, Tokyo, Japan; 4K Ultra HD (3840 × 2160), 29.8 mm ZEISS Vario-Sonnar T* lens, Oberkochen, Germany), using the NightShot infrared recording mode. The video cameras were positioned at the foot of the bed and laterally (left and right of the bed) on tripods (see Figure 3). The camera at the foot of the bed was elevated in order to provide a full body longitudinal view.

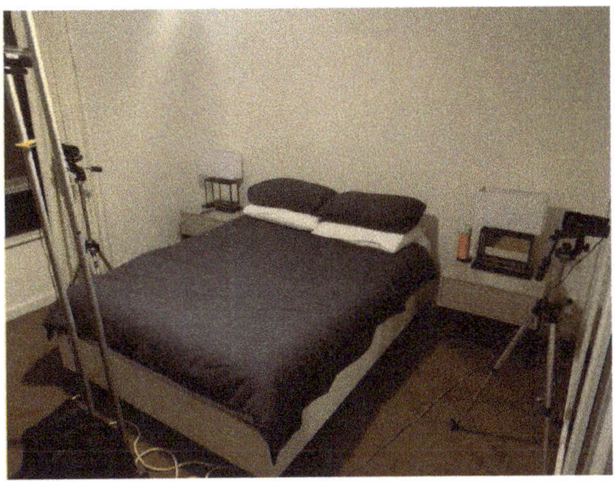

Figure 3. Camera Arrangement for Overnight Recording.

2.4. Data Collection Procedure

Data collection of overnight videography occurred in the participant's native sleeping environment; all participants slept in their usual bed and bedroom. The investigator attended each participant's home and set up the camera array and an Infrared Illuminator (Securview, Edison, NJ, USA) to provide an additional infrared light source to ensure the captured footage was of high enough resolution. The investigator provided each participant with a short training session on how to attach and start recording with the DOTs using the provided smartphone and XSENS DOT app, as well as written instructions (see Supplementary Materials). As the entire body needed to be visualised, participants slept without bedclothes but wore usual sleeping attire. A heater (De'Longhi, Treviso, Italy) was provided to ensure thermal comfort. When participants were ready to sleep for the night, they applied the DOTs, commenced DOT recording via the smartphone app and started recording on the cameras. They then slept, ensuring they took the smartphone with them if they left the bedroom to ensure continuous Bluetooth streaming. Upon waking, participants stopped recording on the DOTs and the cameras. The following morning the investigator attended the participant's home and removed all study equipment.

2.5. Data Processing

2.5.1. Camera Footage

Camera footage was downloaded and edited into a standardised layout using Premiere Pro video editing package (Adobe, San Jose, CA, USA) (Figure 4). Using a custom Labview program (National Instruments, Austin, TX, USA) repositioning throughout the night were identified by changes in DOT orientation, and time-matched clips of approximately 30 s movement duration (with 10 s buffer of footage prior to and after movement) were extracted from the video footage. For each participant, a 10-clip reel was prepared, consisting of six repositionings, two clips of the participant lying in a stationary position, one repeated repositioning clip, and one repeated stationary clip. The order of these clips was randomised for each clip reel. One hundred clips in total were extracted (10 clip reel for each of the 10 participants).

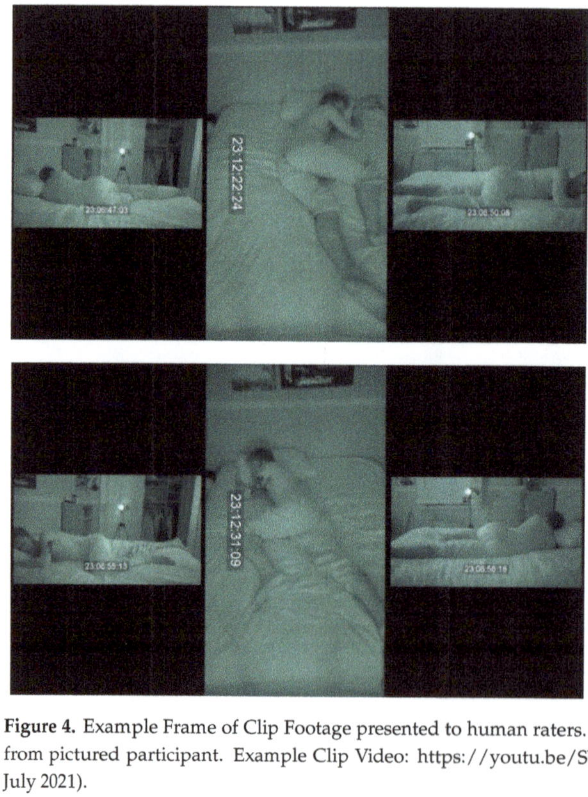

Figure 4. Example Frame of Clip Footage presented to human raters. * Reproduced with consent from pictured participant. Example Clip Video: https://youtu.be/SbKXkGrbrak (accessed on 4 July 2021).

2.5.2. Rating of Camera Footage

Prior to rating, each rater was provided with a single 60 min training session. This consisted of a pair of training videos on how to rate according to the BODS framework (see Supplementary Materials) and three practice clips to rate. Following this session, raters were provided with the clip reel for each of the 10 participants. Raters provided a rating for each body segment (chest, pelvis, left and right thighs) independently, reporting the BODS section for each body segment at both the beginning and the end of the clip. To ensure consistency between raters, only body segment position in the first and last frame of the video was assessed. Raters entered BODS data before playing the clip, then observed the footage of the movement (if any) that occurred, and then at the concluding frame of the clip, entered the BODS data for the body segment positions in that still image. Data were entered into a standard form (see Supplementary Materials).

2.5.3. XSENS Data

After being downloaded from the smartphone, quaternion recordings were converted to Euler angles using a ZXY decomposition. The quaternion method of representing sensor orientation was selected during recording due to smaller storage size of files and convenience of data handling; however, for ease of clinical interpretation, data were ultimately output to the Euler angle format commonly used in biomechanics. Each sensors' pitch angle (corresponding to rotation in the transverse plane for the given segment) was then coded using the BODS framework, giving each body segment an orientation from 1–12 (see Figure 3). The BODS section for each body segment (chest, pelvis, L and R thighs) was identified at the beginning and end of each clip.

2.6. Statistical Analysis

2.6.1. Intra-Rater Reliability

To examine intra-rater reliability for each human rater, difference scores were calculated for the two ratings provided by each rater for each of the repeated clips, represented as the maximum difference in number of sections between the two ratings. For example, if the first BODS rating was Section 5, and the second was Section 7, this would be a difference score of 2 (the difference in BODS sections). The maximum difference score possible was 6 (e.g., a DOT classification of 12 and a rater classification of 6). A difference score was calculated for each of the four dots in each repeated video clip (sternum/pelvis/left leg/right leg). Proportions of the differences (1–6) were calculated to determine highest percentage accuracy within the raters.

2.6.2. Inter-Rater Reliability

To examine agreement between human raters, Cohen's Kappa and Bennett et al.'s S-Score were used to compare BODS classifications between the six raters for each of the 100 clips. Bennet's score was included in addition to the standard Cohen's Kappa due to the potential for small differences between raters resulting in very low Kappa values, the high agreement/low Kappa paradox [20]. Cohen's Kappa could result in an underestimation of inter-rater reliability if used in isolation; Bennett's S score was therefore included as this measure is better able to handle smaller marginal differences.

2.6.3. Raters vs. DOTS

To compare the level of agreement between the raters and the DOTs, difference scores (how many BODS sections two ratings differ by) were calculated for the corresponding DOT and human ratings for each clip. For example, a DOT classification of 12 and a rater classification of 12 would give a difference score of 0; a DOT classification of 12 and a rater classification of 11 would give a difference score of 1. A difference score was calculated for each of the four dots in each video clip (sternum/pelvis/left leg/right leg).

3. Results

3.1. Participant Characteristics

All 10 participants completed data collection and no difficulties or adverse events were reported. There were seven males, and age ranged from 20 to 59 years (mean 29.4 years, median 27.5 years).

3.1.1. Intra-Rater Reliability

All six raters demonstrated a high level of intra-rater reliability, with >48% of ratings with an error score of 0 and >90% of ratings with an error score of $\leq$1, for all body segments

(Table 1). There was slightly higher agreement for chest, pelvis and left leg ratings (mean difference score of ≤1 segment across all raters of 97%, 99%, 98%, respectively) compared with right leg ratings (93%).

Table 1. Frequency and percent of Intra-Rater Reliability of Human Raters (by Difference Score for each body segment).

		Sternum		Pelvis		Left Leg		Right Leg	
		Frequency	Percent	Frequency	Percent	Frequency	Percent	Frequency	Percent
Rater A Difference Scores	0	21	53%	26	65%	23	58%	19	48%
	1	15	38%	11	28%	15	38%	17	43%
	2	1	3%	2	5%	1	3%	2	5%
	3	1	3%	0	0%	0	0%	1	3%
	4	1	3%	0	0%	0	0%	0	0%
	5	0	0%	0	0%	0	0%	0	0%
	6	1	3%	1	3%	1	3%	1	3%
	Total	40	100%	40	100%	40	100%	40	100%
Rater B Difference Scores	0	24	60%	33	83%	26	65%	29	73%
	1	16	40%	7	18%	13	33%	9	23%
	2	0	0%	0	0%	1	3%	2	5%
	3	0	0%	0	0%	0	0%	0	0%
	4	0	0%	0	0%	0	0%	0	0%
	5	0	0%	0	0%	0	0%	0	0%
	6	0	0%	0	0%	0	0%	0	0%
	Total	40	100%	40	100%	40	100%	40	100%
Rater C Difference Scores	0	22	55%	37	93%	27	68%	28	70%
	1	17	43%	3	8%	12	30%	9	23%
	2	0	0%	0	0%	1	3%	3	8%
	3	1	3%	0	0%	0	0%	0	0%
	4	0	0%	0	0%	0	0%	0	0%
	5	0	0%	0	0%	0	0%	0	0%
	6	0	0%	0	0%	0	0%	0	0%
	Total	40	100%	40	100%	40	100%	40	100%
Rater D Difference Scores	0	27	68%	34	85%	26	65%	32	80%
	1	12	30%	6	15%	13	33%	7	18%
	2	0	0%	0	0%	1	3%	1	3%
	3	1	3%	0	0%	0	0%	0	0%
	4	0	0%	0	0%	0	0%	0	0%
	5	0	0%	0	0%	0	0%	0	0%
	6	0	0%	0	0%	0	0%	0	0%
	Total	40	100%	40	100%	40	100%	40	100%
Rater E Difference Scores	0	22	55%	37	93%	27	68%	27	68%
	1	17	43%	3	8%	13	33%	10	25%
	2	0	0%	0	0%	0	0%	3	8%
	3	1	3%	0	0%	0	0%	0	0%
	4	0	0%	0	0%	0	0%	0	0%
	5	0	0%	0	0%	0	0%	0	0%
	6	0	0%	0	0%	0	0%	0	0%
	Total	40	100%	40	100%	40	100%	40	100%
Rater F Difference Scores	0	30	75%	31	78%	27	68%	26	65%
	1	10	25%	9	23%	12	30%	11	28%
	2	0	0%	0	0%	0	0%	2	5%
	3	0	0%	0	0%	1	3%	1	3%
	4	0	0%	0	0%	0	0%	0	0%
	5	0	0%	0	0%	0	0%	0	0%
	6	0	0%	0	0%	0	0%	0	0%
	Total	40	100%	40	100%	40	100%	40	100%

3.1.2. Inter-Rater Reliability

Calculation of Cohen's kappa for comparisons between each rater resulted in a range from 0.254 to 0.470, indicating a low to fair level of agreement. Calculation of Bennett et al.'s S-score [20] gave a range of 0.466 to 0.632, indicating moderate agreement between raters (Table 2).

Table 2. Inter-Rater Reliability of Human Raters.

Cohen's Kappa						
	A	B	C	D	E	F
A		0.254	0.350	0.336	0.310	0.264
B			0.433	0.413	0.344	0.397
C				0.482	0.378	0.352
D					0.470	0.351
E						0.364
F						
Bennett's S Score						
	A	B	C	D	E	F
A		0.487	0.525	0.565	0.493	0.466
B			0.576	0.606	0.509	0.563
C				0.632	0.553	0.508
D					0.622	0.539
E						0.518
F						

3.1.3. Raters vs. DOTS

Overall, the human raters demonstrated a high level of agreement with the DOTs, with >81% of ratings with a maximum difference of 1 section (Table 3). The chest and pelvis ratings displayed a higher level of agreement (mean difference score of 0 segment difference 38% and 53%, and maximum difference of 1 segment of 97% and 96%, respectively, across all raters) when compared to leg ratings. The left and right leg ratings were considerably lower (mean difference score of 0 segment difference 28% and 33%, and maximum difference of 1 segment of 88% and 89%, respectively, across all raters). The raters reported occasional difficulty with confusing left and right legs during rating; visual inspection of clips where there were particularly high difference scores (5 and 6) confirmed that this was the most common cause of rater error.

Table 3. Results of Human Raters as compared to DOTs (by Difference Score for each body segment).

		Sternum		**Pelvis**		**Left Leg**		**Right Leg**	
		Frequency	**Percent**	**Frequency**	**Percent**	**Frequency**	**Percent**	**Frequency**	**Percent**
Rater A Difference Scores	0	73	37%	89	45%	49	25%	62	31%
	1	122	61%	104	52%	126	63%	99	50%
	2	1	1%	4	2%	23	12%	33	17%
	3	1	1%	2	1%	1	1%	5	3%
	4	2	1%	0	0%	0	0%	0	0%
	5	1	1%	1	1%	1	1%	1	1%
	6	0	0%	0	0%	0	0%	0	0%
	Total	200	100%	200	100%	200	100%	200	100%

Table 3. *Cont.*

		Sternum		Pelvis		Left Leg		Right Leg	
		Frequency	Percent	Frequency	Percent	Frequency	Percent	Frequency	Percent
Rater B Difference Scores	0	89	37%	111	56%	51	26%	63	32%
	1	93	61%	81	41%	118	59%	114	57%
	2	15	1%	6	3%	26	13%	18	9%
	3	2	1%	0	0%	3	2%	3	2%
	4	1	1%	1	1%	1	1%	0	0%
	5	0	1%	0	0%	1	1%	1	1%
	6	0	0%	0	0%	0	0%	0	0%
	Missing	0	0%	1	1%	0	0%	1	1%
	Total	200	100%	200	100%	200	100%	200	100%
Rater C Difference Scores	0	61	31%	109	55%	55	28%	60	30%
	1	135	68%	86	43%	118	59%	123	62%
	2	3	2%	4	2%	24	12%	14	7%
	3	1	1%	1	1%	3	2%	3	2%
	4	0	0%	0	0%	0	0%	0	0%
	5	0	0%	0	0%	0	0%	0	0%
	6	0	0%	0	0%	0	0%	0	0%
	Total	200	100%	200	100%	200	100%	200	100%
Rater D Difference Scores	0	61	31%	104	52%	60	30%	56	28%
	1	136	68%	91	46%	121	61%	122	61%
	2	1	1%	3	2%	12	6%	18	9%
	3	0	0%	0	0%	3	2%	0	0%
	4	1	1%	1	1%	1	1%	3	2%
	5	1	1%	0	0%	3	2%	1	1%
	6	0	0%	1	1%	0	0%	0	0%
	Total	200	100%	200	100%	200	100%	200	100%
Rater E Difference Scores	0	75	38%	104	52%	51	26%	68	34%
	1	118	59%	90	45%	130	65%	113	57%
	2	6	3%	6	3%	15	8%	17	9%
	3	1	1%	0	0%	4	2%	2	1%
	4	0	0%	0	0%	0	0%	0	0%
	5	0	0%	0	0%	0	0%	0	0%
	6	0	0%	0	0%	0	0%	0	0%
	Total	200	100%	200	100%	200	100%	200	100%
Rater F Difference Scores	0	106	53%	124	62%	66	33%	88	44%
	1	83	42%	61	31%	113	57%	97	49%
	2	11	6%	15	8%	19	10%	13	7%
	3	0	0%	0	0%	1	1%	2	1%
	4	0	0%	0	0%	1	1%	0	0%
	5	0	0%	0	0%	0	0%	0	0%
	6	0	0%	0	0%	0	0%	0	0%
	Total	200	100%	200	100%	200	100%	200	100%

4. Discussion

This study first aimed to establish the intra- and inter-rater reliability of the current standard clinical tool for assessing sleep positioning, overnight videography rated by clinicians, as codified through the novel BODS framework. Based on the results of this study, we found a high level of intra- rater reliability and moderate level of inter-rater reliability. This study also found high levels of agreement on body position measured by clinician rated overnight videography and XSENS DOTs.

The relatively high levels of agreement demonstrated between and within human raters is encouraging, as it indicates that the existing clinical standard of overnight videography is reliable and so it is appropriate to use it as a benchmark with which to compare new assessments, such as the XSENS DOTs. The good agreement lends further credence to previous studies that have utilised overnight videography to assess sleep position [16,18,21]. One reason may be due to the high level of clinical skill in the human raters, all of whom have 15+ years of experience working in the disability field, routinely performing postural assessments of individuals with neuroimpairments. This specialised experience is not always available in clinical settings, and so use of overnight videography by less experienced clinicians may result in less consistent results. An objective tool such as the XSENS DOTs is likely superior in this respect as it does not rely on the clinical skill of its user and can be easily implemented to accurately measure sleep biomechanics regardless of the user's breadth of experience.

In general, the accuracy of the human raters compared well to that of the XSENS DOTs. While a high proportion of human ratings were a maximum of 1 section different to the corresponding DOT rating, the majority of the sections are large (42.5°) and so variability at a granular level could be greater. Narrower (5°) sections could be used for the cardinal positions, as in these positions the body tends to be more symmetrical and so the position of segments more easily rated. The wider range for the non-cardinal sections of the BODS were necessary due to the possible visual limitations of human raters. Smaller non-cardinal sections would have offered more specific data, but were deemed unrealistically small for even skilled, experienced raters to be able to distinguish. These limitations of human raters have been evidenced in other studies of visually assessed segment position. For example, Abbot et al. demonstrated in a group of physiotherapists that the smallest visually detectable change in range of various dynamic joint angles (lumbar flexion, knee flexion, shoulder abduction) was 9° to 12° [22]. This theory was further borne out by some of the difficulties experienced by the human raters in our study, even with the wider sections of the BODS. As seen in Table 3, there was less agreement for left leg/right leg positions compared to the sternum and pelvis positions, likely due to the greater range of movement at the hip (compared to the spine, which is primarily responsible for sternum and pelvis positioning) resulting in a wider variety of positions being possible for the thigh segments, as compared to the potential positions of the sternum and pelvis. Further, raters reported occasional confusion when distinguishing between left and right, which may account for some of the 5 and 6 difference scores that were present.

Despite being previously unfamiliar with the BODS, following the brief training session raters were able to effectively use the BODS framework to rate body orientation during sleep. The use of this system demonstrates a unique advantage over other classification systems, as the orientation of each body segment can be described, and a composite of each segment describes the entire body, a capacity absent from other systems. For example, Brown et al. assessed only gross body position and coded only in cardinal positions (supine/prone/left side lying/right side lying) [23]. Further, because the DOTs performed well against both a lab-based standard reference system (VICON motion analysis) [24] and the current clinical standard of overnight videography, future studies utilising the DOTs alone need not be constrained by human perception, and different versions of the BODS with finer gradations can be used. While this study focused primarily on classification of static positions, the BODS (with data captured by the DOTs) also allows for recording the number of repositionings/night by registering the number of transitions between sections. The BODS/DOTs combination also allows for exposure analysis of the duration participants rest in each section. These outcome measures can be used in future research to investigate sleep biomechanical phenotypes for clinical populations (e.g., cerebral palsy) and contrast this with the sleep biomechanics of the general population. Moreover, when paired with an objective, computerised system such as the XSENS DOTs the BODS allows for streamlined, automated data analysis and simplified interpretation of findings, putatively lowering the threshold for adoption into clinical practice and research methodology. In the field of neurodisability, simplified assessment of sleep biomechanics would enable easier and more effective prescription of supported lying equipment, improving sleep comfort and quality of life for people with neurodisability [25].

There are several strengths in this study. Raters were highly experienced allied health clinicians from a variety of clinical backgrounds. The study design captured full variability of sleep biomechanics, testing accuracy of classification in a variety of situations including moving, stationary and repeated clips. This study leveraged a large data set relative to its modest sample size (n = 10) by extracting a wide variety of clips (100 per participant) and rating each of the four body segments' positions at the beginning and end of each clip, resulting in 800 individual ratings (100 clips × 2 ratings per clip × 4 body segments) from each of our six raters, resulting in 4800 total ratings. We are confident that this provided an adequate data set with which to compare the DOTs to the clinical standard of overnight videography. This was accompanied by a relatively simple and easily interpreted metric of percentage agreement between the two systems, which clearly demonstrated the high level of intra- rater reliability and high levels of agreement on body position measured by clinician-rated overnight videography and XSENS DOTs.

A limitation of this study was that head orientation was not recorded, as it has been in other studies [14]. The investigators chose not to measure head orientation in this study as trunk and leg position was the primary focus, and out of concern for comfort and unduly influencing naturalistic sleep biomechanics [26]. The inclusion of other XSENS DOTs (e.g., on the forehead to measure head orientation, or on the upper limbs) and the utility of these additional data to the holistic assessment of sleep biomechanics could be a feature of future study designs. Additionally, as previously discussed, the BODS sections in between the cardinal position sections were wide (42.5°), which proved to be a barrier to more granular comparisons of findings between the systems. While this was deemed necessary to allow for visual assessment by human raters, future studies utilising DOTs-captured, BODS-rated data to assess sleep biomechanics could use smaller section sizes (e.g., 5° or 10°) to allow for more detailed description of sleep position and movement. In addition, future studies could use different configurations of the BODS (i.e., a greater or lesser number of sections) depending on the research questions and purpose of analysis.

Compared to current systems, the XSENS/BODS system has a number of distinct advantages. It is easily implemented in the ecological sleeping environment of each participant; this is not always feasible with systems that require large, cumbersome equipment, such as overnight videography (e.g., as proposed by Cary et al. [16]). Further, the data analysis process is far simpler using the BODS; this stands in contrast to the onerous process of manually reviewing hours of video footage, or else using a complex system of classification and analysis as is used in current assessments that utilized accelerometry or IMUs. Further, we are confident that the system presented in this study will yield results that are more easily integrated into current clinical practice due to the superior usability and ease of interpretation of findings (by families and clinicians) as opposed to current solutions (for example, Wrzus et al. [19]).

5. Conclusions

Based on the results of this study, we recommend the use of the XSENS DOTs in future studies examining sleep biomechanics—they are more accurate than human raters and allow for more detailed analysis of sleep biomechanics in a far less labour-intensive manner. Future studies could focus on further development of the BODS framework and trialling of both it and the DOTs in diverse clinical populations.

Supplementary Materials: The following supporting information can be downloaded at: https://www.mdpi.com/article/10.3390/bioengineering10040408/s1, Table S1: Participant Instructions; Table S2: BODS Rating Form; Videos S1–S2: Training Videos for Raters.

Author Contributions: Conceptualization, N.B., P.D., L.J., K.B., A.J., B.J., A.C. and J.D.; methodology, N.B., P.D., L.J., K.B., B.J., A.C. and J.D.; software, P.D.; validation, N.B., P.D., L.J., K.B., A.J., B.J., A.C. and J.D.; formal analysis, A.J. investigation, N.B.; resources, N.B.; data curation, N.B.; writing—original draft preparation, N.B.; writing—review and editing, N.B., P.D., L.J., K.B., A.J., B.J., A.C. and J.D. visualization, N.B., P.D., L.J., K.B., A.J., B.J., A.C. and J.D. supervision, L.J., K.B., B.J.,

A.C. and J.D. project administration, N.B., L.J., K.B., B.J., A.C. and J.D. funding acquisition, N.B. All authors have read and agreed to the published version of the manuscript.

Funding: The authors declare that no funds, grants, or other support was received during the preparation of this manuscript, with the exception of the living expenses stipend received by Nicholas Buckley as part of the Research Training Program scholarship (administered by Curtin University).

Institutional Review Board Statement: This study was approved by Human Research Ethics Committee at Curtin University (protocol code HRE2020-0138).

Informed Consent Statement: Informed consent was obtained from all subjects involved in the study.

Data Availability Statement: The data presented in this study are available on request from the corresponding author. The data are not publicly available due to the participants being readily identifiable (videography).

Conflicts of Interest: The authors declare no conflict of interest.

References

1. Joosten, S.A.; O'Driscoll, D.M.; Berger, P.J.; Hamilton, G.S. Supine position related obstructive sleep apnea in adults: Pathogenesis and treatment. *Sleep Med. Rev.* **2014**, *18*, 7–17. [CrossRef] [PubMed]
2. Sommerauer, M.; Werth, E.; Poryazova, R.; Gavrilov, Y.; Hauser, S.; Valko, P.O. Bound to supine sleep: Parkinson's disease and the impact of nocturnal immobility. *Park. Relat. Disord.* **2015**, *21*, 1269–1272. [CrossRef] [PubMed]
3. Fulford, F.E.; Brown, J.K. Position as a cause of deformity in children with cerebral palsy. *Dev. Med. Child Neurol.* **1976**, *18*, 305–314. [CrossRef]
4. Palisano, R.J.; Rosenbaum, P.; Bartlett, D.; Livingston, M.H. Content validity of the expanded and revised Gross Motor Function Classification System. *Dev. Med. Child Neurol.* **2008**, *50*, 744–750. [CrossRef] [PubMed]
5. Sato, H.; Iwasaki, T.; Yokoyama, M.; Inoue, T. Monitoring of body position and motion in children with severe cerebral palsy for 24 hours. *Disabil. Rehabil.* **2014**, *36*, 1156–1160. [CrossRef]
6. Hill, S.; Goldsmith, J. Biomechanics and prevention of body shape distortion. *Tizard Learn. Disabil. Rev.* **2010**, *15*, 15–32. [CrossRef]
7. McIntyre, S.; Morgan, C.; Walker, K.; Novak, I. Cerebral Palsy—Don't Delay. *Dev. Disabil. Res. Rev.* **2011**, *17*, 114–129. [CrossRef]
8. Poirot, I.; Laudy, V.; Rabilloud, M.; Roche, S.; Ginhoux, T.; Kassaï, B.; Vuillerot, C. Prevalence of pain in 240 non-ambulatory children with severe cerebral palsy. *Ann. Phys. Rehabil. Med.* **2017**, *60*, 371–375. [CrossRef]
9. Littleton, S.R.; Heriza, C.B.; Mullens, P.A.; Moerchen, V.A.; Bjornson, K. Effects of Positioning on Respiratory Measures in Individuals with Cerebral Palsy and Severe Scoliosis. *Pediatr. Phys. Ther.* **2011**, *23*, 159–169. [CrossRef]
10. Novak, I. Evidence-Based Diagnosis, Health Care, and Rehabilitation for Children with Cerebral Palsy. *J. Child Neurol.* **2014**, *29*, 1141–1156. [CrossRef]
11. Casey, J.; Rosenblad, A.; Rodby-Bousquet, E. Postural asymmetries, pain, and ability to change position of children with cerebral palsy in sitting and supine: A cross-sectional study. *Disabil. Rehabil.* **2020**, *44*, 2363–2371. [CrossRef] [PubMed]
12. Gordon, S.J.; Grimmer, K.A.; Trott, P. Self-Reported versus Recorded Sleep Position: An Observational Study. *Internet J. Allied Health Sci. Pract.* **2004**, *2*, 7. [CrossRef]
13. Zahradka, N.; Jeong, I.C.; Searson, P.C. Distinguishing positions and movements in bed from load cell signals. *Physiol. Meas.* **2018**, *39*, 125001. [CrossRef] [PubMed]
14. Sato, H.; Ikura, D.; Tsunoda, M. Assessing head and trunk symmetry during sleep using tri-axial accelerometers. *Disabil. Rehabil. Assist. Technol.* **2015**, *10*, 113–117. [CrossRef] [PubMed]
15. Russo, K.; Bianchi, M.T. How Reliable Is Self-Reported Body Position during Sleep? *J. Clin. Sleep Med.* **2016**, *12*, 127–128. [CrossRef]
16. Cary, D.; Collinson, R. Examining the Relationship between Sleep Posture and Morning Spinal Symptoms in the Habitual Environment Using Infrared Cameras. *J. Sleep Disord. Treat. Care* **2016**, *5*, 2. [CrossRef]
17. Masek, M.; Lam, C.P.; Tranthim-Fryer, C.; Jansen, B.; Baptist, K. Sleep monitor: A tool for monitoring and categorical scoring of lying position using 3D camera data. *SoftwareX* **2018**, *7*, 341–346. [CrossRef]
18. Aaronson, S.T.; Rashed, S.; Biber, M.P.; Hobson, J.A. Brain State and Body Position: A Time-lapse Video Study of Sleep. *Arch. Gen. Psychiatry* **1982**, *39*, 330–335. [CrossRef]
19. Wrzus, C.; Brandmaier, A.; Von Oertzen, T.; Müller, V.; Wagner, G.G.; Riediger, M. A New Approach for Assessing Sleep Duration and Postures from Ambulatory Accelerometry. *PLoS ONE* **2012**, *7*, e48089. [CrossRef]
20. Warrens, M.J. The effect of combining categories on Bennett, Alpert and Goldstein's S. *Stat. Methodol.* **2012**, *9*, 341–352. [CrossRef]
21. DelRosso, L.M.; Jackson, C.V.; Trotter, K.; Bruni, O.; Ferri, R. Video-polysomnographic characterization of sleep movements in children with restless sleep disorder. *Sleep* **2019**, *42*, zsy269. [CrossRef] [PubMed]
22. Abbott, E.; Campbell, A.; Wise, E.; Tidman, S.J.; Lay, B.S.; Kent, P. Physiotherapists could detect changes of 12 degrees or more in single-plane movement when observing forward bending, squat or hand-over-head: A cross-sectional experiment. *Musculoskelet. Sci. Pract.* **2022**, *61*, 102594. [CrossRef] [PubMed]

23. Brown, D.L.; Lisabeth, L.D.; Zupancic, M.J.; Concannon, M.; Martin, C.; Chervin, R.D. High Prevalence of Supine Sleep in Ischemic Stroke Patients. *Stroke* **2008**, *39*, 2511–2514. [CrossRef]
24. Buckley, N.; Davey, P.; Jensen, L.; Baptist, K.; Jansen, B.; Campbell, A.; Downs, J. Can Wearable Inertial Measurement Units Be Used to Measure Sleep Biomechanics? Establishing Initial Feasibility and Validity. *Biomimetics* **2023**, *8*, 2. [CrossRef] [PubMed]
25. Humphreys, G.; King, T.; Jex, J.; Rogers, M.; Blake, S.; Thompson-Coon, J.; Morris, C. Sleep positioning systems for children and adults with a neurodisability: A systematic review. *Br. J. Occup. Ther.* **2019**, *82*, 5–14. [CrossRef]
26. McCambridge, J.; Witton, J.; Elbourne, D.R. Systematic review of the Hawthorne effect: New concepts are needed to study research participation effects. *J. Clin. Epidemiol.* **2014**, *67*, 267–277. [CrossRef]

bioengineering

MDPI

Article

Lumbar Kinematics Assessment of Patients with Chronic Low Back Pain in Three Bridge Tests Using Miniaturized Sensors

Athanasios Triantafyllou [1,2,*], Georgios Papagiannis [1,2], Sophia Stasi [3], Panagiotis Gkrilias [1], Maria Kyriakidou [1], Effrosyni Kampouroglou [4], Apostolos-Zacharias Skouras [2], Charilaos Tsolakis [2,5], George Georgoudis [6], Olga Savvidou [2], Panayiotis Papagelopoulos [2] and Panagiotis Koulouvaris [2]

1 Biomechanics Laboratory, Department of Physiotherapy, University of the Peloponnese, 23100 Sparta, Greece
2 Sports Excellence, 1st Department of Orthopaedic Surgery, National and Kapodistrian University of Athens, 12462 Athens, Greece
3 Laboratory of Neuromuscular and Cardiovascular Study of Motion, Physiotherapy Department, Faculty of Health and Care Science, University of West Attica, 12243 Egaleo, Greece
4 2nd Department of Surgery, Aretaieio Hospital, National and Kapodistrian University of Athens, 11528 Athens, Greece
5 Sports Performance Laboratory, School of Physical Education & Sports Science, National and Kapodistrian University of Athens, 17237 Athens, Greece
6 Department of Physiotherapy, University of West Attica, 12243 Athens, Greece
* Correspondence: athanat@gmail.com; Tel.: +30-6947897190

Abstract: Lumbar muscle atrophy, diminished strength, stamina, and increased fatigability have been associated with chronic nonspecific low back pain (LBP). When evaluating patients with LBP, trunk or core stability, provided by the performance and coordination of trunk muscles, appears to be essential. Several clinical tests have been developed to identify deficiencies in trunk performance, demonstrating high levels of validity and reproducibility. The most frequently prescribed tests for assessing the core body muscles are the prone plank bridge test (PBT), the side bridge test (SBT), and the supine bridge test (SUBT). However, quantitative assessments of the kinematics of the lumbar spine during their execution have not yet been conducted. The purpose of our study was to provide objective biomechanical data for the assessment of LBP patients. The lumbar spine ranges of motion of 22 healthy subjects (Group A) and 25 patients diagnosed with chronic LBP (Group B) were measured using two inertial measurement units during the execution of the PBT, SUBT, and SBT. Statistically significant differences between the two groups were found in all three tests' kinematic patterns. This quantitative assessment of lumbar spine motion transforms the three bridge tests into an objective biomechanical diagnostic tool for LPBs that may be used to assess the efficacy of applied rehabilitation programs.

Keywords: lumbar kinematics; bridge tests; IMUs; miniaturized sensors; low back patients

1. Introduction

Long-lasting low back pain (LBP) of undefined cause has been associated with muscle atrophy, decreased strength, endurance, and excessive fatigability of the lumbar muscles [1–7]. In addition, prospective studies suggest that lumbar muscle deconditioning may be a common risk factor for acute LBP [6,7].

Trunk or core stability quantification—the strength, endurance, and coordination of trunk muscles—with a gold-standard method has yet to be introduced [8,9]. However, that specific parameter seems important when assessing patients with LBP [10]. Furthermore, an objective determination of trunk function can provide valuable information concerning the progression of the pathology in decision making about the optimum rehabilitation program and in evaluating its outcome [11].

Various clinical tests have been proposed to help identify deficits in trunk performance, showing excellent validity and repeatability [12,13]. In addition, reduced trunk muscular endurance has been correlated with nonspecific LBP [12,14,15] and identified as a risk factor for recurrent bouts of the condition [16,17]. The most commonly referred tests for core body musculature assessment are the prone plank bridge test (PBT) for abdominal core muscles, the side bridge test (on both sides) (SBT), and the supine bridge test (SUBT) [18]. Such field tests can be easily applied in a clinical environment without specific equipment, allowing multiple patient evaluations simultaneously [16].

IMUs have been validated and proven to be accurate instruments for the objective assessment of a variety of pathological conditions, such as asymmetrical locomotion; consequently, they are gaining popularity among clinicians for everyday practice outside of the laboratory [19]. The literature supports their established reliability and validity when used to evaluate the lower back. More specifically, the PBT is a valid and reliable measure for assessing abdominal performance, showing an ICC between testing sessions of 0.915. The SUBT presents good to excellent reliability (ICC > 0.836), while the SBT presents high to very high reliability (ICC 0.74–0.96) [20,21].

Even though these tests provide significant information for assessing LBP patients, quantitative measurements of lumbar spine kinematics during their execution have yet to be performed. Miniaturized sensors (inertial measurement units—IMUs) can offer reliable kinematic data on the corresponding kinematic pattern of the aforementioned clinical tests, hence adding a significant quantitative biomechanical component to the testing [22].

Since the prone plank bridge, supine bridge, and side bridge tests are the most commonly used functional tests for assessing patients with low back pain in daily clinical practice, the purpose of this study was to observe/measure the actual kinematics of the lumbar spine for healthy and low back pain subjects. Additionally, we examined possible differences in lumbar ROMs between two groups (as correspondingly recorded for time/endurance) to quantify the lumbar kinematics during the execution of the previously described valuable clinical tools. Eventually, the previously mentioned tests could integrate the objective biomechanical behavior of the lumbar spine, a valuable clinical parameter in low back pain patient evaluation.

2. Materials and Methods

The study's methodological approach and procedure are depicted in the following flow chart (Figure 1).

2.1. Subjects

A total of 53 (30 male and 23 female) patients diagnosed with chronic low back pain due to spondyloarthropathy were initially examined. The inclusion criteria were the occurrence of at least Modic type II changes in magnetic resonance imaging (MRI) and at least grade 5 interverbal disc degeneration changes according to Modified Pfirrmann grading in the absence of neurological signs. Modic changes (MC) are injury signs in the bone marrow of the vertebral body, depicted in MRI, that are related to low back pain (LBP) [23]. Similarly, the Pfirrmann classification is the most widely used categorization system for disc degenerative assessment in rehabilitation and academic settings [24,25]. Chronic low back pain due to anatomical–pathological spine alterations (spondylolysis, spondylolisthesis, scoliosis, bone fractures, neurological symptoms) and non-musculoskeletal pathological conditions such as cancer or renal disease with referral lumbar spine pain constituted the exclusion criteria. A total of 7 patients were eliminated because of sciatica, 2 because of spondylolysis, 1 because of spondylolisthesis, 3 due to radiological scoliosis abnormalities, 8 due to a history of spinal fracture, and 7 because of osteoporosis.

Finally, 22 healthy subjects (12 men and 10 women) (Group A), as well as 25 patients diagnosed with chronic low back pain (10 male and 15 female) (Group B), were included in this study. The mean age was 48.5 ± 9.3 for Group A and 49.4 ± 11.2 years for Group B (p-value = 0.12). The mean body mass index (BMI) was 23.3 ± 1.7 and 24.6 ± 2.4 for Groups A and B, respectively (p-value = 0.18). The measured parameter was the lumbar spine position, which was obtained during the execution of each of the three tests, compared to the neutral position for all subjects when they performed the PBT, the SUBT, and the SBT (Table 1).

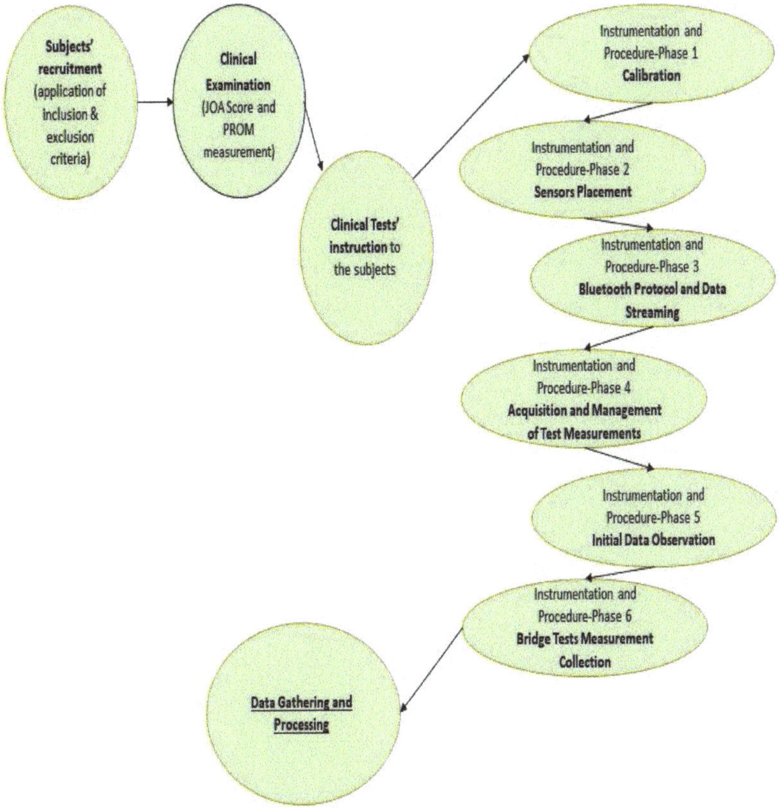

Figure 1. Flow Chart.

Table 1. Demographic data and JOA scores.

Item		Healthy (Mean/±SD)	Low Back Pain (Mean/±SD)	*p*-Value
Total Number		22	25	
Gender	Male	12	10	
	Female	10	15	
Age		48.5/±9.3	49.4/±11.2	0.12
BMI		23.3/±1.7	24.6/±2.4	0.18
JOA Score		27.15/±0.73	22.2/±1.01	0.0003

2.2. Clinical Examination

Various scales for measuring physical impairment are utilized to quantify a patient's state before and after therapy. The JOA score, created by the Japanese Orthopaedic Association in 1975, is the most frequently used measure to assess patients with low back pain. [26]. Our research evaluated both groups with a JOA score before the test execution (Table 1).

All participants' passive flexion–extension, abduction–adduction, and left–right lumbar spine rotation were assessed prior to the clinical testing to guarantee appropriate passive ROM in all three planes and the absence of pain, hence allowing all patients to participate in the clinical tests. The passive ROMs were measured using the IMUs following the instrumentation and procedure mentioned below according to the positions described in the manual muscle test (MMT) for normal muscle strength, but the motion was executed passively by the clinician [27].

2.3. Clinical Tests

Prone Bridge

Each subject was placed in the prone position on a firm surface, propped on the elbows. The elbows were separated and placed shoulder-width apart, and the feet had a narrow base but were not touching. The subject then lifted the pelvis until only the forearms and ankles touched the bed, keeping a horizontal line between the shoulders, pelvis, and ankles (Figure 2A). The test pose was maintained until fatigue or discomfort prohibited its continuation [20].

Supine Bridge

Each subject started in a supine position with their knees flexed 90 degrees and their feet on the bed close to each other but not touching. The arms were placed next to the torso. The subject lifted their pelvis from the bed, maintaining a horizontal line between the shoulders, hips, and knees (Figure 2B). The test position was sustained until fatigue or discomfort prohibited its continuation. The dominant leg was straightened in the air if the subject achieved two minutes in the test position, eliminating one support point. This was intended to reduce the duration of the bridge by adding a torque moment to the bridge's center. In the occurrence of a previous pathology to the dominant support leg (e.g., knee pain), the opposite leg was instead moved forward [28].

Side Bridge Test

For the side bridge test, the participant was directed to recline on one side on the same examination bed. The lower supporting arm was flexed 90 degrees at the elbow, and the upper arm was folded across the torso. The subject was instructed to elevate the hips off the bed surface and keep an extended straight position with a flexed forearm directly beneath the shoulder (Figure 2C). Both sides were subjected to examination [29].

2.4. Instrumentation and Procedure

Throughout the prone plank bridge, supine bridge, and side bridge examinations, lumbar spine ranges of motion (ROMs) were measured. To evaluate the kinematics of the lumbar spine, two MetaMotionR+ inertial measurement units (IMUs) were utilized. MetaMotionR+ (MMR) is designed to record and stream sensor data and has CE approval. Unprocessed sensor information was recorded and transmitted at 400 Hz and 100 Hz, respectively, via Bluetooth. The researcher obtained and examined a CSV file containing data on a local PC. Data fusion integrates information from a three-dimensional gyroscopic sensor, a three-dimensional magnetometer, and a three-dimensional accelerometer to produce a stable constant direction coordinate expressed as Quaternion or Euler angles. Moreover, sophisticated software effectively integrates the unprocessed instrument data to improve each instrument's performance. This method includes techniques for offset correction of each sensor, standardization status monitoring, and Kalman filter integration to produce corrected and usable orientation coordinates. MMR+ is an established device for recording human motion data and monitoring gestures. A list of its technological components is as follows:

- BMI160 6-Axis Accelerometer + Gyroscope;
- LTR-329ALS Luminosity/Ambient Light;
- BMM150 3-Axis Magnetometer;
- BOSCH 9-Axis Sensor Fusion;
- 8 MB memory;
- Lithium-ion rechargeable battery;
- Vibrating coin motor;
- Low-energy Bluetooth, CPU, button, LED, and GPIOs.

A Bluetooth radio embedded in each IMU delivers data wirelessly to a researcher's smartphone. IMUs and Bluetooth radios are battery-powered with 3.6 V cells. The data collection procedure comprises six distinct phases.

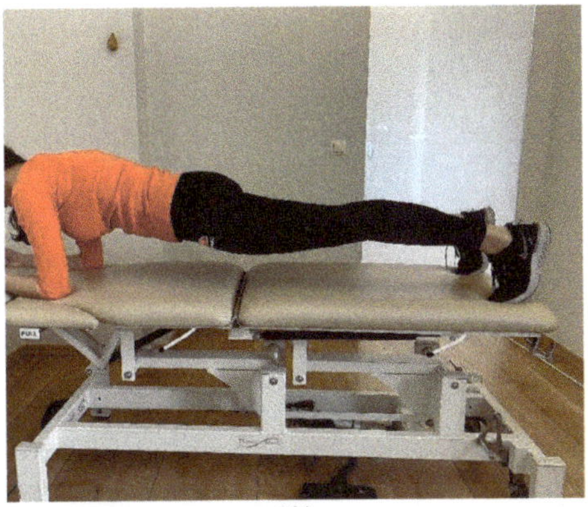

(A)

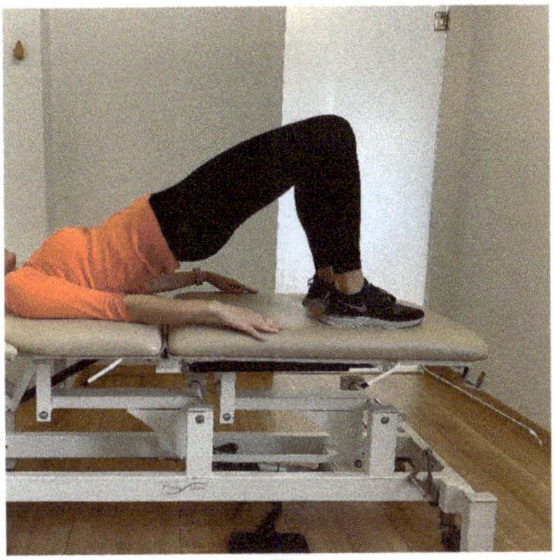

(B)

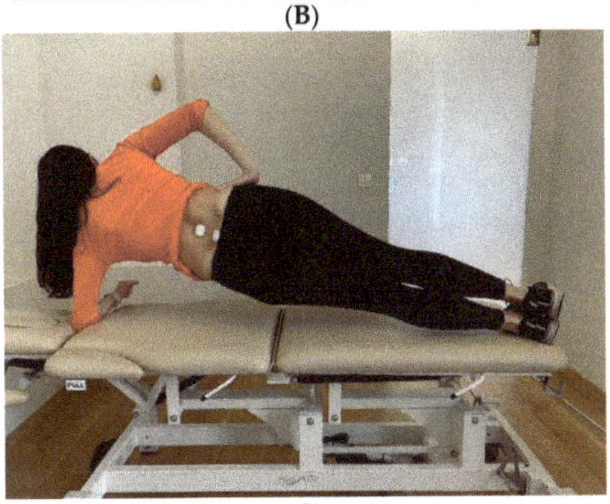

(C)

Figure 2. (**A**) Prone bridge test end position. (**B**) Supine bridge test end position. (**C**) Left-side bridge test end position.

2.4.1. Phase One—Calibration

For human movement assessment using an inertial sensing system, it is necessary to determine the instrument reference and body orientation frame correspondence [21]. Prior to attaching and activating the sensors, the IMUs were adjusted on a flat, horizontal plane to assure that each unit had the same initial position as the coordinate system. Therefore, we assumed that the first and fifth lumbar vertebral segments are in the same plane. This enables the collection of measurements with the lumbar section coordinated with a designated axis of the global reference. It is vital to adhere to a reliable calibration process to acquire reliable data for motion assessment. The calibration was conducted on a smartphone running the Metawear application developed by mbientlab INC (software version: 2.0.1).

2.4.2. Phase Two—Sensor Placement

The positioning of the sensors was carefully carried out to precisely determine the respective orientation and location of the device's frame in relation to the plane of physical motion [30,31]. The first IMU was mounted directly above the spinous process of the first lumbar vertebra, while the second was placed directly above the spinous process of the fifth lumbar vertebra. Using hypoallergenic double-sided adhesive, both sensors were adhered to the epidermis (Figure 3).

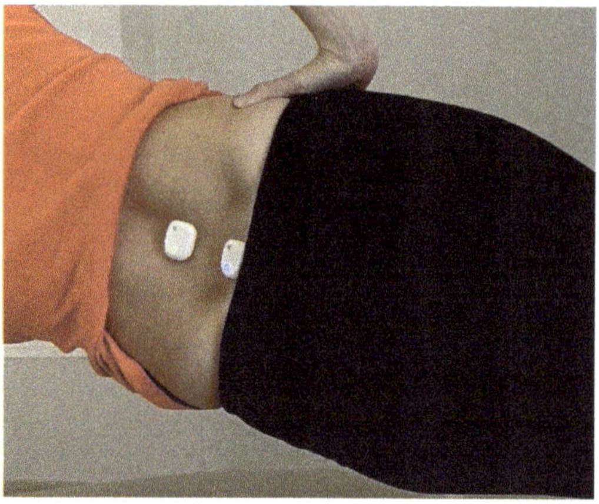

Figure 3. IMUs' placement on L1 and L5 vertebrae.

2.4.3. Phase Three—Bluetooth Protocol and Data Streaming

These IMU sensors interacted via Bluetooth with a smartphone. Metawear, mbientlab INC's application (software version: 2.0.1), was loaded on the smartphone to capture and save data. After each session, the collected data were streamed over Bluetooth to a PC for further analysis. The analysis included pre- and post-filtering of three-axis acceleration, geomagnetic tracking and alignment (roll, pitch, and yaw), and three-dimensional angular acceleration in the local sensor coordinate system.

2.4.4. Phase Four—Acquisition and Management of Test Measurements

Before collecting clinical test data, the same clinician performed passive lumbosacral section flexion–extension and left–right lateral flexion to validate the method's repeatability and ensure that both wearable sensors performed as intended and acquired ROM data. Extension passive range of motion (PROM) was measured with the patient lying in the prone position on an examination bed. A special belt stabilized the patient's pelvis at the bed, and one examiner stabilized the same anatomical region with his hands. At this position, the IMU data showed 0 degrees of ROM. A second examiner wrapped his hands around the subject's chest and executed lumbar spine extension till he felt a firm "end feel" and no more motion could be produced. The "End Feel" is a type of sensation or feeling that examiners experience when the joint is at the end of its available passive range of motion in assessment [32]. At that point, the overall passive lumbar extension ROM was obtained.

Flexion and lateral flexion PROMs were examined with the patient lying in a supine position on an examination bed. A special belt stabilized the patient's pelvis at the bed, and one examiner stabilized the same anatomical region with his hands. At this position, the IMU data showed 0 degrees of ROM. The second examiner wrapped his hands around the subject's thoracic spine and executed lumbar spine flexion until he felt a firm "end feel" and no more motion could be produced. At that point, the overall passive flexion ROM was obtained. As for the right and left lateral flexion, the same methodology was applied regarding pelvis stabilization and the IMU's reference position of 0 degrees. Following this, the second examiner wrapped his hands around the subject's thoracic spine and executed lumbar spine lateral flexion (first to the left, then to the right) till he felt a firm "end feel" and no more motion could be produced. At that point, the overall passive lateral flexion ROM was obtained for both sides.

These records were saved as a CSV file and transmitted directly to the PC's local storage (one for each sensor). All subjects were instructed and prepped for the technique described above. This experiment was performed three times for each ROM to acquire representative motion data.

2.4.5. Phase Five—Initial Material Observation

Even if the wearables' precision is high and the root mean square error (RMS) is employed, a computerized body representation enables the researcher to determine whether movement reconstruction and data acquisition were managed effectively. After the passive ROM measurement experiment was completed, the collected data were examined for irrelevant outcomes. If errors or improper motions were detected due to magnetic field interference, the calibration was examined to eliminate the disturbance while the participants were still present so the measurement could be repeated if necessary.

2.4.6. Phase Six—Bridge Test Measurement Collection

After a successful test session, the patients were asked to perform the prone plank, supine bridge, and side bridge positions. All patients were given clear instructions about the procedure, and they performed two trials for familiarization before data measurements [28]. In addition, they were instructed to carry the smartphone next to them throughout the assessment to prevent signal connectivity problems during the data capture and transmission from the IMU to the smartphone. After the measurements were complete, the clinician removed the sensors from the patients and transferred the collected data from the smartphone to the PC.

2.5. Data Gathering and Processing

Two nine-dimensional inertial units were used to evaluate lumbar spine motion ranges. Mounted on the subject's body, the sensors can remotely stream, via Bluetooth, a 3D vector of the gyroscope's angular velocity (deg/s) in the three planes (x, y, z). Likewise, a 3D vector of the accelerometer and the magnetometer elements are transmitted. Combining the information collected from the three aforementioned elements of the sensors, which eliminates potential errors [33], the orientation of the body section and accompanying Euler angles may be appropriately determined.

The MMR+ NDoF fusion algorithm calibrated the sensor's background automatically. The accelerometer, gyroscope, and magnetometer provide the combined precise position values in this 9-axis setting. The benefits of integrating all three sensors include rapid computation, leading to an increased output data stream, and enhanced resistance to geomagnetic distortion. In this mode, the option for rapid magnetometer calibration was enabled, resulting in more precise output values. NDoF option implemented the following frequency content: The fusion technique uses the accelerometer sensor's output to adjust for gyroscope disturbance and measurement variations. When the subject's target section is in motion, the fusion promptly dismisses accelerometer sensor readings in favor of gyroscope data for pitch and roll. If accelerometer readings are ignored for a prolonged time, pitch and roll values may fluctuate (due to continual movement or vibration). The same will happen if the fluctuation affects the magnetic measurements; the program will, by default, overlook it.

Let x = [a x, a y, a z, g x, g y, g z, m x, m y, m z] correspond to one inertial unit's measurement. Calculating the Euler angles using the x data is the initial stage. Then, the L1 and L5 direction vectors are calculated using information from all three elements (accelerometer, gyroscope, magnetometer). Therefore, the variables a x, g x, and m x are converted to Euler angles of the pitch plane since they correspond to the lumbar region ROM angles [34]. To this end, the method proposed by Qifan Zhou et al. 2021 [35] was implemented, allowing a Kalman filter to determine the sensor's exact direction [36]. The Kalman filter is a system used to depict nonlinear systems ruled by nonlinear differential equations. The IMU data are provided during the update phase, and after four defined steps based on the filter components are completed, the outcome is a position prediction [34,36]. Lastly, typical Euler angles [36] were employed to compute the lower back ROM angles relative to the L1-L5 coordinate system using a 5 Hz data frequency.

3. Results

The independent t-test, one-tailed distribution, and two sample unequal variance were used for the data statistical analysis. The statistical power of our study was calculated using G*Power 3.1.9.7 software for Windows (Heinrich-Heine-Universität Düsseldorf, Düsseldorf, Germany). The analysis was conducted for each dependent variable, which tested lumbar spine kinematics during the execution of the three performed tests. A power analysis for two independent means was employed with a given alpha = 0.05. The power of the study's sample size and observed effect size was higher than 80% for each variable (96.5% for the prone bridge test, 88.2% for the left-side bridge test, close to its maximum of 1 for the supine bridge test, and the right-side bridge test). An intraclass correlation coefficient (ICC; two-way random, absolute agreement) and respective 95% confidence interval were used for relative reliability analysis and to interpret results for within-session measurements in all bridge tests and passive ROM clinical examinations (ICC > 0.90).

3.1. *Clinical Examination*

3.1.1. Passive Range of Motion

No statistically significant differences were found regarding the passive ROM of flexion (Group A: mean = 49.33°, SD = 0.94 and Group B: mean = 48.83°, SD = 1.12, *p*-value = 0.24), the passive ROM of extension (Group A: mean = 14.66°, SD = 0.94 and Group B: mean = 14.16°, SD = 0.68, *p*-value = 0.18), the passive ROM of right lateral flexion (Group A: mean = 18.67°, SD = 0.74 and Group B: mean = 17.83°, SD = 1.06, *p*-value = 0.09), or the left lateral flexion (Group A: mean = 18.34°, SD= 0.74 and Group B: mean = 18.5°, SD = 0.95, *p*-value = 0.38) (Table 2).

Table 2. Passive range of motion measurements in Group A and Group B.

Item	Group A (Mean/±SD)	Group B (Mean/±SD)	*p*-Value
Lumbar flexion	49.33°/±0.94	48.83°/±1.12	0.24
Lumbar extension	14.66°/±0.94	14.16°/±0.68	0.18
Lumbar right lateral flexion	18.67°/±0.74	17.83°/±1.06	0.09
Lumbar left lateral flexion	18.34°/±0.74	18.05°/±0.95	0.38

3.1.2. The Japanese Orthopaedic Association (JOA) Score

The JOA score was used to analyze leg pain, low back pain, and everyday activities in both groups, healthy and LBP patients. This method has a maximum score of 29 points, and higher JOA scores indicate better outcomes for the analyzed criteria [37]. Statistically significant differences were found between the two groups (p-value = 0.0003). The average healthy subjects' JOA score was 27.15 (SD) = 0.73) (Group A), while the corresponding values for LBP patients were evaluated at 22.2 (SD = 1.01) (Group B).

3.2. *Wearable Sensors—IMU Data*

All measured tests presented statistically significant differences between the examined groups, as the p-values mentioned in each case indicate.

Supine Bridge Test

The position obtained during the execution of the supine bridge test was extension (compared to the neutral position), with patients m: mean = 15.27° of extension SD = 1.42 for Group A and mean = 12.96° of extension SD = 2.10 for Group B (p-value = 0.00004) (Figure 4).

Prone Bridge Test

The position obtained during the execution of the prone bridge test was extension (compared to the neutral position), with the patients measured at: mean = 4.45° of extension SD = 1.07 for Group A and mean = 6.07° of extension SD = 1.97 for Group B (p-value = 0.0001) (Figure 5).

Left-Side Bridge Test

The position obtained during the execution of the left-side bridge test was right lateral flexion (compared to the neutral position), with patients achieving the following values: mean = 2.72° of right lateral flexion SD = 1.10 for Group A and mean = 3.64° of right lateral flexion SD = 1.09 for Group B (p-value = 0.0004) (Figure 6).

Right-Side Bridge Test

The position obtained during the execution of the right-side bridge test was left lateral flexion (compared to the neutral position), with the patients measured at: mean = 2.45° of left lateral flexion SD = 0.58 for Group A and mean = 3.44° of left lateral flexion SD = 0.85 for Group B (p-value = 0.00002) (Figure 7).

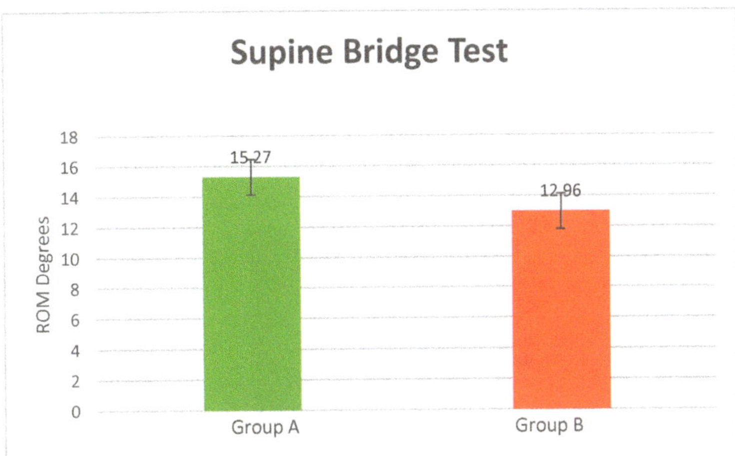

Figure 4. Supine bridge test results (p-value = 0.00004).

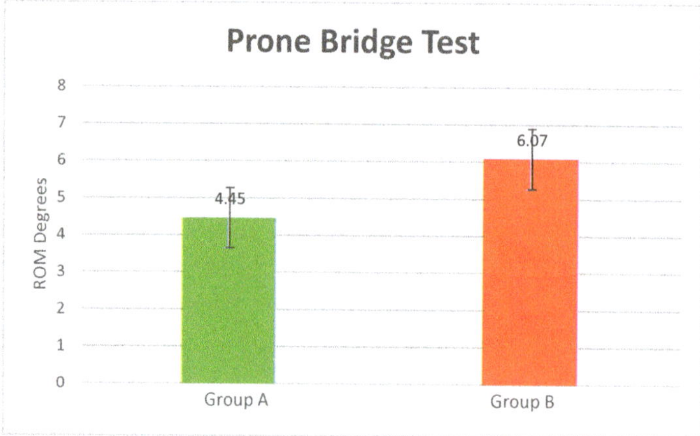

Figure 5. Prone bridge test results (p-value = 0.0001).

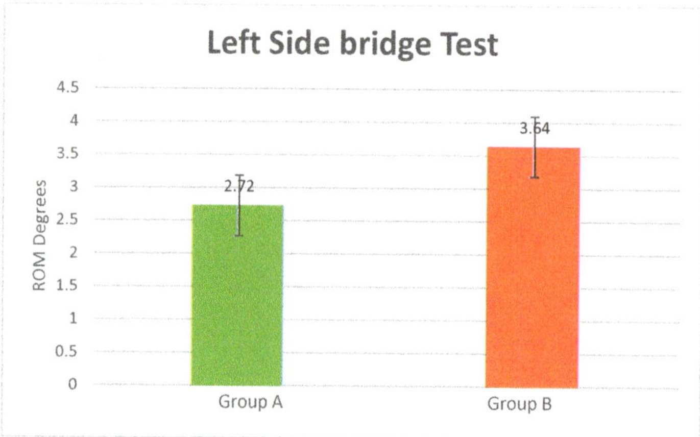

Figure 6. Left-side bridge test results (p-value = 0.0004).

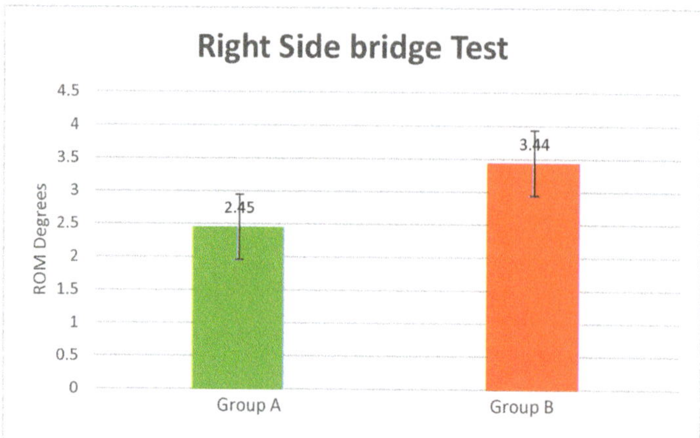

Figure 7. Right-side bridge test results (p-value = 0.00002).

We present some indicative diagrams for the lumbar spine kinematics behavior for both groups in the three tests, as shown in Figures 8–10.

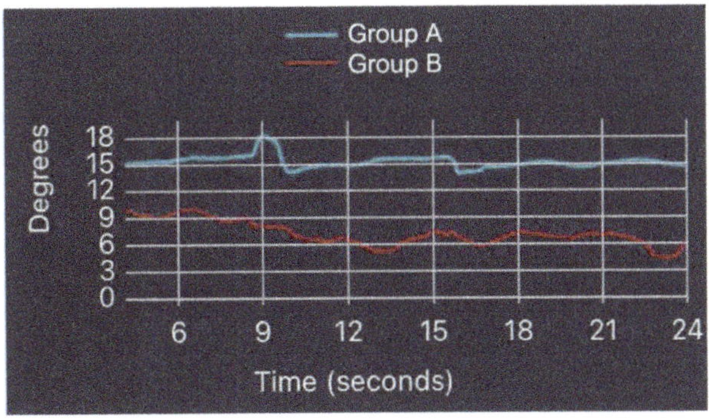

Figure 8. SUBT flexion–extension diagram for Groups A and B.

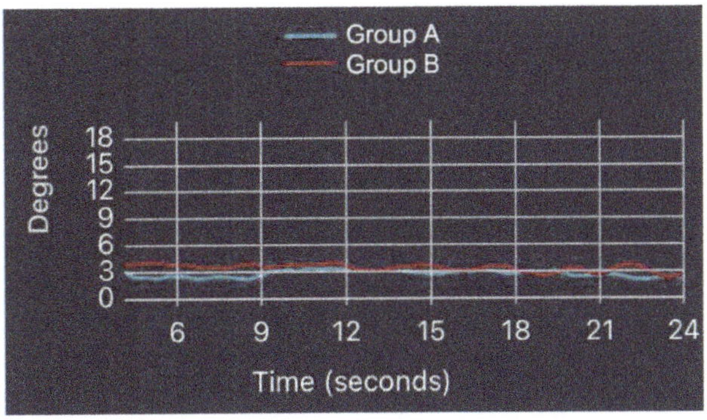

Figure 9. PBT flexion–extension diagram for Groups A and B.

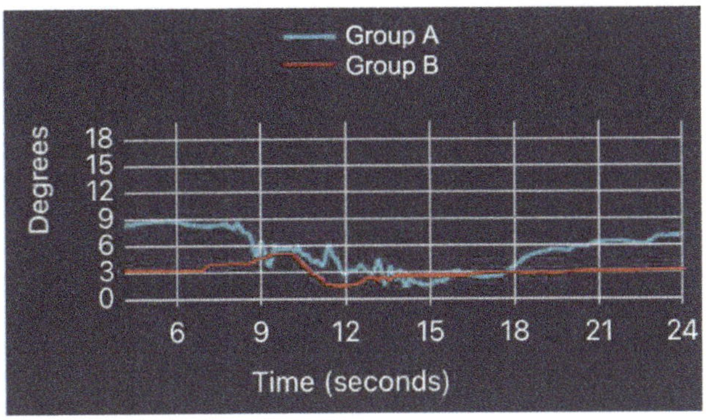

Figure 10. Left-SBT lateral flexion diagram for Groups A and B.

4. Discussion

The clinical assessment of patients with lumbar spine dysfunction includes testing for an abnormal gross range of motion at the three axes of motion [38]. Prone plank bridge, supine bridge, and side bridge tests are the most commonly used functional tests for assessing patients with low back problems in daily clinical practice. However, they do not evaluate possible kinematic impairments for LBP patients compared to healthy individuals [39,40]. In our study, we introduced and measured for the first time, to our knowledge, the kinematic components of the most widely used clinical tests for low back pain assessment. The measured parameter was the lumbar spine position obtained during the execution of each of the three tests compared to the neutral position. The supine bridge test evaluated lumbar extension, the prone bridge test evaluated lumbar flexion, the left-side bridge test evaluated right lateral flexion, and the right-side bridge test evaluated left lateral flexion. We identified statistically significant differences for all measured tests between the examined groups.

Researchers report significant losses in the range of lumbar spine movement in LBP subjects in all directions, for example, loss of hip flexion and altered hip and lumbar spine kinematics while performing trunk movements [41] and between LBP subgroups, some of which involve the action of lumbar spine extension [42,43]. Their results agree with our data when kinematics are measured through clinical tests.

Despite the lack of information about the kinematics of the lumbar spine during these three bridge tests, a number of other experiments examining lumbar spine ROMs during the execution of comparable exercises have been described. Milosavljevic et al. (2008) report mean peak values of angular displacement of the lumbar spine at 17.5 $\pm$ 5.6 degrees when their healthy young subjects performed trunk bending backward and returning to the upright position [38]. These values for peak angular displacement for the lumbar spine and hip are also consistent with those obtained in other studies [41,44]. Our study measured the mean peak values of angular displacement at the supine bridge test for Group A (healthy subjects) at 15.27 degrees.

Our results show less ROM in LBP patients compared to healthy individuals and a shorter duration of the test execution (the time at which the test stopped because of pain). This might suggest that the statistically significant differences found in the ROMs in all three planes and the reduced duration for which patients could maintain the test position could result from muscle strength deficits (since all subjects had a normal passive ROM and could potentially perform similar active ROM scores). Thus, a kinesiotherapy exercise program targeting these muscle groups to increase their strength and endurance could help LBP patients achieve better active ROMs and time scores for our tests and, as a result, reduce symptoms and improve functionality [45–49].

Vanti et al. 1 [50] discovered an improvement in results in symptomatic lumbar spondylolisthesis patients prior to and following treatment (time duration). In addition, they demonstrated the sensitivity of bridge tests since their results were substantially correlated with discomfort and functional changes. Changes in bridge test scores also appeared to be associated with the degree of perceived progress as evaluated by the Global Perceived Effect questionnaire and were consistent with other quality indicators (Oswestry Disability Index—Italian version and the Pain Numerical Rating Scale). In the literature, bridge movements have primarily been investigated as a treatment technique to increase muscle strength and performance of the lower back area in patients with nonspecific LBP [51–53], progressing from reduced-intensity exercises to high-intensity [54].

In the past, physicians evaluated a patient's success in bridge tests (BTs) based on the length of time the patient could hold the relevant posture. With our study, we emphasize the need to correlate these findings with kinematic data to determine whether the improvement observed after rehabilitation protocols also reflects improvement in the functional capacity (kinematics improvement) of these patients, which is a crucial factor in treatment decision making. This quantitative assessment of lumbar spine motion in all three planes converts the prone plank test, supine bridge test, and side bridge test into an objective biomechanical diagnostic tool for LPBs that may be used to evaluate the success of applied rehabilitation programs. However, no study has yet been conducted on the response to the clinical change (kinematics) over time of these tests in patients with LBP. In clinical practice, the clinician evaluates the patients subjectively by visually controlling the correct posture but is not involved in any way in helping patients maintain the position during the test execution [50]. Our study introduces an objective component for the assessment of LBP patients by measuring kinematic parameters, which also reflect the functional ability of LPB patients. Thus, BTs can additionally be utilized to identify clinical and quantitative shifts in chronic LBP patients following rehabilitation treatment. In addition, information on kinematics may enable the physiotherapist to determine the importance of a variation in BTs between the reference point (typically the first session) and each successive phase of treatment. Therefore, additional research should be conducted on using BTs during and after the completion of a physical therapy program for chronic LBP, and not only as an assessment tool to evaluate the fitness level of the core lower back musculature. Furthermore, the advancement in BTs scores, in lumbar kinematics, and the overall improvement in low back discomfort and disability, is significantly clinically relevant, as these easy tests that can be conducted daily in a clinical environment, can assist rehabilitation professionals in objectively evaluating their patients' improvement.

5. Limitations

Conventional motion capture with reflector skin markers is widely used to quantify joint kinematics; nevertheless, the relative movement occurring at the biological tissue between the bones and markers produces a source of measurement error called soft tissue artifacts (STAs). STAs are also prevalent when IMUs are attached to the skin of the lumbar spine to capture the lumbar spine's range of motion. Xin HI et al. employed dual fluoroscopic techniques to assess STAs in lumbar spine motion in healthy adult participants. During extension, they discovered that the lower lumbar region (L4–L5: 2.7 ± 0.7 mm) had considerably fewer STAs than the upper lumbar region (L1–L3: 6.1 ± 3.3 mm) [55]. Likewise, Zemp et al. report a mean STA of 10.7 ± 4.8 mm in lumbar extended postures when comparing skin marker motion to MRI images [56]. Given the fact that IMUs are mounted to the skin in the same manner as skin markers of optoelectronic motion capture systems and that lumbar spinous process mean height dimensions vary from 18 to 27 mm in adults [57], it appears that even though STAs occur and present a potential source of inaccuracy in such measurements, the surface equipment's skin position (markers and IMUs) should still coincide with the underlying spinous process when a full range of motion is executed.

In an effort to further examine the phenomenon in which the motion of the skin does not reflect the motion of the underlying vertebrae perfectly, W.K. Chiou et al. aimed to establish a relationship between skin surface motion and intervertebral motion [58]. The researchers computed and compared the intersegmental joint angles of the lumbar spine during sagittal plane motion using a digitized and transformed data model. In their investigation, the non-invasive and invasive ISA differences varied from 0.29 to 2.08 degrees of the complete range of flexion ROM (0.58 to 5.6% of the full ROM).

Consistent with previous results, Yang et al. report estimation errors of surface-attached sensors in monitoring flexion movement of the lumbar region of approximately 5% of the full range of motion compared to those attained with computed tomography in capturing the entire lumbar spine position (used as the "gold" standard), therefore concluding that kinematic measurements with skin-mounted sensors are sufficiently accurate [59].

Similarly, Ha, Tshui-Hung, and colleagues sought to validate the use of IMUs in measuring the three-dimensional spinal range of motion using an electromagnetic tracking system as a benchmark. They discovered that measurements acquired with the inertial measuring system were strongly correlated with the electromagnetic tracking system, exhibited great agreement, and did not have any major differences from the electromagnetic tracking system. Thus, they concluded that inertial measurement systems containing a gyroscope, an accelerometer, and magnetometer sensors (IMUs with these components were used in our study) are accurate instruments for assessing the three-dimensional spinal range of motion and that their cost-effectiveness, compact footprint, and ease of use offer significant advantages in such measurements [60].

Leroy reports that soft tissue and skin movement can induce IMUs to change their positions relative to the body's bony prominence. However, these artifacts' impact is minor during low-intensity activities (such as the three-bridge test assessed in our study) [61].

6. Conclusions

The development of miniature sensors has created new opportunities for simultaneous and long-term recording and the quantification of human body kinematics, including objective evaluation of motor abnormalities that spontaneously emerge and are recreated by individuals in real-world settings [62,63]. Their lightness, compact size, relatively inexpensive cost, energy efficiency, and mobility characteristics make them appropriate for several applications, providing an objective assessment component for various clinical tests. Spatiotemporal parameters (angular velocity, acceleration) that can also be recorded with IMUs could provide more detailed information about muscular performance, and thus further research in that direction should be promoted.

Author Contributions: Conceptualization, A.T. and G.P.; methodology, A.T., G.P., S.S., P.G. and M.K.; software, A.-Z.S. and E.K.; validation, C.T., O.S., P.P. and P.K.; formal analysis, G.G.; investigation, A.T. and G.P.; resources, A.T., G.P., C.T., O.S., P.P. and P.K.; data curation, A.-Z.S. and E.K.; writing—original draft preparation, A.T. and G.P.; writing—review and editing, A.T., G.P., S.S., P.G. and M.K.; visualization, A.T. and G.P.; supervision, A.T. and G.P.; project administration, A.T. and G.P. All authors have read and agreed to the published version of the manuscript.

Funding: This research received no external funding.

Institutional Review Board Statement: The study was conducted in accordance with the Declaration of Helsinki, and approved by the Institutional Review Board (or Ethics Committee) of the Department of Medicine, National and Kapodistrian University of Athens (67079/7 July 2022).

Informed Consent Statement: Informed consent was obtained from all subjects involved in the study. Written informed consent has been obtained from the patient to publish this paper.

Data Availability Statement: All data supporting the study's reported results are stored in the local computer data network of the Biomechanics Laboratory Department of Physiotherapy, University of the Peloponnese, and are available on request from the corresponding author. The data are not publicly available due to the Laboratory's personal data privacy policy.

Conflicts of Interest: The authors declare no conflict of interest.

References

1. Kolář, P.; Šulc, J.; Kynčl, M.; Šanda, J.; Čakrt, O.; Andel, R.; Kumagai, K.; Kobesová, A. Postural function of the diaphragm in persons with and without chronic low back pain. *J. Orthop. Sports Phys. Ther.* **2012**, *42*, 352–362. [CrossRef] [PubMed]
2. Kalichman, L.; Carmeli, E.; Been, E. The association between imaging parameters of the paraspinal muscles, spinal degeneration, and low back pain. *BioMed Res. Int.* **2017**, *2017*, 2562957. [CrossRef]
3. Hildebrandt, M.; Fankhauser, G.; Meichtry, A.; Luomajoki, H. Correlation between lumbar dysfunction and fat infiltration in lumbar multifidus muscles in patients with low back pain. *BMC Musculoskelet. Disord.* **2017**, *18*, 12. [CrossRef] [PubMed]
4. Freeman, M.D.; Woodham, M.A.; Woodham, A.W. The Role of the Lumbar Multifidus in Chronic Low Back Pain: A Review. *Phys. Med. Rehabil.* **2010**, *2*, 142–146. [CrossRef] [PubMed]
5. Padwal, J.; Berry, D.B.; Hubbard, J.C.; Zlomislic, V.; Allen, R.T.; Garfin, S.R.; Ward, S.R.; Shahidi, B. Regional differences between superficial and deep lumbar multifidus in patients with chronic lumbar spine pathology. *BMC Musculoskelet. Disord.* **2020**, *21*, 1–9. [CrossRef] [PubMed]
6. Steele, J.; Fisher, J.; Perrin, C.; Conway, R.; Bruce-Low, S.; Smith, D. Does change in isolated lumbar extensor muscle function correlate with good clinical outcome? A secondary analysis of data on change in isolated lumbar extension strength, pain, and disability in chronic low back pain. *Disabil. Rehabil.* **2018**, *41*, 1287–1295. [CrossRef]
7. Steele, J.; Bruce-Low, S.; Smith, D. A reappraisal of the deconditioning hypothesis in low back pain: Review of evidence from a triumvirate of research methods on specific lumbar extensor deconditioning. *Curr. Med. Res. Opin.* **2014**, *30*, 865–911. [CrossRef]
8. Imai, A.; Kaneoka, K. The relationship between trunk endurance plank tests and athletic performance tests in adolescent soccer players. *Int. J. Sports Phys. Ther.* **2016**, *11*, 718–724.
9. Avers, D.; Brown, M. *Daniels and Worthingham's Muscle Testing: Techniques of Manual Examination and Performance Testing*; Elsevier: Philadelphia, PA, USA, 2018; pp. 48–80.

10. Witting, N.; Andersen, L.K.; Vissing, J. Axial myopathy: An overlooked feature of muscle diseases. *Brain* **2016**, *139*, 13–22. [CrossRef]
11. Vlažná, D.; Krkoška, P.; Kuhn, M.; Dosbaba, F.; Batalik, L.; Vlčková, E.; Voháňka, S.; Adamová, B. Assessment of Lumbar Extensor Muscles in the Context of Trunk Function, a Pilot Study in Healthy Individuals. *Appl. Sci.* **2021**, *11*, 9518. [CrossRef]
12. Saal, J.A.; Saal, J.S. Nonoperative treatment of herniated lumbar intervertebral disc with radiculopathy: An outcome study. *Spine* **1989**, *14*, 431–443. [CrossRef] [PubMed]
13. Bullock-Saxton, J.E.; Janda, V.; Bullock, M.I. Reflex Activation of Gluteal Muscles in Walking. *Spine* **1993**, *18*, 704–708. [CrossRef] [PubMed]
14. O'Sullivan, P.; Twomey, L.; Allison, G. Evaluation of specific stabilizing exercise in the treatment of chronic low back pain with radiologic diagnosis of spondylolysis or spondylolysthesis. *Spine* **1997**, *24*, 2959–2967. [CrossRef] [PubMed]
15. Jørgensen, K. Human trunk extensor muscles physiology and ergonomics. *Acta Physiol. Scand. Suppl.* **1997**, *637*, 1–58.
16. Wilder, D.G.; Aleksiev, A.R.; Magnusson, M.L.; Pope, M.H.; Spratt, K.F.; Goel, V.K. Muscular Response to Sudden Load. *Spine* **1996**, *21*, 2628–2639. [CrossRef]
17. McGill, S.M.; Childs, A.; Liebenson, C. Endurance times for low back stabilization exercises: Clinical targets for testing and training from a normal database. *Arch. Phys. Med. Rehabil.* **1999**, *80*, 941–944. [CrossRef]
18. Crawford, R.J.; Cornwall, J.; Abbott, R.; Elliott, J.M. Manually defining regions of interest when quantifying paravertebral muscles fatty infiltration from axial magnetic resonance imaging: A proposed method for the lumbar spine with ana-tomical cross-reference. *BMC Musculoskelet. Disord.* **2017**, *18*, 25. [CrossRef]
19. Glowinski, S.; Blazejewski, A.; Krzyzynski, T. Inertial Sensors and Wavelets Analysis as a Tool for Pathological Gait Identification. In *Innovations in Biomedical Engineering*; Advances in Intelligent Systems and Computing; Springer: Cham, Switzerland, 2016; pp. 106–114.
20. Bohannon, R.W.; Steffl, M.; Glenney, S.S.; Green, M.; Cashwell, L.; Prajerova, K.; Bunn, J. The prone bridge test: Performance, validity, and reliability among older and younger adults. *J. Bodyw. Mov. Ther.* **2018**, *22*, 385–389. [CrossRef]
21. Ikezaki, F.; Krueger, E.; de Souza Guerino Macedo, C. Performance, reliability and fatigue in prone bridge test and supine unilateral bridge test. *J. Bodyw. Mov. Ther.* **2020**, *26*, 238–245. [CrossRef]
22. Triantafyllou, A.; Papagiannis, G.; Stasi, S.; Bakalidou, D.; Kyriakidou, M.; Papathanasiou, G.; Papadopoulos, E.C.; Papagelopoulos, P.J.; Koulouvaris, P. Application of Wearable Sensors Technology for Lumbar Spine Kinematic Measurements during Daily Activities following Microdiscectomy Due to Severe Sciatica. *Biology* **2022**, *11*, 398. [CrossRef]
23. Mok, F.P.; Samartzis, D.; Karppinen, J.; Fong, D.Y.; Luk, K.D.; Cheung, K.M. Modic changes of the lumbar spine: Prevalence, risk factors, and association with disc degeneration and low back pain in a large-scale population-based cohort. *Spine J.* **2016**, *16*, 32–41. [CrossRef] [PubMed]
24. Griffith, J.F.; Wang, Y.X.; Antonio, G.E.; Choi, K.C.; Yu, A.; Ahuja, A.T.; Leung, P.C. Modified Pfirrmann grading system for lumbar intervertebral disc degeneration. *Spine* **2007**, *32*, E708–E712. [CrossRef] [PubMed]
25. Urrutia, J.; Besa, P.; Campos, M.; Cikutovic, P.; Cabezon, M.; Molina, M.; Cruz, J.P. The Pfirrmann classification of lumbar intervertebral disc degeneration: An inde-pendent inter- and intra-observer agreement assessment. *Eur. Spine J.* **2016**, *25*, 2728–2733. [CrossRef] [PubMed]
26. Kato, S.; Oshima, Y.; Oka, H.; Chikuda, H.; Takeshita, Y.; Miyoshi, K.; Kawamura, N.; Masuda, K.; Kunogi, J.; Okazaki, R.; et al. Comparison of the Japanese Orthopaedic Association (JOA) Score and Modified JOA (mJOA) Score for the Assessment of Cervical Myelopathy: A Multicenter Observational Study. *PLoS ONE* **2015**, *10*, e0123022. [CrossRef] [PubMed]
27. Hislop, H.J.; Montgomery, J. *Daniels and Worthingham's Muscle Testing: Techniques of Manual Examination*, 8th ed.; Saunders/Elsevier: St. Louis, MO, USA, 2017.
28. Schellenberg, K.L.; Lang, J.M.; Chan, K.M.; Burnham, R.S. A clinical tool for office assessment of lumbar spine stabilization endurance: Prone and supine bridge maneuvers. *Am. J. Phys. Med. Rehabil.* **2007**, *86*, 380–386. [CrossRef]
29. Juan-Recio, C.; Prat-Luri, A.; Galindo, A.; Manresa-Rocamora, A.; Barbado, D.; Vera-Garcia, F.J. Is the Side Bridge Test Valid and Reliable for Assessing Trunk Lateral Flexor Endurance in Recreational Female Athletes? *Biology* **2022**, *11*, 1043. [CrossRef]
30. Cafolla, D.; Chen, I.-M.; Ceccarelli, M. An experimental characterization of human torso motion. *Front. Mech. Eng.* **2015**, *10*, 311–325. [CrossRef]
31. Chaparro-Rico, B.D.M.; Cafolla, D. Test-Retest, Inter-Rater and Intra-Rater Reliability for Spatiotemporal Gait Parameters Using SANE (an eaSy gAte aNalysis systEm) as Measuring Instrument. *Appl. Sci.* **2020**, *10*, 5781. [CrossRef]
32. Hoffman, S.L.; Johnson, M.B.; Zou, D.; Van Dillen, L.R. Differences in end-range lumbar flexion during slumped sitting and forward bending between low back pain subgroups and genders. *Man Ther.* **2012**, *17*, 157–163. [CrossRef]
33. Borden, W.B.; Chiang, Y.-P.; Kronick, R. Bringing Patient-Centered Outcomes Research to Life. *Value Health* **2015**, *18*, 355–357. [CrossRef] [PubMed]
34. Ludwig, S.A.; Burnham, K.D. Comparison of Euler estimate using extended Kalman filter, Madgwick and Mahony on quadcopter flight data. In Proceedings of the 2018 International Conference on Unmanned Aircraft Systems, Dallas, TX, USA, 12–15 June 2018.
35. Zhou, Q.; Li, Z.; Yu, G.; Li, H.; Zhang, N. A novel adaptive Kalman filter for Euler-angle-based MEMS IMU/magnetometer attitude estimation. *Meas. Sci. Technol.* **2021**, *32*, 045104. [CrossRef]

36. Bakhshi, S.; Mahoor, M.H.; Davidson, B.S. Development of a body joint angle measurement system using IMU sensors. In Proceedings of the 2011 Annual International Conference of the IEEE Engineering in Medicine and Biology Society, Boston, MA, USA, 30 August–3 September 2011.
37. Sakaura, H.; Ikegami, D.; Fujimori, T.; Sugiura, T.; Owaki, H.; Fuji, T. Abdominal Aortic Calcification Is a Significant Poor Prognostic Factor for Clinical Outcomes After Decompressive Laminotomy for Lumbar Spinal Canal Stenosis. *Glob. Spine J.* **2019**, *9*, 724–728. [CrossRef] [PubMed]
38. Milosavljevic, S.; Pal, P.; Bain, D.; Johnson, G. Kinematic and temporal interactions of the lumbar spine and hip during trunk extension in healthy male subjects. *Eur. Spine J.* **2007**, *17*, 122–128. [CrossRef]
39. Arab, A.M.; Salavati, M.; Ebrahimi, I.; Mousavi, M.E. Sensitivity, specificity and predictive value of the clinical trunk muscle endurance tests in low back pain. *Clin. Rehabil.* **2007**, *21*, 640–647. [CrossRef] [PubMed]
40. Carlsson, H.; Rasmussen-Barr, E. Clinical screening tests for assessing movement control in non-specific low-back pain. A systematic review of intra- and inter-observer reliability studies. *Man. Ther.* **2013**, *18*, 103–110. [CrossRef] [PubMed]
41. Wong, T.K.T.; Lee, R.Y.W. Effects of low back pain on the relationship between the movements of the lumbar spine and hip. *Hum. Mov. Sci.* **2004**, *23*, 21–34. [CrossRef]
42. Gombatto, S.P.; Collins, D.R.; Sahrmann, S.; Engsberg, J.R.; Van Dillen, L.R. Patterns of lumbar region movement during trunk lateral bending in 2 subgroups of people with low back pain. *Phys. Ther.* **2007**, *87*, 441–454. [CrossRef]
43. Van Dillen, L.R.; Gombatto, S.P.; Collins, D.R.; Engsberg, J.R.; Sahrmann, S.A. Symmetry of timing of hip and lumbopelvic rotation motion in 2 different subgroups of people with low back pain. *Arch. Phys. Med. Rehabil.* **2007**, *88*, 351–360. [CrossRef]
44. Lee, R.Y.W.; Wong, T.K.T. Relationship between the movements of the lumbar spine and hip. *Hum. Mov. Sci.* **2002**, *21*, 481–494. [CrossRef]
45. García-Vaquero, M.P.; Moreside, J.M.; Brontons-Gil, E.; Peco-González, N.; Vera-Garcia, F.J. Trunk muscle activation during stabilization exercises with single and double leg support. *J. Electromyogr. Kinesiol.* **2012**, *22*, 398–406. [CrossRef]
46. Anders, C.; Wenzel, B.; Scholle, H.C. Activation characteristics of trunk muscles during cyclic upper-body perturbations caused by an oscillating pole. *Arch. Phys. Med. Rehabil.* **2008**, *89*, 1314–1322. [CrossRef] [PubMed]
47. Bjerkefors, A.; Ekblom, M.M.; Josefsson, K.; Thorstensson, A. Deep and superficial abdominal muscle activation during trunk stabilization exercises with and without instruction to hollow. *Man. Ther.* **2010**, *15*, 502–507. [CrossRef] [PubMed]
48. Ekstrom, R.A.; Donatelli, R.A.; Carp, K.C. Electromyo-graphic analysis of core trunk, hip, and thigh muscles during 9 rehabilitation exercises. *J. Orthop. Sports Phys. Ther.* **2007**, *37*, 754–762. Available online: https://www.jospt.org/doi/abs/10.2519/jospt.2007.2471 (accessed on 7 July 2021). [CrossRef] [PubMed]
49. McGill, S.M.; Karpowicz, A. Exercises for spine stabilization: Motion/motor patterns, stability progressions, and clinical technique. *Arch. Phys. Med. Rehabil.* **2009**, *90*, 118–126. [CrossRef] [PubMed]
50. Vanti, C.; Ferrari, S.; Berjano, P.; Villafañe, J.H.; Monticone, M. Responsiveness of the bridge maneuvers in subjects with symptomatic lumbar spondylolisthesis: A prospective cohort study. *Physiother. Res. Int.* **2017**, *22*, e1682. [CrossRef]
51. Kong, Y.-S.; Lee, W.-J.; Park, S.; Jang, G.-U. The effects of prone bridge exercise on trunk muscle thickness in chronic low back pain patients. *J. Phys. Ther. Sci.* **2015**, *27*, 2073–2076. [CrossRef] [PubMed]
52. Guthrie, R.J.; Grindstaff, T.L.; Croy, T.; Ingersoll, C.D.; Saliba, S.A. The effect of traditional bridging or suspension-exercise bridging on lateral abdominal thickness in individuals with low back pain. *J. Sport Rehabil.* **2012**, *21*, 151–160. [CrossRef] [PubMed]
53. Ferrari, S.; Vanti, C.; O'Reilly, C. Clinical presentation and physiotherapy treatment of 4 patients with low back pain and isthmic spondylolisthesis. *J. Chiropr. Med.* **2012**, *11*, 94–103. [CrossRef]
54. Ekstrom, R.A.; Osborn, R.W.; Hauer, P.L. Surface electromyographic analysis of the low back muscles during rehabilitation exercises. *J. Orthop. Sports Phys. Ther.* **2008**, *38*, 736–745. [CrossRef]
55. Xi, X.; Ling, Z.; Wang, C.; Gu, C.; Zhan, X.; Yu, H.; Lu, S.; Tsai, T.Y.; Yu, Y.; Cheng, L. Lumbar segment-dependent soft tissue ar-tifacts of skin markers during in vivo weight-bearing forward-Backward bending. *Front. Bioeng. Biotechnol.* **2022**, *10*, 960063. [CrossRef]
56. Zemp, R.; List, R.; Gülay, T.; Elsig, J.P.; Naxera, J.; Taylor, W.R.; Lorenzetti, S. Soft tissue artefacts of the human back: Comparison of the sagittal curvature of the spine measured using skin markers and an open upright MRI. *PLoS ONE* **2014**, *9*, e95426. [CrossRef] [PubMed]
57. Aylott, C.E.; Puna, R.; Robertson, P.A.; Walker, C. Spinous process morphology: The effect of ageing through adulthood on spinous process size and relationship to sagittal alignment. *Eur. Spine J.* **2012**, *21*, 1007–1012. [CrossRef] [PubMed]
58. Chiou, W.-K.; Lee, Y.-H.; Chen, W.-J.; Lee, M.-Y.; Lin, Y.-H. A non-invasive protocol for the determination of lumbar spine mobility. *Clin. Biomech.* **1996**, *11*, 474–480. [CrossRef]
59. Yang, Z.; Ma, H.T.; Wang, D.; Lee, R. Error analysis on spinal motion measurement using skin mounted sensors. *Annu. Int. Conf. IEEE Eng. Med. Biol. Soc.* **2008**, *2008*, 4740–4743. [PubMed]
60. Ha, T.H.; Saber-Sheikh, K.; Moore, A.P.; Jones, M.P. Measurement of lumbar spine range of movement and coupled motion using inertial sensors—A protocol validity study. *Man Ther.* **2013**, *18*, 87–91. [CrossRef]
61. Eve, L. Analysis of the Spine through a Multibody Model and IMU Technology. Master's Thesis, Université Catholique de Louvain, Ottignies-Louvain-la-Neuve, Belgium, 2019.

62. Triantafyllou, A.; Papagiannis, G.; Nikolaou, V.S.; Papagelopoulos, P.J.; Babis, G.C. Similar Biomechanical Behavior in Gait Analysis between Ceramic-on-Ceramic and Ceramic-on-XLPE Total Hip Arthroplasties. *Life* **2021**, *11*, 1366. [CrossRef]
63. Papagiannis, G.; Triantafyllou, A.; Konstantina, Y.G.; Koulouvaris, P.; Anastasiou, A.; Papadopoulos, E.C.; Papagelopoulos, P.J.; Babis, G.C. Biomechanical Factors could Affect Lumbar Disc Reherniation after Microdiscectomy. *J. Orthop. Sports Med.* **2019**, *1*, 46–50. [CrossRef]

bioengineering

MDPI

Article

Pelvic Floor Pressures Differ Based on Location in the Pelvis and Body Position: A Cadaver Mode

Tova Ablove *,†, Alexandra DeRosa †, Steven Lewis *,†, Katelyn Benson †, Frank Mendel † and Scott Doyle *,†

Jacobs School of Medicine and Biomedical Sciences, University at Buffalo, Buffalo, NY 14203-1121, USA

* Correspondence: tablove@buffalo.edu (T.A.); salewis@buffalo.edu (S.L.); scottdoy@buffalo.edu (S.D.); Tel.: +(716)-323-0715 (T.A.); +(585)-358-1585 (S.L.)

† These authors contributed equally to this work.

Abstract: Background: The pelvic floor is a bowl-shaped complex of multiple muscles and fascia, which functions to support the pelvic organs, and it aids in controlling continence. In pelvic floor disease, this complex becomes weakened or damaged leading to urinary, fecal incontinence, and pelvic organ prolapse. It is unclear whether the position of the body impacts the forces on the pelvic floor. Purpose: The primary objective of this work is to measure force applied to the pelvic floor of a cadaver in sitting, standing, supine, and control positions. The secondary objective is to map the forces across the pelvic floor. Methods: An un-embalmed female cadaver without pelvic floor dysfunction was prepared for pelvic floor pressure measurement using a pressure sensory array placed on top of the pelvic floor, and urodynamic catheters were placed in the hollow of the sacrum, the retropubic space, and at the vaginal apex. Pressure measurements were recorded with the cadaver in the supine position, sitting cushioned without external pelvic floor support, and standing. Pressure array data were analyzed along with imaging of the cadaver. Together, these data were mapped into a three-dimensional reconstruction of the pressure points in pelvic floor and corresponding pelvic organs. Results: pressures were higher at the symphysis than in the hollow of the sacrum in the standing position. Pressure array measurements were lowest in the standing position and highest in the sitting position. Three-dimensional reconstruction confirmed the location and accuracy of our measurements. Conclusions: The findings of increased pressures behind the symphysis are in line with the higher incidence of anterior compartment prolapse. Our findings support our hypothesis that the natural shape and orientation of the pelvis in the standing position shields the pelvic floor from downward forces of the viscera.

Keywords: pelvic organ prolapse; pelvic floor structure; pressure analysis; pelvic floor modeling; biomechanics

1. Introduction

The pelvic floor is a bowl-shaped group of muscles and connective tissue located in the pelvis. It is made up of the levator ani muscle complex, coccygeus muscle, and endopelvic connective tissue [1], coalescing into a diaphragm with a maximum thickness of 3 mm that closes the bottom of the pelvis [2]. The perforations (i.e., from the vagina, urethra, and anus) in the pelvic floor created by these organs inherently weaken the structure as a whole. This complex supports the pelvic organs (bladder, vagina, and rectum) while aiding in controlling continence of both urine and stool [3]. Moreover, expansion and contraction of those organs during urination, defecation, and birthing further stress the structure.

Pelvic floor dysfunction (PFD) occurs when the muscles or connective tissue of the pelvic floor weaken. According to the American Urogynecologic Society, the most common types of PFD are urinary incontinence, pelvic organ prolapse, and fecal incontinence [4]. PFD is more common among older women [3], as well as those with risk factors, including obesity, chronic constipation, chronic cough, childbirth, and prior hysterectomy [5]. PFD is also common in women with high physical activity, such as athletes [6]. It is a very common condition with an overall prevalence of 23.7% [3].

PFD can have a profound impact on quality of life. Patients report social isolation, relationship problems, and sexual dysfunction [7,8] as some of the quality of life issues faced with PFD. Although there are many preventative and corrective therapies including pelvic floor muscle training, weight loss, controlling constipation, and pessaries, the majority of women will eventually opt for surgery. The lifetime risk of surgery for PFD is 20% [2]. In addition, according to a report in 2010, PFD costs over $500 million a year on the healthcare industry for surgeries [9], demonstrating the profound societal impact.

The pelvic floor muscles are thin, and the associated connective tissue is weak as compared to abdominal connective tissue or muscle tendons [1]. The inherent anatomy of the pelvic floor muscles dictate that these skeletal muscles would have to be in constant contraction in order to support the weight of the abdomen and pelvic organs. This tissue does not appear strong enough to withstand large forces over long periods of time, and it does not have the energy available for sustainability. Yet, while PFD is a common condition, the majority of women do not develop dysfunction, despite exhibiting the risk factors listed above (childbirth, gravity, long-term physically strenuous activity) [2,3]. Therefore, the risk factors are likely associative and not causal or deterministic.

We believe that anatomical forces incident on the pelvic floor play a role in the risk of developing PFD. To our knowledge, a direct study of the distribution of these anatomical forces on the pelvic floor has not been done.

In this study, we focus on exploring the nature of the anatomical forces that play across the pelvic floor as a result of different body positions. Our hypothesis is that different body positions will demonstrate differing visceral force loads on the pelvic floor, with the lowest visceral pressures displayed in the standing position. Further, we hypothesize that visceral load will be greater closer to the pubic symphisis, especially in postures reducing the lordotic lumbar curve.

2. Methods

This study has been approved by the Institutional Review Board at the University at Buffalo.

2.1. Cadaver Preparation and Pressure Sensor Placement

A fresh (un-embalmed) 103 lb female cadaver was acquired from the University at Buffalo, Department of Pathology and Anatomical Sciences Anatomical Gift Program. The cadaver was donated by a woman who was 92 years of age at the time of death. No signs of pelvic floor dysfunction were evident upon examination. A low transverse abdominal incision was made to expose the junction between small and large bowels. After the distal ileum was tied off, contrast was injected into the small bowel. A 16 French Foley catheter was inserted into the bladder. Remaining retroperitoneal, blunt dissection was used to access the pelvic floor on the right side without disrupting midline structures. A 3×8 cm array of pressure sensors mounted in cloth-like material (Tactarry Model 5334, Pressure Profile Systems Inc.) was inserted directly on top of the pelvic floor [10]. To reduce force dissipation through the array, a lead backing plate $1/64''$ thick was inserted on the bone side of the array. T-DOC urodynamic catheters were placed in the hollow of the sacrum, in the retropubic space (symphysis), and transvaginally at the vaginal apex. The urodynamic catheter pressure data were recorded and analyzed using the Laborie Goby Portable Urodynamic System (Laborie UDS) [11].

Measurements were taken transvaginally for pressures at the vaginal apex because this is a pressure commonly measured during standard urodynamic testing in women, and there are normal ranges published in the literature that could be compared to our findings as a control. The pressure array was tared and the abdominal incision closed. Lifting straps attached to a hydraulic lift were applied to the cadaver's upper extremities. To simulate abdominal wall tone, a rubber belt was placed snugly around the trunk.

2.2. Cadaver Postures

Data were collected with the cadaver manipulated into four positions: standing, sitting, supine, and a control position where the cadaver was seated on a donut-shaped inflatable hemorrhoid cushion that, in theory, precluded external support of the pelvic floor when seated. For the first three positions we performed urodynamic pressure measurements (Laborie UDS), pressure array readings, and image capture as described below. For the donut-seated control position, we limited our capture to urodynamic pressure and pressure array readings to compare with published in vivo data (i.e., vaginal apex sensor in the sitting position on donut shaped hemorrhoid cushion).

2.3. Force Measurements

The cadaver was first placed in the supine position with the pressure array in place. Pressure measurements from the pressure array and the Laborie UDS (sacrum, symphysis, vaginal apex) were recorded electronically for approximately one minute. Via a hydraulic lift, the cadaver was then lifted into the sitting position where pressure measurements were again recorded for approximately one minute. Next, the cadaver was moved onto the hemorrhoid cushion, and measurements were recorded. Finally, the cadaver was lifted into the standing position (feet on the floor), and the pressure measurements were recorded.

For reproduceability, this series was repeated a total of ten times. During cadaver manipulation, an external video camera was used to record movements and was synchronized to the pressure array; this ensured that the sensor readings were taken when the cadaver was at rest.

Pressure array data were analyzed via Chameleon Tactile Visualization and Recording Software [12]. The total pressure in each position for each experiment was recorded in grams. A visualization of the pressures exerted on the array in each position for each experiment was saved for texture mapping in the three-dimensional reconstruction step Figure 1.

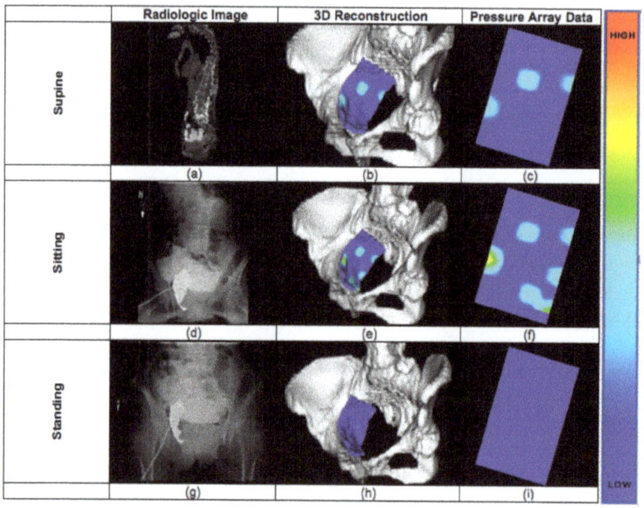

Figure 1. Examples of the body position radiology data with three-dimensional reconstructions of the bones of the pelvis with the pressure array data. (**a**,**d**,**g**) Radiological images of the cadaver with the pressure sensor implanted in supine, sitting and standing positions. (**b**,**e**,**h**) 3D reconstructions of the lumbar and pelvic bones with the pressure sensor mapping along the pelvic floor. (**c**,**f**,**i**) Images of the pressure array data taken without 3D reconstruction. The higher the pressure the more red the color, while the lower the pressure the more blue the color on the map.

2.4. Statistical Analysis

Sacral and symphysis UDS pressures were compared via *t*-test. The effect of cadaver position on total array pressures and UDS vaginal apex pressures were compared using ANOVA, and post hoc tests were conducted using TukeyHSD. Analyses were conducted using the R statistical programming language [13].

2.5. Image Acquisition

Following the force measurement experiments, the cadaver was taken to Buffalo General Hospital for imaging. The Foley catheter, pressure array, and urodynamic catheters remained in place. A CT scan of the supine cadaver was first taken. A standing CT was not available. Therefore, multiple X-ray images were taken. The cadaver was first placed in a seated position where anterior-posterior, right lateral, left lateral, and oblique images were taken. The cadaver was then placed in the standing position (via the hydraulic lift), and the same series of images were again taken. The CT and X-ray images were saved on CDs for analysis.

2.6. Image Analysis and Three-Dimensional Reconstruction

The supine CT images were uploaded into 3D Slicer 4.7 for analysis [14,15]. With use of the segment editor and editor modules, a three-dimensional model of the pelvic floor was constructed (Figure 2).

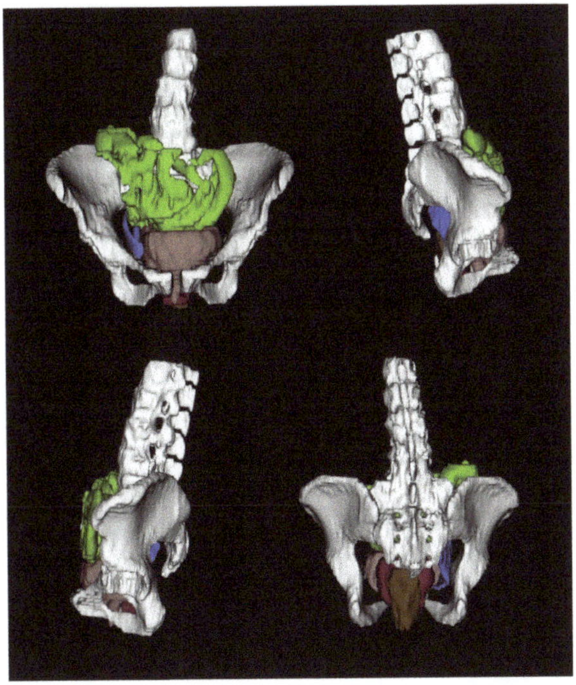

Figure 2. 3D models of the pelvic floor with abdominal structures.

The lumbar spine with sacrum, pelvic bones, bladder, vagina, rectum, pressure array, and bowel were segmented. Each segment was loaded into a scene to create a three-dimensional model of the cadaver in the supine position. The X-ray images were utilized to model the cadaver's pelvic floor in the sitting and standing positions. Each segment was aligned to the X-ray images via the transform module. A linear transform was created for each segment in each position to correctly orient the model with the X-ray images. The left column of Figure 1 shows the original radiologic data sets.

The images from the pressure array collected via Chameleon Tactile Visualization were utilized to create a texture in the MeshLab 3D modeling software [16]. Examples of this texture are shown in the right column of Figure 1, where blue colors correspond to low pressures, and red corresponds to high. The texture was then applied to the pressure array model in 3D Slicer for the various cadaver positions (the middle column of Figure 1). The tactile images of the array allowed for the mapping of pressure points within the context on the pelvic floor and the corresponding pelvic organs.

3. Results

3.1. Force Measurements (UDS and Pressure Array)

The results of the UDS pressure catheter measurements are shown in the plots in Figures 3–5. The pressures recorded by the T-DOC catheters are in cm H_2O whereas those recorded by the array are in gm/cm^2 (Figure 3). For the pressure array, values are reported as mean (gm/cm^2), standard deviation values over the rectangular array area. In each plot, the horizontal line indicates the median recorded value.

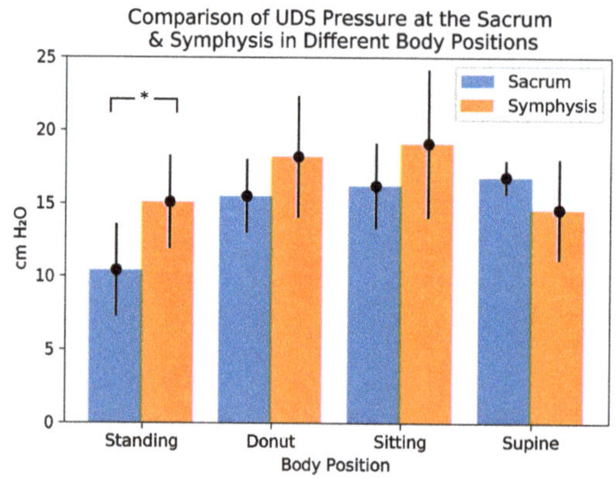

Figure 3. Comparison of the different pressures exerted on the pelvic floor in the different positions in the anterior vs. the posterior compartments (anterior being the symphisis region while posterior being the sacral region). Asterisks indicate statistically significant values.

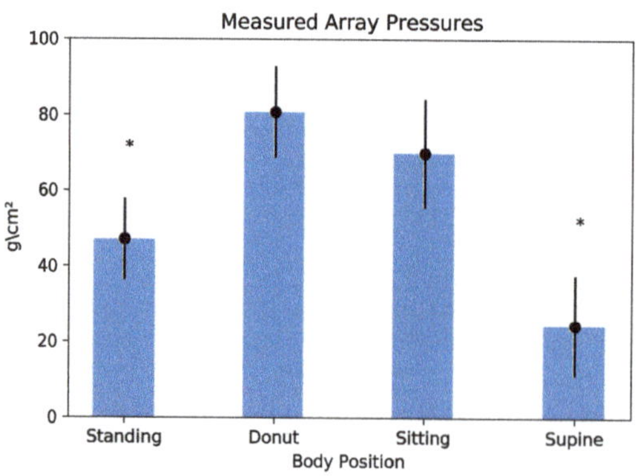

Figure 4. Overall pressures measured via the pressure array. Asterisks indicate statistically significant values.

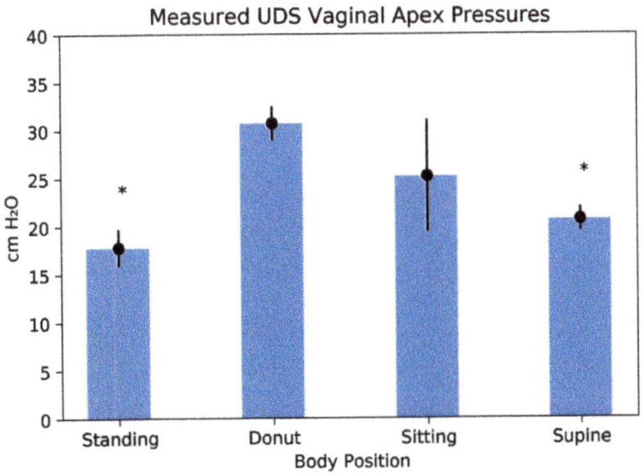

Figure 5. Pressures measured at the vaginal apex in the different positions. Asterisks indicate statistically significant values.

3.1.1. Symphysis vs. Sacrum Comparisons

Pressures at the sacrum were significantly lower than those at the symphysis in the standing position ($p = 0.0037$). There were no significant differences in pressures between sacrum and symphysis in the supine ($p = 0.08112$), sitting ($p = 0.1335$), or donut positions ($p = 0.0956$) (Figure 3).

3.1.2. Array Comparisons

Pressures were lowest and statistically different in the standing position (24.5 gm/cm^2, SD 13.2) when compared to the supine (47.1 gm/cm^2, SD 10.7), sitting (80.8 gm/cm^2, SD 12.1), and donut positions (69.9 gm/cm^2, SD 14.4). Pressure in the supine position was found to be lower and statistically different from those in the sitting and donut positions (Figures 1 and 4).

3.1.3. Vaginal Apex Comparisons

Pressures in the standing and supine positions were similar to each other ($p = 0.21$), but they were lower and statistically different from those in the sitting ($p < 0.01$) and donut positions ($p < 0.01$). Pressures in the sitting and donut position were statistically different from each other ($p < 0.01$) (Figure 5).

3.2. Image Acquisition Results

The images acquired via X-ray and CT are shown in Figure 1. The CT image was acquired in the supine position (top row), whereas X-ray images were acquired in the sitting and standing positions. In all of the imaging modalities, the pressure array was clearly identifiable; there was no observable movement of the array relative to other structures in the pelvic throughout manipulation of the cadaver on the hydraulic lift. Although the pressure array was fixed with a lead backing, the presence of a metal artifact did not preclude our ability to model the pelvis and surrounding soft tissues.

3.3. Three-Dimensional Modelling

The images of the pressure array are shown in Figure 1. Red colors on the array indicate increasing pressures, and blue represents zero pressure. Pressures were not evenly distributed across the array, but instead were specific to geographic locations. Pressure increases were observed where viscera contacted the array.

4. Discussion

The purpose of this study was to directly measure pressure experienced in the pelvic cavity in different postures and anatomic locations. Placing a UDS sensor at the vaginal apex is a common means of measuring abdominal pressures in vivo. To further simulate live urodynamic testing, we placed the cadaver on a hemorrhoid donut removing external support, as would be standard when sitting on a commode in the urodynamic suite. In addition, we placed UDS sensors in locations that cannot be measured in vivo. These were placed behind the pubic symphysis (in the space of Retzius) near the anterior floor of the pelvis, as well as in the hollow of the sacrum (near the roof of the pelvis). We also measured total force on the pelvic floor using the Pressure Profile Systems array positioned directly on top of the levator ani muscles, which also cannot be done in vivo. We hypothesized UDS pressures would be highest anteriorly, and array pressures would be lowest in the standing position

UDS pressures were indeed higher anteriorly, and array pressures were lowest in the standing position. UDS measured sitting and supine measurements, which were consistent with normative in vivo findings, supporting the validity of the model [17,18]. Reported intraabdominal pressure readings obtained similarly through a Foley catheter were 6.5 mm Hg with a range of 0.2–16.2 mm Hg [19], and in various body positions at 9.5 cm H_2O for supine, 11.5 cm H_2O at 30 degrees, and 14 cm H_2O at 45 degrees. In addition, intravaginal measurement of intraabdominal pressures have been reported at 27.5 cm H_2O [20] and in the supine position at 1.5 cm H_2O [21]. Finally, for the morbidly obese, intraabdominal pressures have been reported at 12.0 cm H_2O, which was compared to the control of 0–1.2 cm H_2O.

The way the pressures are generated at the vaginal apex are very different from those in the abdominal cavity, and, for this reason, we did not directly compare them. At the vaginal apex, the UDS sensor is sandwiched between the anterior and posterior vaginal walls. The distal vagina is normally oriented along the horizontal plane and is compressed by downward internal forces. The compression of the distal vagina is likely a protective mechanism.

Noblett et al. [20] reported higher pressures in the sitting position compared to the supine using an intravaginal pressure catheter. Our study also noted higher pressures in the sitting compared to the supine position at the vaginal apex. Interestingly, pressures were higher over the levators and behind the symphysis in the sitting position. At the hollow of the sacrum, pressures in the sitting and supine position were similar and both higher than standing. Shaw et al. [21] measured abdominal pressures using an intravaginal sensor in studies designed to evaluate how exercise affected intra-abdominal pressure. They noted increased abdominal pressures in obese patients and did not report measurements at rest. Several studies measured visceral pressures as a surrogate for abdominal pressures, and they found that obesity increased abdominal pressure [19,22,23]. This effect of increased weight in the viscera, seen in truncal obesity, supports the idea that the small bowel plays a role in pressure applied to the pelvic floor. There are no studies in live subjects or cadavers measuring abdominal pressures at various locations within the pelvis, nor are there any studies showing these pressures as a result of differing body positions.

This research helps explain the higher incidence of anterior compartment prolapse in women with pelvic floor disease. Pressures were higher at the symphysis than in the hollow of the sacrum in the standing position, supporting our hypothesis. Values were lowest in standing position (sacrum has maximum shielding) and highest in sitting position (sacrum has diminished shielding), potentially due to loss of lumbar lordosis when sitting. Pressures measured in the donut position were between the sitting and standing positions.

Imaging and Three-Dimensional Modeling Are Consistent with Pressure Readings

Our experiments were performed on a cadaver, which initially raised concerns about the relevance of our findings for in vivo conditions. In an effort to address this concern, we measured pressures at the vaginal apex using the Laborie Gomi UDS machine, as we would during an in vivo UDS procedure. We positioned the cadaver in the sitting position on a donut to simulate sitting on the UDS chair. Our measurements at the vaginal apex were consistent with in vivo results. We repeated the experiment 10× to confirm its reproducibility. We also had concerns regarding the reliability of our array and its position in the pelvis. We confirmed the position of the array using CT scan, X-ray, and three-dimensional modeling. We found that the array was precisely positioned over the levator ani muscles abutting the midline structures. The small bowel moved with changes in position and generated pressures measured by the array, which was confirmed with our imaging.

The three-dimensional modeling of the pelvic region was performed in 3D Slicer to verify the positions of internal organs, as well as the pressure array (Figure 2). The use of radiology, and specifically of magnetic resonance imaging (MRI), has been well established in the assessment of pelvic floor anatomy, identification of dysfunction, and assessment of surgical outcomes.

The use of non-contrast-enhanced cadaveric CT scanning for generating three-dimensional models presents a set of unique challenges. Lack of contrast between soft tissue organs decreases the fidelity of the structures of interest, and, while cadaveric contrast agents are being developed, they are not yet widely available or well studied. Thus, our segmentation and analysis is limited to tissues with clear boundaries (i.e., bones, bladder, intestines). Thin structures, such as the pelvic floor itself and microvessels, were difficult to visualize and model, and so were inferred from the surrounding anatomy. Additionally, without a standing CT apparatus, the assessment of the mesh locations in non-supine positions needed to be inferred from other imaging methods (X-ray). As far as we are aware, the positioning of the mesh was not significantly altered from the movement of the cadaver, but this should be confirmed by additional imaging.

5. Conclusions

Our findings of increased pressures behind the symphysis are in line with the known higher incidence of anterior compartment prolapse. In addition, the notion that the natural shape and orientation of the pelvis with standing helps to protect the pelvic floor is supported by our findings of lower pressures at the hollow of the sacrum in the standing position.

This study was conducted using a single sample body to generate a set of pilot readings. We were unable to calculate average and variation of pressures across different body morphologies; future work should expand the sample size to look at whether these pressure readings hold across different ages and pelvic floor states (dysfunction vs. normal).

Additionally, due to the nature of the study, we used a human gift cadaver to record pressures directly on the pelvic floor. Such an invasive methodology is not feasible to perform on living patients, and we do not know the extent to which our findings are directly translatable to living individuals. Our specimen was, likewise, from an elderly individual (aged 92 years) and, therefore, may not be translatable to the general condition.

The magnitude of our UDS pressure recordings are in line with previously reported findings, suggesting that the overall findings are at least reasonably comparable with the pressures one could expect from living subjects. More detailed and less invasive pressure recording approaches will be needed before these findings can be replicated on pre-mortem patients [19–23]. The potential applications of these results may demonstrate that lower lumbar lordosis treatment can alleviate pelvic floor dysfunction.

Author Contributions: Methodology, experimentation and formal analysis, T.A.; Experimentation and writing, A.D.; Writing and software, S.L.; Experimentation, K.B.; Conceptualization and experimentation, F.M.; Conceptualization and formal analysis, S.D. All authors have read and agreed to the published version of the manuscript.

Funding: This research was funded by the National Institute of Biomedical Imaging and Bioengineering (NIBIB) grant number 5 F31 EB030904 and the University at Buffalo Impact Grant.

Institutional Review Board Statement: Not applicable.

Informed Consent Statement: Not applicable.

Data Availability Statement: Data are not available at this time.

Conflicts of Interest: The authors declare no conflict of interest.

Abbreviations

The following abbreviations are used in this manuscript:

PFD	Pelvic Floor Dysfunction
UDS	Urodynamic System
ANOVA	Analysis of Variance

References

1. Herschorn, S. Female Pelvic Floor Anatomy: The Pelvic Floor, Supporting Structures, and Pelvic Organs. *Rev. Urol.* **2004**, *6*, S2–S10. [PubMed]
2. Wu, J.M.; Vaughan, C.P.; Goode, P.S.; Redden, D.T.; Burgio, K.L.; Richter, H.E.; Markland, A.D. Prevalence and Trends of Symptomatic Pelvic Floor Disorders in U.S. Women. *Obstet. Gynecol.* **2014**, *123*, 141–148. [CrossRef] [PubMed]
3. Nygaard, I.; Barber, M.D.; Burgio, K.L.; Kenton, K.; Meikle, S.; Schaffer, J.; Spino, C.; Whitehead, W.E.; Wu, J.; Brody, D.J. Prevalence of symptomatic pelvic floor disorders in US women. *JAMA* **2008**, *300*, 1311–1316. [CrossRef] [PubMed]
4. What Are PFDs?–About | Voices for PFD. Available online: https://www.voicesforpfd.org/about/what-are-pfds/ (accessed on 29 August 2022).
5. Good, M.M.; Solomon, E.R. Pelvic Floor Disorders. *Obstet. Gynecol. Clin. N. Am.* **2019**, *46*, 527–540. [CrossRef] [PubMed]
6. Nygaard, I.E.; Shaw, J.M. Physical activity and the pelvic floor. *Am. J. Obstet. Gynecol.* **2016**, *214*, 164–171. [CrossRef] [PubMed]
7. Mazi, B.; Kaddour, O.; Al-Badr, A. Depression symptoms in women with pelvic floor dysfunction: A case-control study. *Int. J. Womens Health* **2019**, *11*, 143–148. [CrossRef] [PubMed]
8. Verbeek, M.; Hayward, L. Pelvic Floor Dysfunction And Its Effect On Quality Of Sexual Life. *Sex. Med. Rev.* **2019**, *7*, 559–564. [CrossRef] [PubMed]
9. Sung, V.W.; Washington, B.; Raker, C.A. Costs of ambulatory care related to female pelvic floor disorders in the United States. *Am. J. Obstet. Gynecol.* **2010**, *202*, 483.e1–483.e4. [CrossRef] [PubMed]
10. Pressure Profile Systems Inc. Systems® | Tactile Pressure Mapping Systems. Available online: https://pressureprofile.com/ (accessed on 30 August 2022).
11. Laborie. Available online: https://www.laborie.com/ (accessed on 30 August 2022).
12. Pressure Profile Systems Inc. Chameleon Visualization Software. Available online: https://pressureprofile.com/sensor-systems/software.Date (accessed on 30 August 2022).
13. R: The R Project for Statistical Computing. v4.1.3. Available online: https://www.r-project.org/ (accessed on 30 August 2022).
14. Fedorov, A.; Beichel, R.; Kalpathy-Cramer, J.; Finet, J.; Fillion-Robin, J.C.; Pujol, S.; Bauer, C.; Jennings, D.; Fennessy, F.; Sonka, M.; et al. 3D Slicer as an Image Computing Platform for the Quantitative Imaging Network. *Magn. Reson. Imaging* **2012**, *30*, 1323–1341. [CrossRef] [PubMed]
15. Kikinis, R.; Pieper, S.D.; Vosburgh, K.G. 3D Slicer: A Platform for Subject-Specific Image Analysis, Visualization, and Clinical Support. In *Intraoperative Imaging and Image-Guided Therapy*; Jolesz, F.A., Ed.; Springer: New York, NY, USA, 2014; pp. 277–289. [CrossRef]
16. Cignoni, P.; Callieri, M.; Corsini, M.; Dellepiane, M.; Ganovelli, F.; Ranzuglia, G. MeshLab: An Open-Source Mesh Processing Tool. In Proceedings of the Eurographics Italian Chapter Conference, Salerno, Italy, 2–4 July 2008; Volume 2008, pp. 129–136. [CrossRef]
17. Nager, C.W.; Albo, M.E.; Fitzgerald, M.P.; McDermott, S.; Wruck, L.; Kraus, S.; Howden, N.; Norton, P.; Sirls, L.; Varner, E.; et al. Reference urodynamic values for stress incontinent women. *Neurourol. Urodyn.* **2007**, *26*, 333–340. [CrossRef] [PubMed]
18. Schäfer, W.; Abrams, P.; Liao, L.; Mattiasson, A.; Pesce, F.; Spangberg, A.; Sterling, A.M.; Zinner, N.R.; van Kerrebroeck, P. Good urodynamic practices: Uroflowmetry, filling cystometry, and pressure-flow studies. *Neurourol. Urodyn.* **2002**, *21*, 261–274. [CrossRef] [PubMed]
19. Sanchez, N.C.; Tenofsky, P.L.; Dort, J.M.; Shen, L.Y.; Helmer, S.D.; Smith, R.S. What is normal intra-abdominal pressure? *Am. Surg.* **2001**, *67*, 243–248. [CrossRef] [PubMed]
20. Noblett, K.L.; Jensen, J.K.; Ostergard, D.R. The relationship of body mass index to intra-abdominal pressure as measured by multichannel cystometry. *Int. Urogynecol. J. Pelvic Floor Dysfunct.* **1997**, *8*, 323–326. [CrossRef] [PubMed]
21. Shaw, J.M.; Hamad, N.M.; Coleman, T.J.; Egger, M.J.; Hsu, Y.; Hitchcock, R.; Nygaard, I.E. Intra-abdominal pressures during activity in women using an intra-vaginal pressure transducer. *J. Sport. Sci.* **2014**, *32*, 1176–1185. [CrossRef] [PubMed]
22. Lambert, D.M.; Marceau, S.; Forse, R.A. Intra-abdominal pressure in the morbidly obese. *Obes. Surg.* **2005**, *15*, 1225–1232. [CrossRef] [PubMed]
23. Chionh, J.J.L.; Wei, B.P.C.; Martin, J.A.; Opdam, H.I. Determining normal values for intra-abdominal pressure. *ANZ J. Surg.* **2006**, *76*, 1106–1109. [CrossRef] [PubMed]

MDPI AG
Grosspeteranlage 5
4052 Basel
Switzerland
Tel.: +41 61 683 77 34

Bioengineering Editorial Office
E-mail: bioengineering@mdpi.com
www.mdpi.com/journal/bioengineering

www.ingramcontent.com/pod-product-compliance
Lightning Source LLC
Chambersburg PA
CBHW061620210926
51850CB00009B/2387
9783725864348